4/08

Diet Information for Teens

Second Edition

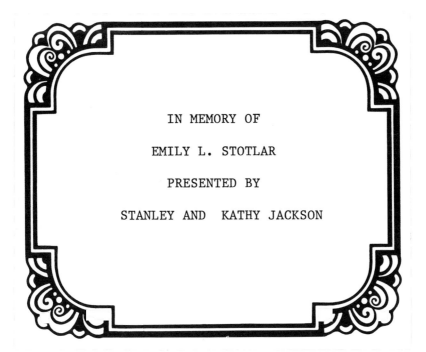

IN MEMORY OF

EMILY L. STOTLAR

PRESENTED BY

STANLEY AND   KATHY JACKSON

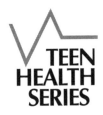

TEEN HEALTH SERIES

Second Edition

Diet Information for Teens

Health Tips about Diet and Nutrition

*Including Facts about Dietary Guidelines,
Food Groups, Nutrients, Healthy Meals,
Snacks, Weight Control, Medical Concerns
Related to Diet, and More*

Edited by Karen Bellenir

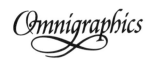

615 Griswold Street • Detroit, MI 48226

Bibliographic Note

Because this page cannot legibly accommodate all the copyright notices, the Bibliographic Note portion of the Preface constitutes an extension of the copyright notice.

Edited by Karen Bellenir

Teen Health Series

Karen Bellenir, *Managing Editor*
David A. Cooke, M.D., *Medical Consultant*
Elizabeth Barbour, *Permissions and Research Coordinator*
Dawn Matthews, *Verification Assistant*
Laura Pleva Nielsen, *Index Editor*
Cherry Stockdale, *Permissions Assistant*
EdIndex, Services for Publishers, *Indexers*

* * *

Omnigraphics, Inc.

Matthew P. Barbour, *Senior Vice President*
Kay Gill, *Vice President—Directories*
Kevin Hayes, *Operations Manager*
Leif Gruenberg, *Development Manager*
David P. Bianco, *Marketing Director*

* * *

Peter E. Ruffner, *Publisher*

Frederick G. Ruffner, Jr., *Chairman*

Copyright © 2006 Omnigraphics, Inc.

ISBN 0-7808-0820-7

Library of Congress Cataloging-in-Publication Data

Diet information for teens : health tips about diet and nutrition including facts about dietary guidelines, food groups, nutrients, healthy meals, snacks, weight control, medical concerns related to diet, and more / edited by Karen Bellenir.-- 2nd ed.
    p. cm. -- (Teen health series)
  Includes bibliographical references and index.
  ISBN 0-7808-0820-7 (hardcover : alk. paper)
  1. Teenagers--Nutrition. 2. Teenagers--Health and hygiene. 3. Diet. 4. Health. I. Bellenir, Karen. II. Series.
  RJ235.D546 2006
  613.20835--dc22
                                                    2006004413

Printed in the United States

Table of Contents

Part Three: Weight Control

Part Four: Medical Concerns And Special Circumstances Related To Diet

Part Five: If You Need More Information

Preface

About This Book

According to the Centers for Disease Control and Prevention, 15% of children and adolescents aged 6 to 19 years—about 9 million young people—are considered overweight. Simply asking them to eat less is not the answer. In fact, teens often need to eat more of specific types of foods because they frequently fail to get enough of several important nutrients. For example, federal agencies estimate that only 19% of girls between the ages of 9 and 19 get as much calcium as is recommended, and fewer than 20% of all teens eat the recommended amounts of fruits and vegetables. Additionally, because of the growth spurt that accompanies adolescence, young people actually need to eat more during the teen years than at other stages of life. Balancing this need to eat more with efforts to avoid excess weight can make dietary planning a complex challenge.

Diet Information For Teens, Second Edition provides updated information about the components of a healthy diet. Tips for food shopping and eating in restaurants, fast food establishments, and school cafeterias are included. Vitamins, minerals, dietary supplements, grains, vegetables, fruits, and protein sources are also discussed, and the book explains why the consumption of some food items—such as caffeine, sugar, fat, and salt—may need to be limited. A special section on weight control provides information for teens who wish to lose or gain weight. The book concludes with cooking tips and directories of resources for dietary and fitness information.

Some topics related to the subject of this book are covered in greater detail in other volumes of the *Teen Health Series*:

- For more information about food allergies, see *Allergy Information For Teens*.

- For more information about diabetes, see *Diabetes Information For Teens*.

- For more information about eating disorders, see *Eating Disorders Information For Teens*.

- For more information about physical fitness, see *Fitness Information For Teens*.

How To Use This Book

This book is divided into parts and chapters. Parts focus on broad areas of interest; chapters are devoted to single topics within a part.

Part One: What You Should Know About Healthy Eating describes the new food guidance system for Americans and dietary guidelines for teens. It explains the information found on food labels and offers suggestions for making healthy food choices in a variety of settings, including eating out, eating in the school cafeteria, and snacking.

Part Two: Nutrients, Foods, And Food Groups discusses vitamins, minerals, dietary supplements, and water and describes the roles they play in maintaining good health. Chapters about individual food groups describe why such items as grains, vegetables, fruits, and proteins are necessary components of a healthy diet. Problems associated with fats, sugars, and salt—nutrients that are sometimes consumed in excessive amounts—are also described.

Part Three: Weight Control provides guidance to people who want to identify and maintain a healthy weight. It describes the body mass index (BMI), discusses body image concerns, and provides suggestions for people seeking to achieve weight-related goals. Facts about how physical activity contributes to the success of weight management efforts are also included.

Part Four: Medical Concerns And Special Circumstances Related To Diet begins with information about how good dietary practices and maintaining a physically active lifestyle can help prevent some chronic diseases. It describes conditions that are commonly associated with dietary choices, including obesity, eating disorders, heart disease, and type 2 diabetes, and it offers specific suggestions for dieters, athletes, and people with food allergies and intolerances. The part concludes with information about foodborne illnesses.

Part Five: If You Need More Information includes tips about working in the kitchen, finding recipes, and planning meals. Directories of dietary and fitness resources are also included.

Bibliographic Note

This volume contains documents and excerpts from publications issued by the following government agencies: Agricultural Research Service; Army Medicine; Center for Food Safety and Applied Nutrition; Center for Nutrition Policy and Promotion; Centers for Disease Control and Prevention; Food Safety and Inspection Service; National Agricultural Library; National Center for Chronic Disease Prevention And Health Promotion; National Heart, Lung, and Blood Institute; National Institute of Allergy and Infectious Diseases; National Institute of Child Health and Human Development; National Institute of Diabetes and Digestive and Kidney Diseases; National Institutes of Health; National Women's Health Information Center; Office of Dietary Supplements; President's Council on Fitness; School Health Policies and Programs Study; U.S. Department of Agriculture; U.S. Department of Health and Human Services; U.S. Federal Trade Commission; and the U.S. Food and Drug Administration.

In addition, this volume contains copyrighted documents and articles produced by the following organizations and individuals: A.D.A.M., Inc.; Akron Children's Hospital; American Academy of Orthopaedic Surgeons; American Dietetic Association; American Heart Association; Baylor College of Medicine; Patrick Bird, Ph.D., Children's Nutrition Research Center; Food Allergy and Anaphylaxis Network; International Food Information Council; Maryland State Department of Education; Michigan Department of Agriculture; Munson Healthcare; National Academy of Sciences; National Dairy Council; Nemours Foundation; Partnership for Food Safety Education;

Thomson Healthcare, Inc.; University of Florida; and the University of Iowa's Virtual Hospital.

The photograph on the front cover is from www.comstock.com.

Full citation information is provided on the first page of each chapter. Every effort has been made to secure all necessary rights to reprint the copyrighted material. If any omissions have been made, please contact Omnigraphics to make corrections for future editions.

Acknowledgements

In addition to the organizations listed above, special thanks are due to editorial assistant Elizabeth Bellenir and permissions specialist Liz Barbour.

About The *Teen Health Series*

At the request of librarians serving today's young adults, the *Teen Health Series* was developed as a specially focused set of volumes within Omnigraphics' *Health Reference Series*. Each volume deals comprehensively with a topic selected according to the needs and interests of people in middle school and high school.

Teens seeking preventive guidance, information about disease warning signs, medical statistics, and risk factors for health problems will find answers to their questions in the *Teen Health Series*. The *Series*, however, is not intended to serve as a tool for diagnosing illness, in prescribing treatments, or as a substitute for the physician/patient relationship. All people concerned about medical symptoms or the possibility of disease are encouraged to seek professional care from an appropriate health care provider.

If there is a topic you would like to see addressed in a future volume of the *Teen Health Series*, please write to:

Editor
Teen Health Series
Omnigraphics, Inc.
615 Griswold Street
Detroit, MI 48226

Locating Information Within The *Teen Health Series*

The *Teen Health Series* contains a wealth of information about a wide variety of medical topics. As the *Series* continues to grow in size and scope, locating the precise information needed by a specific student may become more challenging. To address this concern, information about books within the *Teen Health Series* is included in *A Contents Guide to the Health Reference Series*. The *Contents Guide* presents an extensive list of more than 12,000 diseases, treatments, and other topics of general interest compiled from the Tables of Contents and major index headings from the books of the *Teen Health Series* and *Health Reference Series*. To access *A Contents Guide to the Health Reference Series*, visit www.healthreferenceseries.com.

Our Advisory Board

We would like to thank the following advisory board members for providing guidance to the development of this *Series*:

Dr. Lynda Baker,
Associate Professor of Library and Information Science,
Wayne State University, Detroit, MI

Nancy Bulgarelli, William Beaumont Hospital Library,
Royal Oak, MI

Karen Imarisio, Bloomfield Township Public Library,
Bloomfield Township, MI

Karen Morgan, Mardigian Library,
University of Michigan-Dearborn, Dearborn, MI

Rosemary Orlando, St. Clair Shores Public Library,
St. Clair Shores, MI

Medical Consultant

Medical consultation services are provided to the *Teen Health Series* editors by David A. Cooke, M.D. Dr. Cooke is a graduate of Brandeis University, and he received his M.D. degree from the University of Michigan. He completed residency training at the University of Wisconsin Hospital and Clinics. He is board-certified in internal medicine. Dr. Cooke currently works as part of the University of Michigan Health System and practices in Ann Arbor, MI. In his free time, he enjoys writing, science fiction, and spending time with his family.

Part One

What You Should Know About Healthy Eating

Chapter 1

A New Food Guidance System

The New Food Guide Pyramid

The government has updated the U.S. Food Guide Pyramid. The old pyramid was developed 13 years ago when we didn't know as much about nutrition. For instance, in 1992, there was a lot less emphasis on whole grain foods than there is today. And even experts didn't understand how very important exercise was to staying healthy. To keep up with the times, the U.S. Department of Agriculture (USDA) decided to update the pyramid in April 2005.

The New Food Guide Pyramid Is A Guide To Healthy Living

The food guide pyramid is designed as a symbol to remind people of what they should eat to stay healthy. The old pyramid showed only foods. The new pyramid has been updated to include physical activity as well.

About This Chapter: This chapter begins with "The New Food Guide Pyramid," information provided by TeensHealth, one of the largest resources online for medically reviewed health information written for parents, kids, and teens. For more articles like this one, visit www.TeensHealth.org, or www.KidsHealth.org. © 2005 The Nemours Center for Children's Health Media, a division of The Nemours Foundation. "My Pyramid: Steps To A Healthier You" and "Sample Menus for a 2000 Calorie Food Pattern" are from the Center for Nutrition Policy and Promotion, U.S. Department of Agriculture, April 2005.

The new pyramid shows food groups as a series of differently sized colored bands. The colors are:

- orange for grains;

- green for vegetables;

- red for fruit;

- yellow for fats and oils;

- blue for dairy;

- purple for meats, beans, and fish.

The bands are different widths to show how much of a particular food group a person should eat each day. So the orange band is much wider than the yellow one because people need to eat a lot more grains than fats and oils.

♣ It's A Fact!!
Find Your Balance Between Food And Physical Activity

- Be sure to stay within your daily calorie needs.

- Be physically active for at least 30 minutes most days of the week.

- About 60 minutes a day of physical activity may be needed to prevent weight gain.

- For sustaining weight loss, at least 60 to 90 minutes a day of physical activity may be required.

- Children and teenagers should be physically active for 60 minutes every day; or most days.

Source: U.S. Department of Agriculture, April 2005.

The drawing of a person climbing stairs at the side of the new pyramid is there to remind us that physical activity is as important to healthy living as eating well. Exercise helps all teens stay healthy—it can increase bone strength, for example. And food and exercise are closely linked. A teen needs to eat well to get the nutrients that help the body grow. But teens who are extremely active need additional food so they can fuel their activity levels. That way they satisfy their bodies' needs for both growth and activity.

The new food guide pyramid is supposed to help people remember the following key points:

Combine exercise with eating well: Exercise benefits every part of the body, including the mind. Experts now know that exercise fights off a range of possible health problems like heart disease, diabetes, and even depression. Teens need more than 60 minutes of moderate to vigorous exercise every day to stay healthy.

Eat a variety of foods: The different color bands in the pyramid send the message that it's important to eat lots of different foods. Not only does eating a variety of foods provide people with a good balance of nutrients, it also keeps our taste buds entertained.

Eat foods in moderation: The colored bands that show each food group are wider at the bottom of the pyramid than they are at the top. That's a reminder that some foods in each group can be eaten in large quantities but others should be limited. Foods at the bottom of each section include those with little or no solid fats and little or no added sugars or sweeteners. So a person should eat more whole-wheat bread than regular pasta, for example. Likewise, people should eat whole, fresh apples more often than apple pie and try to get most of their dairy intake from low-fat milk instead of cream cheese or other high-fat dairy products.

A Reminder To Eat Right And Exercise

Why these changes? Americans are getting fatter—kids and teens as well as adults. A lot of this is because we're becoming a nation of couch potatoes. We're spending more time in front of computer screens and TV sets than meeting up with friends and playing sports. We're sitting behind a desk or the wheel of a car instead of working at more active jobs or walking to our destinations.

The government's worried about this trend towards a fatter America. In fact, kids and teens growing up today may be the first generation to die before their parents because of diseases that are related to being overweight. So experts redesigned the food guide pyramid to include messages about getting exercise and eating in moderation.

What Does It Mean to You?

The new food guide pyramid design is just one part of the government's new guidelines for eating and living well. In addition to updating the pyramid, the USDA is providing information on exactly how much of each food group teens should eat compared to adults and younger kids. For example, the daily recommended amount of vegetables for a 13-year-old boy is 2½ cups; for a 13-year-old girl, it's 2 cups. For 14- to 18-year-olds, that number goes up to 2½ cups for girls and 3 cups for guys.

Exercise levels also factor into how much a person should eat. To create a personal profile that shows what you should eat for your age, gender, and activity level, visit the USDA's MyPyramid website (http://www.mypyramid.gov).

My Pyramid: Steps To A Healthier You

Grains

- Make half your grains whole.

- Eat at least 3 oz. of whole-grain cereals, breads, crackers, rice, or pasta every day.

- 1 oz. is about one slice of bread, about 1 cup of breakfast cereal, or ½ cup of cooked rice, cereal, or pasta.

Vegetables

- Vary your veggies.

- Eat more dark-green veggies like broccoli, spinach, and other dark leafy greens.

- Eat more orange vegetables like carrots and sweet potatoes.

- Eat more dry beans and peas like pinto beans, kidney beans, and lentils.

Fruits

- Focus on fruits.

- Eat a variety of fruit

- Choose fresh, frozen, canned, or dried fruit.

- Go easy on fruit juices.

✔ **Quick Tip**
Know The Limits On Fats, Sugars, And Salt (Sodium)

- Make most of your fat sources from fish, nuts, and vegetable oils.

- Limit solid fats like butter, stick margarine, shortening, and lard, as well as foods that contain these.

- Check the Nutrition Facts label to keep saturates fats, *trans* fats, and sodium low.

- Choose food and beverages low in added sugars. Added sugars contribute calories with few, if any, nutrients.

Source: U.S. Department of Agriculture, April 2005.

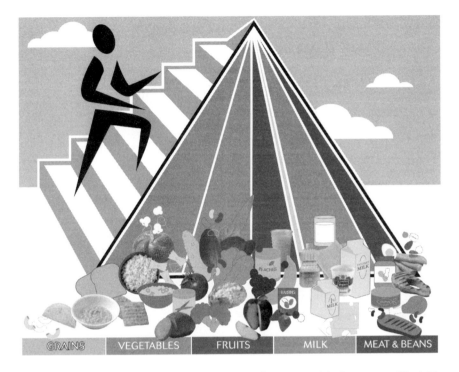

Figure 1.1. The new food guidance graphic (MyPyramid: Steps to a Healthier You, available at http://www.MyPyramid.gov).

Milk

- Get your calcium-rich foods.
- Go low-fat or fat-free when you choose milk, yogurt, and other milk products.
- If you don't or can't consume milk, choose lactose-free products or other calcium sources such as fortified foods and beverages.

Meat and Beans

- Go lean with protein.
- Choose low-fat or lean meats and poultry.
- Bake it, broil it, or grill it.
- Vary your protein routine—choose more fish, beans, peas, nuts, and seeds.

Sample Menus For A 2000 Calorie Food Pattern

Averaged over a week, this sample seven day menu provides all of the recommended amounts of nutrients and food from each food group. The actual number of calories that are appropriate for you will vary based on your gender, age, and level of activity. (See Chapter 2 or visit http://www.mypyramid.gov for more information about how many calories you should eat).

Italicized foods are part of the dish or food that proceeds it. Starred items (*) are foods that are labeled as no-salt-added, low-sodium, or low-salt versions of the foods. They can also be prepared from scratch with little or no added salt. All other foods are regular commercial products which contain variable levels of sodium. Average sodium level of the 7 day menu assumes no salt added during cooking or at the table.

✎ Weird Words

Calorie: A measure of the energy you get from the food you eat. The number of calories you need varies depending on your gender, height, weight, age, and level of activity.

Nutrients: Things in food (like vitamins, minerals, protein, fat & carbohydrates), that help your body function and grow.

Source: From "Dictionary," Powerful Bones, Centers for Disease Control and Prevention (CDC), 2001.

Day 1

Breakfast

Breakfast burrito
1 flour tortilla (7" diameter)
1 scrambled egg (in 1 tsp soft margarine)
*1/3 cup black beans**
2 tbsp salsa
1 cup orange juice
1 cup fat-free milk

Lunch

Roast beef sandwich
1 whole grain sandwich bun
3 ounces lean roast beef
2 slices tomato
1/4 cup shredded romaine lettuce
1/8 cup sautéed mushrooms
(in 1 tsp oil)
1 1/2 ounce part-skim mozzarella cheese
1 tsp yellow mustard
3/4 cup baked potato wedges*
1 tbsp ketchup
1 unsweetened beverage

Dinner

Stuffed broiled salmon
5 ounce salmon filet
1 ounce bread stuffing mix
1 tbsp chopped onions
1 tbsp diced celery
2 tsp canola oil
1/2 cup saffron (white) *rice*
1 ounce slivered almonds
1/2 cup steamed broccoli
1 tsp soft margarine
1 cup fat-free milk

Snacks

1 cup cantaloupe

Day 2

Breakfast
Hot cereal
    1/2 cup cooked oatmeal
    2 tbsp raisins
    1 tsp soft margarine
1/2 cup fat-free milk
1 cup orange juice

Lunch
Taco salad
    2 ounces tortilla chips
    2 ounces ground turkey, sautéed in
    2 tsp sunflower oil
    *1/2 cup black beans**
    1/2 cup iceberg lettuce
    2 slices tomato
    1 ounce low-fat cheddar cheese
    2 tbsp salsa
    1/2 cup avocado
    1 tsp lime juice
1 unsweetened beverage

Dinner
Spinach lasagna
    1 cup lasagna noodles, cooked (2 oz dry)
    2/3 cup cooked spinach
    1/2 cup ricotta cheese
    *1/2 cup tomato sauce tomato bits**
    1 ounce part-skim mozzarella cheese
1 ounce whole wheat dinner roll
1 cup fat-free milk

Snacks
1/2 ounce dry-roasted almonds*
1/4 cup pineapple
2 tbsp raisins

Day 3

Breakfast
Cold cereal
    1 cup bran flakes
    1 cup fat-free milk
    1 small banana
1 slice whole wheat toast
    1 tsp soft margarine
1 cup prune juice

Lunch
Tuna fish sandwich
    2 slices rye bread
    3 ounces tuna (packed in water, drained)
    2 tsp mayonnaise
    1 tbsp diced celery
    1/4 cup shredded romaine lettuce
    2 slices tomato
1 medium pear
1 cup fat-free milk

Dinner
Roasted chicken breast
    *3 ounces boneless skinless chicken breast**
1 large baked sweet potato
1/2 cup peas and onions
    1 tsp soft margarine
1 ounce whole wheat dinner roll
    1 tsp soft margarine
1 cup leafy greens salad
    3 tsp sunflower oil and vinegar dressing

Snacks
1/4 cup dried apricots
1 cup low-fat fruited yogurt

Table 1.1. Food Groups Represented In The Sample Menus For A 2000 Calorie Food Pattern.

Food Group Over One Week	Daily Average	
Grains	Total Grains (oz eq.)	6.0
	Whole Grains	3.4
	Refined Grains	2.6
Vegetables	Total Vegetables* (cups)	2.6
Fruits	Fruits (cups)	2.1
Milk	Milk (cups)	3.1
Meat and Beans	Meat/ Beans (oz eq.)	5.6
Oils	Oils (teaspoon/grams)	7.2 tsp/32.4 g

*Vegetable subgroups (weekly totals)

Dark Green Vegetables = 3.3 cups

Orange Vegetables = 2.3 cups

Beans/Peas = 3.0 cups

Starchy Vegetables = 3.4 cups

Other Vegetables = 6.6 cups

oz eq = ounce equivalents

Day 4

Breakfast

1 whole wheat English muffin

   2 tsp soft margarine
   1 tbsp jam or preserves

1 medium grapefruit

1 hard-cooked egg

1 unsweetened beverage

Lunch

White bean-vegetable soup

   1 1/4 cup chunky vegetable soup
   *1/2 cup white beans**

2 ounce breadstick

8 baby carrots

1 cup fat-free milk

Dinner

Rigatoni with meat sauce

   1 cup rigatoni pasta (2 ounces dry)
   *1/2 cup tomato sauce tomato bits**
   2 ounces extra lean cooked ground beef
   (sautéed in 2 tsp vegetable oil)
   3 tbsp grated Parmesan cheese

Spinach salad

   1 cup baby spinach leaves
   1/2 cup tangerine slices
   1/2 ounce chopped walnuts
   3 tsp sunflower oil and vinegar dressing

1 cup fat-free milk

Snacks

   1 cup low-fat fruited yogurt

   1 tbsp chopped onions

Day 5

Breakfast

Cold cereal

   1 cup puffed wheat cereal
   1 tbsp raisins
   1 cup fat-free milk

1 small banana

1 slice whole wheat toast

   1 tsp soft margarine
   1 tsp jelly

Lunch

Smoked turkey sandwich

   2 ounces whole wheat pita bread
   1/4 cup romaine lettuce
   2 slices tomato
   *3 ounces sliced smoked turkey breast**
   1 tbsp mayo-type salad dressing
   1 tsp yellow mustard

1/2 cup apple slices

1 cup tomato juice*

Dinner

Grilled top loin steak

   5 ounces grilled top loin steak

3/4 cup mashed potatoes

   2 tsp soft margarine

1/2 cup steamed carrots

   1 tbsp honey

2 ounces whole wheat dinner roll

   1 tsp soft margarine

1 cup fat-free milk

Snacks

1 cup low-fat fruited yogurt

Table 1.2. Nutrients Provided In The Sample Menus For A 2000 Calorie Food Pattern

Nutrient	Daily Average Over One Week	Nutrient	Daily Average Over One Week
Calories	1994	Magnesium	432 mg
Protein	98 g	Copper	1.9 mg
Protein	20% kcal	Iron	21 mg
Carbohydrate	264 g	Phosphorus	1830 mg
Carbohydrate	53 % kcal	Zinc	14 mg
Total fat	67 g	Thiamin	1.9 mg
Total fat	30% kcal	Riboflavin	2.5 mg
Saturated fat	16 g	Niacin equivalents	24 mg
Saturated fat	7.0% kcal	Vitamin B_6	2.9 mg
Monounsaturated fat	23 g	Vitamin B_{12}	18.4 mcg
Polyunsaturated fat	23 g	Vitamin C	190 mg
Linoleic Acid	21 g	Vitamin E	
Alpha-linolenic Acid	1.1 g	(alpha-tocopheryl)	18.9 mg
Cholesterol	207 mg	Vitamin A	
Total dietary fiber	31 g	(retinol activity	
Potassium	4715 mg	equivalents)	1430 mcg
Sodium*	1948 mg	Dietary folate	
Calcium	1389 mg	equivalents, mcg	558 mcg

* = assuming no salt was added during cooking or at the table
g = grams
% kcal = percent of calories
mg = milligram
mcg = microgram

Day 6

Breakfast
French toast
> *2 slices whole wheat French toast*
> *2 tsp soft margarine*
> *2 tbsp maple syrup*

1/2 medium grapefruit

1 cup fat-free milk

Lunch
Vegetarian chili on baked potato
> *1 cup kidney beans**
> *1/2 cup tomato sauce w/tomato tidbits**
> *3 tbsp chopped onions*
> *1 ounce low-fat cheddar cheese*
> *1 tsp vegetable oil*
> *1 medium baked potato*

1/2 cup cantaloupe

3/4 cup lemonade

Dinner
Hawaiian pizza
> *2 slices cheese pizza*
> *1 ounce Canadian bacon*
> *1/4 cup pineapple*
> *2 tbsp mushrooms*
> *2 tbsp chopped onions*

Green salad
> *1 cup leafy greens*
> *3 tsp sunflower oil and vinegar dressing*

1 cup fat-free milk

Snacks
5 whole wheat crackers*

1/8 cup hummus

1/2 cup fruit cocktail (in water or juice)

Day 7

Breakfast
Pancakes
> *3 buckwheat pancakes*
> *2 tsp soft margarine*
> *3 tbsp maple syrup*

1/2 cup strawberries

3/4 cup honeydew melon

1/2 cup fat-free milk

Lunch
Manhattan clam chowder
> *3 ounces canned clams (drained)*
> *3/4 cup mixed vegetables*
> *1 cup canned tomatoes**

10 whole wheat crackers*

1 medium orange

1 cup fat-free milk

Dinner
Vegetable stir-fry
> *4 ounces tofu (firm)*
> *1/4 cup green and red bell peppers*
> *1/2 cup bok choy*
> *2 tbsp vegetable oil*

1 cup brown rice

1 cup lemon-flavored iced tea

Snacks
1 ounce sunflower seeds*

1 large banana

1 cup low-fat fruited yogurt

Chapter 2

Dietary Guidelines And Nutrition For Teens

What Is Nutrition?

Before we can talk about nutrition, try to answer this question: What is food?

It might sound like a silly question, but food is many things to people. Basically, food provides building blocks for growth and repair, and it is the fuel for your body to keep it going. Just as you need to put gas in a car to make it run, you need to put food in your body to keep it going. However, many people see food as a comfort, a way to reduce stress, a status symbol, a reward or punishment, or as an enemy. While it's normal to take pleasure in food and to eat it in a social atmosphere, there are many unhealthy attitudes about food that you should avoid. Food should never be a substitute for feelings other than hunger.

Nutrition involves using food to nourish your body. To have a healthy body, you must give it all the nutrients it needs to grow and develop. But how do you do that? First of all, you need to understand that there are no good or bad foods. Foods supply nutrients your body needs to grow, have energy, and stay healthy, and all foods can be part of a healthy diet. A healthy diet includes grain products, vegetables, fruits, low-fat milk products, lean meats, fish, poultry, and dry beans.

About This Chapter: This chapter begins with "What Is Nutrition?" from Bodywise (http://www.girlpower.gov/girlarea/bodywise), U.S. Department of Health and Human Services, 2004; "An Overview Of The Dietary Guidelines For Americans 2005," "Key Recommendations for the General Population," and "What Are Discretionary Calories?" are from the U.S. Department of Agriculture, 2005.

Choose fewer foods that are high in salt, sugar, or saturated fat. The fats from meat, milk, and milk products are the main sources of saturated fats in most diets. Many bakery products are also sources of saturated fats. Vegetable oils supply smaller amounts of saturated fat. For example, non-fat milk, lean meat, and low-fat cheese have lower saturated fat than fatty meat, whole milk, and regular cheese. It's the total amount and types of foods you eat over several days that make up a healthy or unhealthy diet. So eat a variety of foods to get the energy, protein, vitamins, minerals, and fiber you need for good health.

An Overview Of The Dietary Guidelines For Americans 2005

What are the Dietary Guidelines for Americans 2005?

The *Dietary Guidelines* are the cornerstone of federal nutrition policy and education. They are based on what experts have determined to be the best scientific knowledge about diet, physical activity and other issues related to what we should eat and how much physical activity we need.

The *Dietary Guidelines* answer the questions, "What should Americans eat, how should we prepare our food to keep it safe and wholesome, and how should we be active to be healthy?" The *Dietary Guidelines* are designed to help Americans choose diets that will meet nutrient requirements, promote health, support active lives and reduce risks of chronic disease.

Why are the Dietary Guidelines important?

The *Dietary Guidelines* will help Americans make smart choices about food and physical activity, so they can have healthier lives.

The *Dietary Guidelines* allow government to speak with one voice to the public when presenting advice about proper dietary habits for healthy Americans older than two years of age and how to make food and physical activity choices to promote health and prevent chronic disease. All federal dietary guidance for the public is required to be consistent with the *Dietary Guidelines*.

The *Dietary Guidelines* provide the foundation for food and nutrition policy and the government's position for debating standards and international reports.

✎ Weird Words

Basic Food Groups: In the U.S. Department of Agriculture food intake patterns, the basic food groups are:

- grains;
- fruits;
- vegetables;
- milk, yogurt, and cheese; and
- and meat, poultry, fish, dried peas and beans, eggs, and nuts.

Cholesterol: A type of bodily chemical present in all animal tissues. Free cholesterol is a component of cell membranes and serves as a precursor for steroid hormones, including estrogen, testosterone, aldosterone, and bile acids. Humans are able to make sufficient cholesterol to meet biologic requirements, and there is no evidence for a dietary requirement for cholesterol. "Dietary cholesterol" is cholesterol that is consumed from foods of animal origin, including meat, fish, poultry, eggs, and dairy products. "Serum cholesterol" travels in the blood.

Daily Food Intake Pattern: Identifies the types and amounts of foods that are recommended to be eaten each day and that meet specific nutritional goals.

Nutrient-Dense Foods: Nutrient-dense foods are those that provide substantial amounts of vitamins and minerals and relatively fewer calories.

Ounce-Equivalent: In the grains food group, the amount of a food counted as equal to a one-ounce slice of bread; in the meat, poultry, fish, dry beans, eggs, and nuts food group, the amount of food counted as equal to one ounce of cooked meat, poultry, or fish.

Source: Excerpted from "Appendix C: Glossary of Terms," *Dietary Guidelines for Americans 2005*, U.S. Department of Agriculture, 2005.

The *Dietary Guidelines* influence the direction of government nutrition programs, including research, labeling, and nutrition promotion. This includes the U.S. Department of Agriculture's (USDA) Food Guidance System—what's now known as the Food Guide Pyramid—and which has been updated to reflect the new *Dietary Guidelines*.

Federal nutrition assistance programs such as USDA's School Meal and Food Stamp Programs, and the WIC Program (Supplemental Food Program for Women, Infants and Children) use the principles in the *Dietary Guidelines* as the scientific underpinning for designing benefit structures and nutrition education programs.

Key Recommendations For The General Population

Adequate Nutrients Within Calorie Needs

• Consume a variety of nutrient-dense foods and beverages within and among the basic food groups while choosing foods that limit the intake of saturated and trans fats, cholesterol, added sugars, salt, and alcohol.

Teen Nutrition   ♣ It's A Fact!!

Adolescents need extra nutrients to support the adolescent growth spurt, which begins in girls at ages 10 or 11, reaches its peak at age 12 and is completed by about age 15. In boys, it begins at 12 or 13 years of age, peaks at age 14 and ends by about age 19.

In addition to other nutrients, adequate amounts of iron and calcium are particularly important as the adolescent body undergoes this intensive growth period. From ages 9 to 18 years, both males and females are encouraged to consume a calcium-rich diet (1,300 milligrams daily) in order to ensure adequate calcium deposits in the bones. This may help reduce the incidence of osteoporosis in later years. By eating at least three servings of dairy products daily, the recommended calcium intake can be achieved. For persons who don't wish to consume dairy products, a variety of other calcium sources are available such as green, leafy vegetables, calcium-fortified soy products and other calcium-fortified foods and beverages.

Teens' caloric needs vary depending on their growth rate, degree of physical maturation, body composition and activity level. Overweight is one of the most serious nutrition problems of adolescents, particularly among Native Americans, Hispanics and African-Americans.

- Meet recommended intakes within energy needs by adopting a balanced eating pattern, such as the U.S. Department of Agriculture (USDA) Food Guide or the Dietary Approaches to Stop Hypertension (DASH) Eating Plan.

Weight Management

- To maintain body weight in a healthy range, balance calories from foods and beverages with calories expended.

- To prevent gradual weight gain over time, make small decreases in food and beverage calories and increase physical activity.

Eating disorders also are common among teens, whose food choices are often influenced by social pressure to achieve cultural ideals of thinness, gain peer acceptance or assert independence from parental authority. Eating disorders may be classified as anorexia, bulimia, compulsive overeating or binge-eating disorder and eating disorders not otherwise specified (any combination of the previous disorders mentioned). Each eating disorder is based on specific diagnostic criteria. According to the National Center for Health Statistics, one in 100 females between the ages of 12 and 18 has anorexia nervosa, a disorder causing people to severely limit their food intake. Both anorexia and bulimia (a disorder in which people binge and purge by vomiting or using laxatives) can lead to convulsions, kidney failure, irregular heartbeats, osteoporosis and dental erosion. Those suffering from compulsive overeating or binge-eating disorder are at risk for heart attack, developing high blood pressure and high cholesterol, kidney disease and/or failure, arthritis, bone deterioration and stroke.

Source: From "Background on Nutrition, Health, and Physical Activity During Childhood and Early Adolescence," © 2005 International Food Information Council. All rights reserved. Reprinted with permission.

Table 2.1. How many calories should you eat? It depends on your gender, age, and level of physical activity. For more detailed information, visit http://www.mypyramid.gov.

Gender	Age	Physical Activity	Daily Calories
Male	12	Less than 30 minutes	1800
Male	12	30 to 60 minutes	2200
Male	12	More than 60 minutes	2400
Female	12	Less than 30 minutes	1600
Female	12	30 to 60 minutes	2000
Female	12	More than 60 minutes	2200
Male	14	Less than 30 minutes	2000
Male	14	30 to 60 minutes	2400
Male	14	More than 60 minutes	2800
Female	14	Less than 30 minutes	1800
Female	14	30 to 60 minutes	2000
Female	14	More than 60 minutes	2400
Male	16	Less than 30 minutes	2400
Male	16	30 to 60 minutes	2800
Male	16	More than 60 minutes	3200
Female	16	Less than 30 minutes	1800
Female	16	30 to 60 minutes	2000
Female	16	More than 60 minutes	2400
Male	18	Less than 30 minutes	2400
Male	18	30 to 60 minutes	2800
Male	18	More than 60 minutes	3200
Female	18	Less than 30 minutes	2400
Female	18	30 to 60 minutes	2000
Female	18	More than 60 minutes	2400

Source: U.S. Department of Agriculture, 2005.

Physical Activity

- Engage in regular physical activity and reduce sedentary activities to promote health, psychological well-being, and a healthy body weight.

  - To reduce the risk of chronic disease in adulthood: Engage in at least 30 minutes of moderate-intensity physical activity, above usual activity, at work or home on most days of the week.

  - For most people, greater health benefits can be obtained by engaging in physical activity of more vigorous intensity or longer duration.

  - To help manage body weight and prevent gradual, unhealthy body weight gain in adulthood: Engage in approximately 60 minutes of moderate- to vigorous-intensity activity on most days of the week while not exceeding caloric intake requirements.

  - To sustain weight loss in adulthood: Participate in at least 60 to 90 minutes of daily moderate-intensity physical activity while not exceeding caloric intake requirements. Some people may need to consult with a healthcare provider before participating in this level of activity.

- Achieve physical fitness by including cardiovascular conditioning, stretching exercises for flexibility, and resistance exercises or calisthenics for muscle strength and endurance.

Food Groups To Encourage

- Consume a sufficient amount of fruits and vegetables while staying within energy needs. Two cups of fruit and 2½ cups of vegetables per day are recommended for a reference 2,000-calorie intake, with higher or lower amounts depending on the calorie level.

- Choose a variety of fruits and vegetables each day. In particular, select from all five vegetable subgroups (dark green, orange, legumes, starchy vegetables, and other vegetables) several times a week.

- Consume three or more ounce-equivalents of whole-grain products per day, with the rest of the recommended grains coming from enriched

✔ **Quick Tip**
Meal Patterns

To meet energy needs, children and teens should eat at least three meals a day, beginning with breakfast. Studies show eating breakfast affects both cognitive and physical performance; that is, if a child eats breakfast, he or she may be more alert in school and better able to learn and to perform sports or other physical activities.

Snacks also form an integral part of meal patterns for children and teens. Young children generally cannot eat large quantities of food at one sitting and get hungry long before the next regular mealtime. Mid-morning and mid-afternoon snacks are generally advised for this age.

Fast-growing, active teens may have tremendous energy needs. Even though their regular meals can be substantial, they still may need snacks to supply energy between meals and to meet their daily nutrient needs.

Source: From "Background on Nutrition, Health, and Physical Activity During Childhood and Early Adolescence," © 2005 International Food Information Council. All rights reserved. Reprinted with permission.

or whole-grain products. In general, at least half the grains should come from whole grains.

- Consume 3 cups per day of fat-free or low-fat milk or equivalent milk products.

Fats

- Consume less than 10 percent of calories from saturated fatty acids and less than 300 mg/day of cholesterol, and keep trans fatty acid consumption as low as possible.

- Keep total fat intake between 20 to 35 percent of calories, with most fats coming from sources of polyunsaturated and monounsaturated fatty acids, such as fish, nuts, and vegetable oils.

- When selecting and preparing meat, poultry, dry beans, and milk or milk products, make choices that are lean, low-fat, or fat-free.

- Limit intake of fats and oils high in saturated and/or trans fatty acids, and choose products low in such fats and oils.

Carbohydrates

- Choose fiber-rich fruits, vegetables, and whole grains often.

- Choose and prepare foods and beverages with little added sugars or caloric sweeteners, such as amounts suggested by the USDA Food Guide and the DASH Eating Plan.

- Reduce the incidence of dental caries by practicing good oral hygiene and consuming sugar- and starch-containing foods and beverages less frequently.

Sodium And Potassium

- Consume less than 2,300 mg (approximately 1 teaspoon of salt) of sodium per day.

- Choose and prepare foods with little salt. At the same time, consume potassium-rich foods, such as fruits and vegetables.

✔ **Quick Tip**

The *Dietary Guidelines* talk about a 2,000 calorie diet but is that the right calorie level for me? How can I find out how many calories I should eat in a day?

Many times throughout the *Guidelines* publication, a 2,000 calorie level is used in examples. This was done for consistency purposes but the recommended calorie level will differ for individuals depending on age, sex, and activity level. See Table 2.1 for more information about recommended calorie levels for teens or visit http://www.mypyramid.gov for an interactive version of the new food guidance system.

Source: U.S. Department of Agriculture (http://www.nutrition.gov), 2005.

Table 2.2. This information can help you choose the foods and amounts that are right for you.

Daily Calories	Grains[1]	Vegetables[2]	Fruits	Milk	Meat and Beans	Oils	Discretionary Calories[3]
1600	5 ounces	2 cups	1.5 cups	3 cups	5 ounces	5 teaspoons	130
1800	6 ounces	2.5 cups	1.5 cups	3 cups	5 ounces	5 teaspoons	195
2000	6 ounces	2.5 cups	2 cups	3 cups	5.5 ounces	6 teaspoons	265
2200	7 ounces	3 cups	2 cups	3 cups	6 ounces	6 teaspoons	290
2400	8 ounces	3 cups	2 cups	3 cups	6.5 ounces	7 teaspoons	360
2800	10 ounces	3.5 cups	2.5 cups	3 cups	7 ounces	7 teaspoons	360
3200	10 ounces	4 cups	2.5 cups	3 cups	7 ounces	8 teaspoons	425

[1] Half of your grains should be whole grains.

[2] Vary your vegetables throughout the week. Include dark green vegetables, orange vegetables, dry beans and peas, starchy vegetables, and other vegetables.

[3] Limit extra calories from fats and sugars to this amount.

Source: U.S. Department of Agriculture, 2005.

Food Safety

- To avoid microbial foodborne illness:

  - Clean hands, food contact surfaces, and fruits and vegetables. Meat and poultry should not be washed or rinsed.

  - Separate raw, cooked, and ready-to-eat foods while shopping, preparing, or storing foods.

  - Cook foods to a safe temperature to kill microorganisms.

  - Chill (refrigerate) perishable food promptly and defrost foods properly.

  - Avoid raw (unpasteurized) milk or any products made from unpasteurized milk, raw or partially cooked eggs or foods containing raw eggs, raw or undercooked meat and poultry, unpasteurized juices, and raw sprouts.

Note: The *Dietary Guidelines for Americans 2005* contains additional recommendations for specific populations. The full document is available at www.healthierus.gov/dietaryguidelines.

What Are Discretionary Calories?

You need a certain number of calories to keep your body functioning and provide energy for physical activities. Think of the calories you need for energy like money you have to spend. Each person has a total calorie "budget." This budget can be divided into "essentials" and "extras."

With a financial budget, the essentials are items like rent and food. The extras are things like movies and vacations. In a calorie budget, the "essentials" are the minimum calories required to meet your nutrient needs. By selecting the lowest fat and no-sugar-added forms of foods in each food group you would make the best nutrient "buys." Depending on the foods you choose, you may be able to spend more calories than the amount required to meet your nutrient needs. These calories are the "extras" that can be used on luxuries like solid fats, added sugars, and alcohol, or on more food from any food group. They are your "discretionary calories."

Each person has an allowance for some discretionary calories. But, many people have used up this allowance before lunch-time. Most discretionary calorie allowances are very small, between 100 and 300 calories, especially for those who are not physically active. For many people, the discretionary calorie allowance is totally used by the foods they choose in each food group, such as higher fat meats, cheeses, whole milk, or sweetened bakery products.

You can use your discretionary calorie allowance to:

- Eat more foods from any food group than the food guide recommends.

- Eat higher calorie forms of foods—those that contain solid fats or added sugars. Examples are whole milk, cheese, sausage, biscuits, sweetened cereal, and sweetened yogurt.

- Add fats or sweeteners to foods. Examples are sauces, salad dressings, sugar, syrup, and butter.

- Eat or drink items that are mostly fats or caloric sweeteners, such as candy or soda.

For example, assume your calorie budget is 2,000 calories per day. Of

> ## ♣ It's A Fact!!
> ## Why so many fruits and vegetables?
>
> Eating more fruits and vegetables is associated with a lower risk of stroke and possibly other cardiovascular diseases as well as a lower risk of type 2 diabetes and certain cancers (cancers of the oral cavity and pharynx, larynx, lung, esophagus, stomach, and colon-rectum). Fruit and vegetable consumption can also give you a feeling of fullness and help you eat fewer calories. In these ways, fruit and vegetables may help with weight control.
>
> Source: U.S. Department of Agriculture (http://www.nutrition.gov), 2005.

these calories, you need to spend at least 1,735 calories for essential nutrients, if you choose foods without added fat and sugar. Then you have 265 discretionary calories left. You may use these on "luxury" versions of the foods in each group, such as higher fat meat or sweetened cereal. Or, you can spend them on sweets, sauces, or beverages. Many people overspend their discretionary calorie allowance, choosing more added fats and sugars than their budget allows.

Chapter 3

Reading And Understanding Food Labels

People look at food labels for different reasons. But whatever the reason, many consumers would like to know how to use this information more effectively and easily. The following label-building skills are intended to make it easier for you to use nutrition labels to make quick, informed food choices that contribute to a healthy diet.

The Nutrition Facts Label: An Overview

The information in the main or top section (see Figure 3.1: the main section includes everything except the footnote, #5) can vary with each food product; it contains product-specific information (serving size, calories, and nutrient information). The bottom part (see #5 in Figure 3.1) contains a footnote with Daily Values (DVs) for 2,000 and 2,500 calorie diets. This footnote provides recommended dietary information for important nutrients, including fats, sodium, and fiber. The footnote is found only on larger packages and does not change from product to product.

The Serving Size

The first place to start when you look at the Nutrition Facts label is the serving size and the number of servings in the package (#1 in Figure 3.1.).

About This Chapter: "How to Understand and Use the Nutrition Facts Label," U.S. Food and Drug Administration, November 2004.

Serving sizes are standardized to make it easier to compare similar foods; they are provided in familiar units, such as cups or pieces, followed by the metric amount, for example, the number of grams.

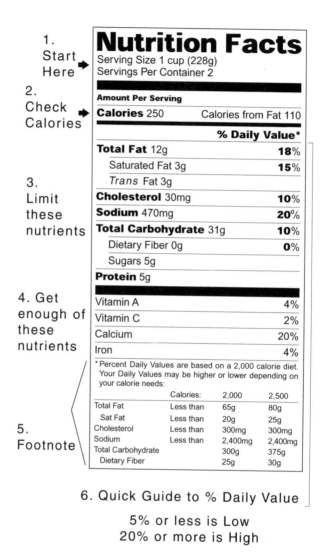

Figure 3.1. Sample Nutrition Facts Label For Macaroni And Cheese (Source: U.S. Food and Drug Administration, 2004).

The size of the serving on the food package influences the number of calories and all the nutrient amounts listed on the top part of the label. Pay attention to the serving size, especially how many servings there are in the food package. Then ask yourself, "How many servings am I consuming"? (for example, ½ serving, 1 serving, or more) In the sample label, one serving of macaroni and cheese equals one cup. If you ate the whole package, you would eat two cups. That doubles the calories and other nutrient numbers, including the %Daily Values as shown in the sample label. Table 3.1. illustrates the differences between a single serving and a double serving.

Table 3.1. Example Nutrition Facts For A Single *vs.* Double Serving

	Single Serving	%DV	Double Serving	%DV
Serving Size	1 cup (228g)		2 cups (456g)	
Calories	250		500	
Calories from Fat	110		220	
Total Fat	12g	18%	24g	36%
Trans Fat	1.5g		3g	
Saturated Fat	3g	15%	6g	30%
Cholesterol	30mg	10%	60mg	20%
Sodium	470mg	20%	940mg	40%
Total Carbohydrate	31g	10%	62g	20%
Dietary Fiber	0g	0%	0g	0%
Sugars	5g		10g	
Protein	5g		10g	
Vitamin A		4%		8%
Vitamin C		2%		4%
Calcium		20%		40%
Iron		4%		8%

Calories And Calories From Fat

Calories provide a measure of how much energy you get from a serving of this food. Many Americans consume more calories than they need without meeting recommended intakes for a number of nutrients. The calorie section of the label can help you manage your weight (that is, gain, lose, or maintain body weight) Remember: the number of servings you consume determines the number of calories you actually eat (your portion amount).

In the example shown in Figure 3.1, there are 250 calories in one serving of this macaroni and cheese (#2 on the sample label). How many calories from fat are there in one serving? Answer: 110 calories, which means almost half the calories in a single serving come from fat. What if you ate the whole package content? Then, you would consume two servings, or 500 calories, and 220 would come from fat.

The Nutrients: How Much?

Look at the top of the nutrient section in the sample label (#3 and #4 in Figure 3.1). It shows you some key nutrients that impact on your health and separates them into two main groups:

Limit These Nutrients (#3 on sample label): The nutrients listed first are the ones Americans generally eat in adequate amounts, or even too much. They are identified "Limit these Nutrients." Eating too much fat, saturated fat, *trans* fat, cholesterol, or sodium may increase your risk of certain chronic diseases, like heart disease, some cancers, or high blood pressure.

Get Enough of These (#4 on sample label): Most Americans don't get enough dietary fiber, vitamin A, vitamin C, calcium, and iron in their diets. They are identified as "Get Enough of these Nutrients." Eating enough of these nutrients can improve your health and help reduce the risk of some diseases and conditions. For example, getting enough calcium may reduce the risk of osteoporosis, a condition that results in brittle bones as one ages. Eating a diet high in dietary fiber promotes healthy bowel function.

✎ What's It Mean?

We see these terms all the time, but what do they mean? (These definitions are based on one serving of a food. If you eat more than one serving, you will go over these levels of calories, fat, cholesterol, and sodium.)

Calorie-Free: Fewer than 5 calories.

Low Calorie: 40 calories or fewer.

Reduced Calorie: At least 25% fewer calories than the regular food item has.

Fat Free: Less than ½ gram of fat.

Low Fat: 3 Grams of fat or fewer.

Reduced Fat: At least 25% less fat than the regular food item has.

Cholesterol Free: Fewer than 2 milligrams cholesterol and no more than 2 grams of saturated fat.

Low Cholesterol: 20 milligrams or fewer cholesterol and 2 grams or less saturated fat.

Sodium Free: Fewer than 5 milligrams sodium.

Very Low Sodium: Fewer than 35 milligrams sodium.

Low Sodium: Fewer than 140 milligrams sodium.

High Fiber: 5 grams or more fiber.

Source: Excerpted from "Healthy Eating," National Women's Health Information Center, August 2004.

Additionally, a diet rich in fruits, vegetables, and grain products that contain dietary fiber, particularly soluble fiber, and low in saturated fat and cholesterol may reduce the risk of heart disease.

Understanding the Footnote

Note the * used after the heading "%Daily Value" on the Nutrition Facts label. It refers to the Footnote in the lower part of the nutrition label (#5 on sample label shown in Figure 3.1) which tells you "%DVs are based on a 2,000 calorie diet." This statement must be on all food labels. But the remaining information in the full footnote may not be on the package if the size of the label is too small. When the full footnote does appear, it will always be the same. It doesn't change from product to product, because it shows recommended dietary advice for all Americans—it is not about a specific food product.

Look at the amounts in the footnote—these are the Daily Values (DV) for each nutrient listed and are based on public health experts' advice. DVs are recommended levels of intakes. DVs in the footnote are based on a 2,000 or 2,500 calorie diet. Note how the DVs for some nutrients change, while others (for cholesterol and sodium) remain the same for both calorie amounts.

Remember!!

You can use the Nutrition Facts label not only to help limit those nutrients you want to cut back on but also to increase those nutrients you need to consume in greater amounts.

Source: U.S. Food and Drug Administration, 2004.

How the Daily Values Relate to the %DVs: Look at the example in Table 3.2 for another way to see how the Daily Values (DVs) relate to the %DVs and dietary guidance. For each nutrient listed there is a DV, a %DV, and dietary advice or a goal. If you follow this dietary advice, you will stay within public health experts' recommended upper or lower limits for the nutrients listed, based on a 2,000 calorie daily diet.

Upper Limit—Eat "Less Than": The nutrients that have "upper daily limits" are listed first on the footnote of larger labels and on the example in Table 3.2. Upper limits means it is recommended that you stay below (eat "less than") the Daily Value nutrient amounts listed per day. For example, the DV for Saturated fat is 20g. This amount is 100% DV for this nutrient. What is the goal or dietary advice? To eat "less than" 20 g or 100%DV for the day.

Lower Limit—Eat "At Least": Now look at the section of the label show in Figure 3.1 where dietary fiber is listed. The DV for dietary fiber is 25g, which is 100% DV. This means it is recommended that you eat "at least" this amount of dietary fiber per day.

The DV for Total Carbohydrate is 300g or 100%DV. This amount is recommended for a balanced daily diet that is based on 2,000 calories, but can vary, depending on your daily intake of fat and protein.

Table 3.2. Examples of DVs versus %DVs Based on a 2,000 Calorie Diet

Nutrient	DV	%DV	Goal
Total Fat	65g	= 100%DV	Less than
Sat Fat	20g	= 100%DV	Less than
Cholesterol	300mg	= 100%DV	Less than
Sodium	2400mg	= 100%DV	Less than
Total Carbohydrate	300g	= 100%DV	At least
Dietary Fiber	25g	= 100%DV	At least

The Percent Daily Value (%DV)

The % Daily Values (%DVs) are based on the Daily Value recommendations for key nutrients but only for a 2,000 calorie daily diet—not 2,500 calories. You, like most people, may not know how many calories you consume in a day. But you can still use the %DV as a frame of reference whether you consume more or less than 2,000 calories.

The %DV helps you determine if a serving of food is high or low in a nutrient. Note: a few nutrients, like *trans* fat, do not have a %DV—they will be discussed later.

Do you need to know how to calculate percentages to use the %DV? No, the label (the %DV) does the math for you. It helps you interpret the numbers (grams and milligrams) by putting them all on the same scale for the day (0–100%DV). The %DV column doesn't add up vertically to 100%. Instead each nutrient is based on 100% of the daily requirements for that nutrient (for a 2,000 calorie diet). This way you can tell high from low and know which nutrients contribute a lot, or a little, to your daily recommended allowance (upper or lower).

✎ What's It Mean?

<u>Milligram (mg):</u> A unit of measure used on nutrition labels to show the amount of minerals in foods. A milligram is a little itty-bit of a gram (there are 1,000 milligrams in a gram).

<u>Ounce:</u> A unit of weight. There are 16 ounces in one pound. Ounces can be used to measure liquids (like 8 fluid ounces in a cup), or they can be used to measure solid things (a slice of cheese is a little less than one ounce).

<u>Percent Daily Value (%DV):</u> The "%DV" on the Nutrition Facts food labels is a number that tells you if there's a lot or a little of a nutrient in a serving of food. 5% DV or less of a nutrient in a serving is low; 20% DV or more is high. Your needs may be different from the illustrations used on food labels. For example, the percentage for calcium is calculated for a person who needs 1,000 mg of calcium in a day. Girls aged 9–18 need more calcium than most adults, so strive to get 130% DV for calcium.

<u>Portion:</u> A helping of food. Portions and servings are different. For example, "one cheese sandwich" is a portion (probably made up of 2 servings of bread and 1 serving of cheese).

<u>Serving Size:</u> A serving size (shown on a Nutrition Facts food label) is an amount of food that people typically eat. All of the nutrition information found on a food label (like %DV of calcium) is for one serving only. Serving sizes can be shown in different ways for different foods—like "slices" of cheese or "ounces" of juice, for example.

Source: From "Dictionary," Powerful Bones, Centers for Disease Control and Prevention (CDC), 2001.

Quick Guide to %DV: 5%DV or less is low and 20%DV or more is high (#6 on sample label show in Figure 3.1). This guide tells you that 5%DV or less is low for all nutrients, those you want to limit (for example, fat, saturated fat, cholesterol, and sodium) or for those that you want to consume in greater amounts (fiber, calcium, etc.). As the Quick Guide shows, 20%DV or more is high for all nutrients.

Look at the amount of Total Fat in one serving listed on the sample nutrition label. Is 18%DV contributing a lot or a little to your fat limit of 100% DV? Check the Quick Guide to %DV. 18%DV, which is below 20%DV, is not yet high, but what if you ate the whole package (two servings)? You would double that amount, eating 36% of your daily allowance for Total Fat. Coming from just one food, that amount leaves you with 64% of your fat allowance (100% - 36% = 64%) for all of the other foods you eat that day, snacks and drinks included.

The %DV can help you with the following tasks:

- **Comparisons:** The %DV makes it easy for you to make comparisons. You can compare one product or brand to a similar product. Just make sure the serving sizes are similar, especially the weight (for example, gram, milligram, ounces) of each product. It's easy to see which foods are higher or lower in nutrients because the serving sizes are generally consistent for similar types of foods, except in a few cases like cereals.

- **Nutrient Content Claims:** Use the %DV to help you quickly distinguish one claim from another, such as "reduced fat" *vs.* "light" or "non-fat." Just compare the %DVs for Total Fat in each food product to see which one is higher or lower in that nutrient—there is no need to memorize definitions. This works when comparing all nutrient content claims, for example, less, light, low, free, more, high, etc.

✔ Quick Tip

The % Daily Value column of the Nutrition Facts label shows you how different foods fit into your diet. (Remember, daily value is the amount needed for a healthy diet.) You want to make sure the total amount of fat, saturated fat, cholesterol, and sodium that you eat in one day doesn't go over 100 percent of your daily value. For nutrients like fiber or vitamins and minerals, you should try to eat foods that will add up to at least 100 percent.

Source Excerpted from "Food Labels," BodyWise (http://www.girlpower.gov/girlarea/bodywise), U.S. Department of Health and Human Services.

- **Dietary Trade-Offs:** You can use the %DV to help you make dietary trade-offs with other foods throughout the day. You don't have to give up a favorite food to eat a healthy diet. When a food you like is high in fat, balance it with foods that are low in fat at other times of the day. Also, pay attention to how much you eat so that the total amount of fat for the day stays below 100%DV.

Nutrients With A %DV But No Weight Listed

Calcium: Look at the %DV for calcium on food packages so you know how much one serving contributes to the total amount you need per day. Remember, a food with 20%DV or more contributes a lot of calcium to your daily total, while one with 5%DV or less contributes a little.

Experts advise adult consumers to consume adequate amounts of calcium, that is, 1,000 mg or 100%DV in a daily 2,000 calorie diet. This advice is often given in milligrams (mg), but the Nutrition Facts label only lists a %DV for calcium.

For certain populations, they advise that adolescents, especially girls, consume 1,300 mg (130%DV) and post-menopausal women consume 1,200 mg (120%DV) of calcium daily. But, the DV for calcium on food labels is 1,000 mg.

Don't be fooled—always check the label for calcium because you can't make assumptions about the amount of calcium in specific food categories. Example: the amount of calcium in milk, whether skim or whole, is generally the same per serving, whereas the amount of calcium in the same size yogurt container (8 oz.) can vary from 20 to 45 %DV.

Trans **Fats, Protein, and Sugars:** Note that *Trans* fat, Sugars and, Protein do not list a %DV on the Nutrition Facts label.

- *Trans* **Fat:** Experts could not provide a reference value for *trans* fat nor any other information that the U.S. Food and Drug Administration (FDA) believes is sufficient to establish a Daily Value or %DV. Scientific reports link *trans* fat (and saturated fat) with raising blood LDL ("bad") cholesterol levels, both of which increase your risk of coronary heart disease, a leading cause of death in the U.S.

☞ **Remember!!**

- Use food labels to make smart choices. The "Nutrition Facts" label tells you the calories, fat, and other nutrients in one serving. (Double the numbers for two servings.)

- The "Serving Size" section of a food label tells you how big the typical portion is. This isn't always the same as a Food Guide Pyramid serving, but it helps you calculate the calories, fat, and other nutrients. Serving size is expressed in common household measurements like cups or teaspoons, as well as metric measurements like grams and milligrams.

- The "Calories" section tells you how many calories are in one serving. "Calories From Fat" tells you how many of the calories in a single serving come from fat. It is recommended that no one get more than 30 percent of calories from fat.

- The "Daily Value Percentages" part of the label tells you how nutritious the food is by showing how much of each nutrient is contained in each serving. Some of the items listed include total and saturated fat, cholesterol, sodium, total carbohydrates (including dietary fiber and sugars), and protein.

Source: Excerpted from "Food Labels," BodyWise (http://www.girlpower.gov/girlarea/bodywise), U.S. Department of Health and Human Services.

- **Protein:** A %DV is required to be listed if a claim is made for protein, such as "high in protein." Otherwise, unless the food is meant for use by infants and children under 4 years old, none is needed. Current scientific evidence indicates that protein intake is not a public health concern for adults and children over 4 years of age.

- **Sugars:** No daily reference value has been established for sugars because no recommendations have been made for the total amount to eat in a day. Keep in mind, the sugars listed on the Nutrition Facts label include naturally occurring sugars (like those in fruit and milk) as well as those added to a food or drink. Check the ingredient list for specifics on added sugars. If you are concerned about your intake of sugars, make sure that added sugars are not listed as one of the first few ingredients. Other names for added sugars include: corn syrup, high-fructose corn syrup, fruit juice concentrate, maltose, dextrose, sucrose, honey, and maple syrup.

To limit nutrients that have no %DV, like *trans* fat and sugars, compare the labels of similar products and choose the food with the lowest amount.

Chapter 4

What Is The Difference Between Portions And Servings?

Have you noticed that the size of muffins, candy bars, and soft drinks has grown over the years? How about portions of restaurant foods like pasta dishes, steaks, and french fries? As portion sizes grow, people tend to eat more-often more than they need to stay healthy.

Larger food portions have more calories. Eating more calories than you need may lead to weight gain. Too much weight gain can put you at risk for weight-related diseases like type 2 diabetes, heart disease, and some cancers.

Managing your weight calls for more than just choosing a healthful variety of foods like vegetables, fruits, grains (especially whole grains), beans, and low-fat meat, poultry, and dairy products. It also calls for looking at how much and how often you eat. This chapter shows you how to use serving sizes to help you eat just enough for you.

What's the difference between a portion and a serving?

A "portion" is how much food you choose to eat, whether in a restaurant, from a package, or in your own kitchen. A "serving" is a standard amount set

About This Chapter" "Just Enough for You: About Food Portion," National Institute of Diabetes and Digestive and Kidney Diseases, NIH Pub. No. 03-5287, June 2005.

by the U.S. government, or sometimes by others for recipes, cookbooks, or diet plans. There are two commonly used standards for serving sizes:

MyPyramid Plan can help you make healthier food choices from every food group and find your balance between food and physical activity. MyPyramid replaces the Food Guide Pyramid. Available from the U.S. Department of Agriculture (USDA) at http://www.mypyramid.gov.

The **Food and Drug Administration (FDA) Nutrition Facts Label** is printed on most packaged foods. It tells you how many calories and how much fat, carbohydrate, sodium, and other nutrients are in one serving of the food. The serving size is based on the amount of food people say they usually eat in one sitting. This size is often different than the serving sizes in the Food Guide Pyramid.

> ### ✎ What's It Mean? Portions and servings, what's the difference?
>
> A **portion** is the amount of food you choose to eat. There is no standard portion size and no single right or wrong portion size.
>
> A **serving** is a standard amount used to help give advice about how much to eat, or to identify how many calories and nutrients are in a food.
>
> Source: From "How Much Are You Eating," Center for Nutrition Policy and Promotion, U.S. Department of Agriculture, March 2002.

How do I know how big my portions are?

For foods that don't have a Nutrition Facts label, such as ground beef, use a kitchen scale to measure the food in ounces (according to the Food Guide Pyramid, one serving of meat, chicken, turkey, or fish is 2 to 3 ounces).

The portion size that you are used to eating may be equal to two or three standard servings. Take a look at this Nutrition Facts label for cookies. The serving size is two cookies, but if you eat four cookies, you are eating two servings—and double the calories, fat, and other nutrients in a standard serving.

To see how many servings a package contains, check the "servings per container" listed on the Nutrition Facts label. You may be surprised to find that small containers often have more than one serving inside.

Table 4.1. What Size Is Your Serving?

Milk Group

8 oz glass of milk = size of a small milk carton

1½ oz of natural cheese = size of two 9-volt batteries

8 oz cup of yogurt = size of a baseball

Meat and Beans Group

2–3 oz of meat, poultry, or fish = size of a deck of cards

2 tablespoons or peanut butter counts as 1 oz = size of a roll of film

1 cup of beans counts as 2 oz = size of a baseball

Vegetable Group

1 cup of raw, leafy vegetables = size of a baseball

10 french fries = size of a deck of cards

½ cup of peas or other vegetables = size of a small computer mouse

Fruit Group

3/4 cup of fruit juice = size of a 6 oz can

1/2 cup of sliced fruit = size of a small computer mouse

1 medium fruit = size of a baseball

Grains Group

1 slice of bread = size of a computer floppy disk

1 cup of dry cereal = size of a baseball

½ cup of pasta = size of a small computer mouse

Source: From Kids Nutrition, U.S. Department of Agriculture, 2002.

Learning to recognize standard serving sizes can help you judge how much you are eating. When cooking for yourself, use measuring cups and spoons to measure your usual food portions and compare them to standard serving sizes from Nutrition Facts labels for a week or so. Put the measured food on a plate before you start eating. This will help you see what one standard serving of a food looks like compared to how much you normally eat.

Another way to keep track of your portions is to use a food diary. Writing down when, what, how much, where, and why you eat can help you be aware of the amount of food you are eating and the times you tend to eat too much. Table 4.2 shows what 1 day of a person's food diary might look like.

After reading the food diary, you can see that this person chose sensible portion sizes for breakfast and lunch—she ate to satisfy her hunger. She had a large chocolate bar in the afternoon for emotional reasons—boredom, not in response to hunger. If you tend to eat when you are not hungry, try doing something else, like taking a break to walk around the block or call a friend, instead of eating.

By 8 p.m., this person was very hungry and ate large portions of higher-fat, higher-calorie foods. If she had made an early evening snack of fruit or pretzels, she might have been less hungry at 8 p.m. and eaten less. She also may have eaten more than she needed because she was at a social event, and was not paying attention to how much she was eating. Through your diary, you can become aware of the times and reasons you eat too much, and try to make different choices in the future.

How can I control portions at home?

You do not need to measure and count everything you eat for the rest of your life—just long enough to recognize standard serving sizes. Try these other ideas to help you control portions at home:

- Take a standard serving out of the package and eat it off a plate instead of eating straight out of a large box or bag.

- Avoid eating in front of the TV or while busy with other activities. Pay attention to what you are eating and fully enjoy the smell and taste of your foods.

Table 4.2. Sample Food Diary

Thursday

Time	Food	Amount	Place	Hunger/Reason
8 am	Coffee, black Banana Low-fat yogurt	6 fl. oz. 1 medium 1 cup	Home	Slightly hungry
1 pm	Turkey and cheese sandwich on whole wheat bread with mustard, tomato, and lettuce	3 oz. turkey, 1 slice American cheese, 2 slices bread	Work	Hungry
	Potato chips, baked	1 small bag, ½ oz.		
	Water	16 fl. oz.		
3 pm	Chocolate bar King size (4 oz.)		Work	Not hungry/bored
8 pm	Fried mozzarella sticks	4	Restaurant	Very hungry/out with friends
	Chicken Caesar Salad	2 cups lettuce, 6 oz. chicken, 6 tbs. dressing, ¾ cups croutons		
	Breadsticks	2 large		
	Apple pie with vanilla ice cream	1/8 of 9-inch pie, 1 cup ice cream		
	Soft drink	12 fl. oz.		

- Eat slowly so your brain can get the message that your stomach is full.

- Take seconds of vegetables or salads instead of higher-fat, higher-calorie parts of a meal such as meats or desserts.

✔ Quick Tip
Tips to help you choose sensible portions

When eating out:

- Choose a "small" or "medium" portion. This includes main dishes, side dishes, and beverages as well. Remember that water is always a good option for quenching your thirst.

- If main dish portions are larger than you want, order an appetizer or side dish instead, or share a main dish with a friend.

- Resign from the "clean your plate club"—when you've eaten enough, leave the rest. If you can chill the extra food right away, take it home in a "doggie bag."

- Ask for salad dressing to be served "on the side" so you can add only as much as you want.

- Order an item from the menu instead of the "all-you-can-eat" buffet.

At home:

- Once or twice, measure your typical portion of foods you eat often. Use standard measuring cups. This will help you estimate the portion size of these foods and similar foods.

- Be especially careful to limit portions of foods high in calories, such as cookies, cakes, other sweets, and fats, oils, and spreads.

- Try using a smaller plate for your meal.

- Put sensible portions on your plate at the beginning of the meal, and don't take "seconds."

Source: From "How Much Are You Eating," Center for Nutrition Policy and Promotion, U.S. Department of Agriculture, March 2002.

- When cooking in large batches, freeze food that you will not serve right away. This way, you won't be tempted to finish eating the whole batch before the food goes bad. And you'll have ready-made food for another day. Freeze in single-meal-sized containers.

- Try to eat three sensible meals at regular times throughout the day. Skipping meals may lead you to eat larger portions of high-calorie, high-fat foods at your next meal or snack. Eat breakfast every day.

- Keep snacking to a minimum. Eating many snacks throughout the day may lead to weight gain.

- When you do have a treat like chips, cookies, or ice cream, eat only one serving, eat it slowly, and enjoy it!

Is getting more food for your money always a good value?

Have you noticed that it only costs a few cents more to get a larger size of fries or soft drink? Getting a larger portion of food for just a little extra money may seem like a good value, but you end up with more food and calories than you need.

Before you buy your next "value combo," be sure you are making the best choice for your health and your wallet. If you are with someone else, share the large-size meal. If you are eating alone, skip the special deal and just order what you need.

How can I control portions when eating out?

Research shows that the more often a person eats out, the more body fat he or she has. Try to prepare more meals at home. Eat out and get take-out foods less often. When you do eat away from home, try these tips to help you control portions:

- Share your meal, order a half-portion, or order an appetizer as a main meal.

- Take half or more of your meal home. You can even ask for your half-meal to be boxed up before you begin eating so you will not be tempted to eat more than you need.

Table 4.3. Sample food portions larger than one serving. This list shows the size of a portion you may choose or be served. They are *not* recommendations. This table compares these portions to Pyramid servings so that you can judge how they might fit into your overall daily eating plan.

Food	Sample portion you receive	Compare to Pyramid serving size	Approximate Pyramid servings in this portion
Grains Group			
Bagel	1 bagel 4½" in diameter (4 ounces)	½ bagel 3" in diameter (1 ounce)	4
Muffin	1 muffin 3½" in diameter (4 ounces)	1 muffin 2½" in diameter (1½ ounces)	3
English-muffin	1 whole muffin	½ muffin	2
Sweet roll or cinnamon bun	1 large from bakery (6 ounces)	1 small (1½ ounces)	4
Pancakes	4 pancakes 5" in diameter (10 ounces)	1 pancake 4" in diameter (1½ ounces)	6
Burrito-sized flour tortilla	1 tortilla 9" in diameter (2 ounces)	1 tortilla 7" in diameter (1 ounce)	2
Individual bag of tortilla chips	1¾ ounces	12 tortilla chips (¾ ounce)	2
Popcorn	16 cups (movie theatre, medium)	2 cups	8

Food	Sample portion you receive	Compare to Pyramid serving size	Approximate Pyramid servings in this portion
Grains Group, continued			
Bun	1 hamburger bun	½ bun	2
Spaghetti	2 cups (cooked)	½ cup (cooked)	4
Rice	1 cup (cooked)	½ cup (cooked)	2
Vegetable Group			
Baked potato	1 large (7 ounces)	1 small (2¼ ounces)	3
French fries	1 medium order (4 ounces)	½ cup, 10 French fries (1 ounce)	4
Meat and Beans Group			
Broiled chicken breast	6 ounces	2 to 3 ounces	2
Fried chicken	3 pieces (7 to 8 ounces)	2 to 3 ounces	3
Broiled fish	6 to 9 ounces	2 to 3 ounces	3
Sirloin steak	8 ounces (cooked, trimmed)	2 to 3 ounces	3
Porterhouse steak or prime rib	13 ounces (cooked, trimmed)	2 to 3 ounces	5
Ham or roast beef*	5 ounces	2 to 3 ounces	2
Tuna salad*	6 ounces	2 to 3 ounces	2

*in deli sandwich

Source: From "How Much Are You Eating," Center for Nutrition Policy and Promotion, U.S. Department of Agriculture, March 2002.

- Stop eating when you begin to feel full. Focus on enjoying the setting and your friends or family for the rest of the meal.

- Avoid large beverages, such as "supersize" soft drinks. They have a large number of calories. Order the small size, choose a calorie-free beverage, or drink water with a slice of lemon.

- When traveling, bring along nutritious foods that will not spoil such as fresh fruit, small cans of fruit, peanut butter and jelly (spread both thin) sandwiches, whole grain crackers, carrot sticks, air-popped popcorn, and bottled water. If you stop at a fast food restaurant, choose one that serves salads, or order the small burger with lettuce and tomato. Have water or nonfat milk with your meal instead of a soft drink. If you want french fries, order the small size.

☞ Remember!!

The amount of calories you eat affects your weight and health. In addition to selecting a healthful variety of foods, look at the size of the portions you eat. Choosing nutritious foods and keeping portion sizes sensible may help you reach and stay at a healthy weight.

Source: National Institute of Diabetes and Digestive and Kidney Diseases, June 2005.

Chapter 5

Healthy Eating Starts With Healthy Shopping

The Power Of Choice

We have the power of choice to decide which foods we will bring home from the grocery store. Making the healthiest food choices when shopping is the key for a well-balanced diet.

Guidelines For A Healthy You

Healthy food choices are important for good health and well-being. Eating well means eating a variety of nutrient-packed foods and beverages from the basic food groups. Make your goal to choose foods low in saturated and trans fats, cholesterol, added sugars, salt, and alcohol.

Basic Healthy Shopping Skills

Keys for making your shopping the most healthful:

• Know your store

• Take a list

• Read the facts

About This Chapter: "Build a Healthy Diet with Smart Shopping," U.S. Department of Agriculture (USDA), May 2005.

Know Your Store

Grocery stores have thousands of products, with most food items grouped together to make your decision-making easier. Many grocery stores have sections where foods are shelved much like the basic food groups.

The basic food groups put foods with similar nutritional value together. The basic food groups are the following:

- fruits

- vegetables

- grains

- calcium-rich foods

- protein sources

Don't forget that your local farmer's market is a great place for finding healthy foods.

Table 5.1. Where are the basic food groups in your store?

Basic Food Group	Typical Store Location(s)	Choose More Often
Fruits	Produce Aisle, Canned Goods, Freezer Aisle, Salad Bar	Variety! Fresh, Frozen, Canned and Dried
Vegetables	Produce Aisle, Canned Goods, Freezer Aisle, Salad Bar	Variety! Fresh, Frozen or Canned
Grains Bakery	Bread Aisle, Pasta & Rice Aisle(s), Cereal Aisle	Whole Grains for at least half of choices
Calcium-Rich Foods (Milk, Yogurt, & Cheese)	Dairy Case, Refrigerated Aisle, Produce Aisle	Reduced-Fat and Fat-Free Choices
Protein Sources (Meat, Fish, Poultry, Eggs, Soy, Beans &Nuts	Deli, Meat Case, Seafood Counter, Egg Case, Canned Goods, Produce(vegetable proteins), Salad Bar	Lean Meats, Skinless Poultry and reduced-fat choices

✔ Quick Tip
Low-Calorie Shopping List

We live in a fast-moving world. To reduce the time you spend in the kitchen you can improve your organization by using a shopping list and keeping a well-stocked kitchen. Shop for quick, low-fat food items, and fill your kitchen cupboards with a supply of low-calorie basics.

Read labels as you shop. Pay attention to the serving size and the servings per container. All labels list total calories in a serving size of the product. Compare the total calories in the product you choose with others like it; choose the one that is lowest in calories.

Source: From "Low-Calorie Shopping List," National Heart, Lung, and Blood Institute, Obesity Education Initiative, December 2004.

Take A List

And stick to it. Healthy decisions start at home. Planning ahead can improve your health while saving you time and money. Before shopping, take the time to check which foods you need at home, and how much you will need to last throughout your meals.

Consider creating a shopping list based on the basic food groups to include a variety of healthy food choices. Think about your menu ideas when adding items to your list. Write your list to match the groups to the layout of your store.

Have everyone in your family make suggestions for the shopping list. Kids (and adults, too) are more willing to try new foods when they help to pick them.

Read The Facts

The Nutrition Facts that is. The Nutrition Facts label is your guide to learning the information you need for making healthy choices. Learning about the Nutrition Facts label is important when shopping to be able to compare foods before you buy.

When reading the Nutrition Facts consider this:

Keep the following low:

- saturated fats
- trans fats
- cholesterol
- sodium

Look for more of the following:

- fiber
- vitamins A and C
- calcium
- iron

Enjoy

Enjoy food shopping while exploring different foods and learning about their Nutrition Facts. Healthy choice can make a healthy you.

Try *Recipes and Tips for Healthy, Thrifty Meals* (http://www.pueblo.gsa.gov/cic_text/food/rec-thrifty/recipes.htm) for ideas on making healthful food choices and meal preparation with sample shopping lists.

> ### ✔ Quick Tip
>
> Shop for quick low fat food items and fill your kitchen cupboards with a supply of lower calorie basics like the following:
>
> - Fat free or low fat milk, yogurt, cheese, and cottage cheese
> - Light or diet margarine
> - Eggs/Egg substitutes
> - Sandwich breads, bagels, pita bread, English muffins
> - Soft corn tortillas, low fat flour tortillas
> - Low fat, low sodium crackers
> - Plain cereal, dry or cooked
> - Rice, pasta
> - White meat chicken or turkey (remove skin)
> - Fish and shellfish (not battered)
> - Beef: round, sirloin, chuck arm, loin and extra lean ground beef
> - Pork: leg, shoulder, tenderloin
> - Dry beans and peas
> - Fresh, frozen, canned fruits in light syrup or juice
> - Fresh, frozen, or no salt added canned vegetables
> - Low fat or nonfat salad dressings
> - Mustard and catsup
> - Jam, jelly, or honey
> - Herbs and spices
> - Salsa
>
> Source: From "Healthy Eating Starts with Healthy Food Shopping," National Heart, Lung, and Blood Institute, Obesity Education Initiative, May 2005.

All year round, check out *Food, Family and Fun: A Seasonal Guide to Healthy Eating* (http://www.fns.usda.gov/tn/students/food_family/index.html) for tips on seasonal foods and cooking methods with great recipes.

Visit *5 a Day Fruits and Vegetables* (http://www.cdc.gov/nccdphp/dnpa/5aday/recipes) to find delicious Fruit and Vegetable recipes for any meal.

Check *Family Meals- Fast, Healthful!* (http://www.fns.usda.gov/tn/resources/nibbles/family_meals.pdf) for tips on how to create speedy meals that are good for you.

Chapter 6

Eating Well While Eating Out

You know the importance of eating well, but how are you supposed to do so when your schedule is so demanding that you're hardly ever at home? Read this chapter to find out how people make healthy food choices while eating out.

If I Eat Well At Home, What's Wrong With Splurging When I Eat Out?

A slice of pizza once in a while won't do you any harm, but if pizza (or any fast food) is all you eat, that can lead to problems. The most obvious health threat of eating too much fast food is weight gain—or even obesity. Teens are more at risk than ever of developing type 2 diabetes, a disease that's linked to overweight and used to affect only adults. But weight gain isn't the only problem. Too much fast food can drag a person's body down in other ways. Because the food we eat affects all aspects of how the body functions, eating the right (or wrong) foods can influence any number of things, including:

- mental functioning;
- emotional well-being;

About This Chapter: This information was provided by TeensHealth, one of the largest resources online for medically reviewed health information written for parents, kids, and teens. For more articles like this one, visit www.TeensHealth.org, or www.KidsHealth.org. © 2004 The Nemours Center for Children's Health Media, a division of The Nemours Foundation.

- energy;   • strength;
- weight;   • future health.

According to the U.S. Food and Drug Administration (FDA), what's important is a person's average food intake over a few days—not just in a single meal. So if you eat a meal consisting of only junk food, try to balance it with healthier foods the rest of that day and the next.

One thing you may want to watch out for when eating out (or even in) is your soda consumption. Colas and other sodas not only contain a lot of sugar, which can cause you to gain weight, they can also interfere with a person's calcium absorption. Because even the sugar-free versions can cause this problem, it's best to limit soda intake.

Eating On The Go

Eating at a fast-food restaurant, the mall, or even the cafeteria may not sound healthy. But it's actually easier than you think to make good choices in these kinds of situations. Cafeterias and fast-food places now offer healthy choices that are also tasty, like grilled chicken salads.

There are two pointers to remember that can help you make wise choices when eating out:

- Our bodies (and our taste buds) need variety. Look for meals that contain a balance of lean proteins (like fish, chicken, or beans if you're a vegetarian), fruits and vegetables (fries and potato chips don't qualify as veggies), and complex carbohydrates like whole-grain breads. That's why a turkey sandwich on whole wheat (with fixings) is a better choice than a burger on a white bun.

- Watch your portion sizes. The portion sizes of American foods have increased over the past few decades so that we are now eating way more than we need. The average size of a hamburger in the 1950s was just 1.5 ounces, compared to our "supersize" version weighing in at 8 ounces today.

Here are some more suggestions to keep in mind when you're eating away from home.

At A Restaurant

Most restaurant portions are way larger than the average serving of food. Ask for half portions, share an entrée with a friend, or take half of your dish home. Here are some other restaurant survival tips:

- Ask for sauces and salad dressings on the side and use them sparingly.
- Use salsa and mustard instead of mayonnaise or oil.
- Ask for olive or canola oil instead of butter, margarine, or shortening.
- Use nonfat or low-fat milk instead of whole milk or cream.
- Order baked, broiled, or grilled (not fried) lean meats including turkey, chicken, seafood, or sirloin steak.
- Salads and vegetables make healthier side dishes than french fries. Use a small amount of sour cream instead of butter if you order a baked potato.
- Choose fresh fruit instead of sugary, high-fat desserts.

At The Mall Or Fast-Food Place

It's tempting to pig out while shopping, but with a little planning, it's easy to eat healthy foods at the mall. Here are some choices:

- single slice of veggie pizza
- grilled, not fried, sandwiches (for example, a grilled chicken breast sandwich)
- small hamburger
- bean burrito
- baked potato
- side salad
- frozen yogurt

Resist the temptation to supersize your meals. This can add up to 25% more fat and calories. The American Dietetic Association also recommends that when you have a craving for something unhealthy, try sharing the food you crave with a friend.

In The School Cafeteria

The suggestions for eating in a restaurant and at the mall apply to cafeteria food as well. Add vegetables and fruit whenever possible, and opt for leaner, lighter items. Go easy on the high-fat, low-nutrition items, such as mayonnaise, fried foods, and heavy salad dressings.

You might want to consider packing your own lunch occasionally. Here are some lunch items that pack a healthy punch:

✔ Quick Tip

Tips For Eating Healthy When Eating Out

- As a beverage choice, ask for water or order fat-free or low-fat milk, unsweetened tea, or other drinks without added sugars.

- Ask for whole wheat bread for sandwiches.

- In a restaurant, start your meal with a salad packed with veggies, to help control hunger and feel satisfied sooner.

- Ask for salad dressing to be served on the side. Then use only as much as you want.

- Choose main dishes that include vegetables, such as stir fries, kebobs, or pasta with a tomato sauce.

- Order steamed, grilled, or broiled dishes instead of those that are fried or sautéed.

- Choose a "small" or "medium" portion. This includes main dishes, side dishes, and beverages.

- Order an item from the menu instead heading for the "all-you-can-eat" buffet.

- If main portions at a restaurant are larger than you want, try one of these strategies to keep from overeating:

  - Order an appetizer or side dish instead of an entrée.

- sandwiches with lean meats or fish, like turkey, chicken, tuna (made with low-fat mayo), lean ham, or lean roast beef. For variety, try other sources of protein, like peanut butter, hummus, or meatless chili.

- low-fat or nonfat milk, yogurt, or cheese

- any fruit that's in season

- raw baby carrots, green and red pepper strips, tomatoes, or vegetable juice

- whole-grain breads, pita, bagels, or crackers

- Share a main dish with a friend.

- If you can chill the extra food right away, take leftovers home in a "doggy bag."

- When your food is delivered, set aside or pack half of it to go immediately.

- Resign from the "clean your plate club"—when you've eaten enough, leave the rest.

- To keep your meal moderate in calories, fat, and sugars:

  - Ask for salad dressing to be served "on the side" so you can add only as much as you want.

  - Order foods that do not have creamy sauces or gravies.

  - Add little or no butter to your food.

  - Choose fruits for dessert most often.

- On long commutes or shopping trips, pack some fresh fruit, cut-up vegetables, low-fat string cheese sticks, or a handful of unsalted nuts to help you avoid stopping for sweet or fatty snacks.

Source: U.S. Department of Agriculture (www.MyPyramid.gov), 2005.

☞ Remember!!

It can be easy to achieve a healthy diet, even on the run. If you develop the skills to make healthy choices now, your body will thank you later. And the good news is you don't have to eat perfectly all the time. It's OK to splurge every once in a while, as long as your diet is generally good.

Source: © 2004 The Nemours Center for Children's Health Media, a division of The Nemours Foundation.

Chapter 7

Fast Food Choices

Definition: Fast foods are quick, reasonably priced, and readily available alternatives to home cooking. While convenient and inexpensive for a busy lifestyle, fast foods are typically high in calories, fat, saturated fat, sugar, and salt.

Fast food chains and restaurants have responded to the public's increasing awareness about nutrition and have attempted to help people concerned about health. For example, they now make ingredient and nutrition information available on their menus. Despite these changes, however, in order to maintain a healthy diet, it is necessary to choose fast foods carefully.

Function: Most people today have less time to select, prepare and eat food than their grandparents did. Fast foods are very appealing because they are widely available and inexpensive.

Food Sources: Fast food items have been modified to reflect consumers' concern about the fat content of their food. Many fast food restaurants have switched from beef tallow or lard to hydrogenated vegetable oils for frying.

Some restaurants offer low calorie choices like salad bars and assorted take-out salads with low calorie dressing, low-fat milkshakes, whole grain buns, lean meats, and grilled chicken items.

Side Effects: Maintaining nutritional balance is not easy with fast food, because there is no control over how they are cooked. For example, some are cooked with a lot of oil and butter, and there may be no option if you want your selection with reduced fat.

The large portions also encourage overeating. Fast food also tend to lack fresh fruits and vegetables.

In general, people with high blood pressure, diabetes, and heart disease must be much more careful about choosing fast food, due to the high content of fat, sodium, and sugar.

Recommendations: Knowing the number of calories and the amount of fat and salt in the fast food can help you decide which items are better choices. Many fast food restaurants have published the nutrient content of their foods. These are often available on request. You can plan a convenient yet healthful diet with this information.

Make better choices when eating at fast food restaurants. In general eat at places that offer a variety of salads, soups, and vegetables. Consider these general tips:

- *Pizza:* Ask for less cheese, and choose low-fat toppings such as onions, mushrooms, green peppers, tomatoes, and other vegetables.

- *Sandwiches:* Healthier choices include regular or junior-size lean roast beef, turkey, or chicken breast, or lean ham. Extras, such as, bacon, cheese, or mayo will increase the fat and calories of the item. Select whole-grain breads over high-fat croissants or biscuits.

- *Hamburgers:* A single, plain meat patty without the cheese and sauces is the best choice. Ask for extra lettuce, tomatoes, and onions. Limit your intake of french fries.

- *Meat, Chicken, and Fish:* Look for items that are roasted, grilled, baked, or broiled. Avoid meats that are breaded or fried. Ask for heavy sauces, such as gravy, on the side. Better still, avoid heavy sauces and dressings altogether.

♣ It's A Fact!!
Survey Links Fast Food, Poor Nutrition Among U.S. Children

A collaborative study conducted by Agricultural Research Service and Harvard University scientists showed decreased nutritional dietary quality and increased caloric intake among U.S. children on days when they consumed fast food. The study, which appears in the January issue of the journal *Pediatrics*, confirms other similar, previously published studies.

The authors analyzed existing dietary intake data from 6,212 children and adolescents, aged 4 to 19, from a nationally representative USDA Continuing Survey of Food Intakes by Individuals, 1994–1996, and the Supplemental Children's Survey, 1998. The survey data are collected on two non-consecutive days by ARS, the U.S. Department of Agriculture's chief scientific research agency.

U.S. children who ate fast food, compared with those who did not, consumed more total calories, more calories per gram of food, more total and saturated fat, more total carbohydrate, more added sugars and more sugar-sweetened beverages, but less milk, fiber, fruit and non-starchy vegetables. The study also revealed out of the two days surveyed, those children who consumed fast food on only one day showed similar nutrient shortfalls on the day they had fast food. But they did not show these shortfalls on the other day.

The study's coauthors include nutritionist Shanthy A. Bowman with the ARS Community Nutrition Research Group, Beltsville, Maryland.; David S. Ludwig and colleagues with Children's Hospital Boston, Massachusetts; and Steven L. Gortmaker with Boston's Harvard School of Public Health.

Some experts estimate that childhood consumption of fast foods increased fivefold, from 2 percent of daily meals in the late 1970s, to 10 percent of daily meals by the mid-1990s. During that time, the number of fast food restaurants more than doubled to an estimated 250,000 nationwide.

The findings are important because childhood obesity is increasing in prevalence. Inadequate consumption of fruits and vegetables has been associated with obesity-related problems such as cardiovascular disease and diabetes. Fruits and non-starchy vegetables may protect against excessive weight gain because of their low energy density and high fiber content.

Source: By Rosalie Marion Bliss, Agricultural Research Service, U.S. Department of Agriculture, January 5, 2004.

Choose smaller-sized servings. Consider splitting some fast food items to reduce the amount of calories and fat. Ask for a "doggy bag." or simply leave the excess on your plate.

To help supplement and balance the fast food meal, make nutritious options such as fresh fruits, vegetables, and yogurt available as snacks.

When chosen carefully and not used in excess, fast foods can offer reasonably good quality nutrition. By being aware of what and how much you eat, and paying attention to how it affects your health, you can set a good example for your children. As always, variety and moderation are the key principles in providing a healthy diet for children as well as adults.

Chapter 8

Delicious Decisions:
Healthy Tips For Any Cuisine

International Indulgence: So how can you eat at Marcel's and avoid those rich cream sauces? At Luigi's and steer clear of cream cake? At the China Pagoda or Juan's without loading up on fried foods?

It's easy! All you need to know is how to place your order for a low-fat lifestyle. The good news is that almost every cuisine boasts delicious help-your-heart foods.

American Family Restaurants: Avoid dishes with lots of cheese, sour cream, and mayonnaise. Instead of fried oysters, fish, or chicken, choose boiled shrimp, or baked, broiled, or grilled fish or chicken. Choose bread or pita pockets over croissants. Salads make great meals, but be careful of the dressing. If you must have a high-fat entree, split it with another family member. You'll save dollars, and fat.

Cajun: Avoid fried seafood and hush puppies. Blackened entrees are usually dipped in butter or oil, covered with spices and pan-fried; ask the cook to use only a small amount of oil. Ask for all sauces and gravies on the side.

About This Chapter: Excerpted from *Delicious Decisions* and reproduced with permission. American Heart Association. For more information visit www.deliciousdecisions.org. © 1998, American Heart Association.

Chinese: Choose entrees with lots of vegetables—chop suey with steamed rice is an example. Ask to substitute chicken for duck. Skip the crispy fried noodles on the table.

Fast Food: Beware of topping burgers with cheese, special (mayonnaise-based) sauce, and bacon—they add fat and calories. Pickles, onions, lettuce, tomato, mustard, and ketchup add flavor without the fat. Steer clear of fried fish sandwiches. A baked potato can be a healthful option, but have it plain or with yogurt or low-fat cottage cheese.

French: Bypass the rich entrees, desserts, and sauces. Aim for simple dishes with sauces on the side. Nouvelle cuisine or Provençal tomato-and-herb-based entrees are good choices. Ask that margarine instead of butter be used in cooking, or leave it out altogether.

Greek and Middle Eastern: Ask for dishes to be prepared with less oil and served with high-sodium foods, like feta cheese and olives, on the side. Phyllo pastry dishes are usually high in butter, so skip them. Most Greek desserts are high in fat. If you want to splurge, split one with a friend.

Health Food and Vegetarian: Health food and vegetarian food are usually fresh and wholesome. Protein usually comes from chicken or fish, or it may be from combined vegetable proteins (such as rice and beans). But watch out for fats and oils. Sometimes vegetarian recipes compensate for meatless entrees by adding fat to fill you up. There are many great vegetarian sandwiches. Just avoid those with lots of cheese and avocado.

Indian: Start with salads or yogurt with chopped or shredded vegetables. Choose chicken or seafood rather than beef or lamb. Choose dishes prepared without ghee. Order one protein and one vegetable dish to cut down the fat and calories. If sodium is a concern, forgo the soups.

Italian: Enjoy pasta as a main entree rather than as an appetizer. Share foods among your dinner companions. Ask your server to hold the Parmesan (grated) cheese, and the bacon, olives and pine nuts. If you order pizza, choose ingredients like spinach, mushrooms, broccoli and roasted peppers.

✔ Quick Tip

If you're treating yourself to a meal out, here are some tips to help make it a dining experience that is both tasty and good for you.

Ask

Will the restaurant:

• serve margarine rather than butter with the meal?

• serve fat free (skim) milk rather than whole milk or cream?

• trim visible fat from poultry or meat?

• leave all butter, gravy or sauces off a dish?

• serve salad dressing on the side?

• accommodate special requests?

• use less cooking oil when cooking?

Act

Select foods which are:

• steamed

• garden fresh

• broiled

• baked

• roasted

• poached

• lightly sautéed or stir-fried

Source: "Eating Healthy When Dining Out," an undated *Tipsheet* produced by the National Heart, Lung, and Blood Institute in cooperation with the National Institute of Diabetes and Digestive and Kidney Diseases, December 2004.

Japanese: Ask the cook to prepare your food without high-sodium marinades, sauces and salt. And ask that sauces be served on the side. Avoid deep-fried, battered, or breaded foods.

Mexican: Tell your server not to bring fried tortilla chips to the table. And hold the sour cream and guacamole from entrees—use salsa to add flavor. Vera cruz or other tomato-based sauces are better than creamy or cheesy sauces. If you order a taco salad, don't eat the fried shell.

Steakhouses: Don't order king-sized cuts. About 3 ounces of a thinly sliced cut is perfect, or choose a 6 ounce steak and enjoy non-meat entrees the rest of the day. Steakhouses generally prepare your food to order, so ask them to trim all visible fat before cooking.

Take-Home: It's a challenge to eat tasty, nutritious meals when you're racing against the clock. Many supermarkets and specialty stores now offer prepared entrees and even entire meals to take home when you're not in a rush.

Guess what? The same tips for restaurant foods apply to prepared take-out foods. Here are some low-fat side dishes to add to your prepared entrees:

• Salad with fat-free or low-fat dressing

• Fresh, cut-up, or cooked vegetables

• Bread or rolls

• Fruit for dessert

Thai: Aim for the lighter, stir-fried dishes, and the fresh spring rolls. Steer clear of heavy sauces and deep-fried entrees. Ask that cooking be done with vegetable oil rather than coconut oil or lard. Choose chicken over duck, but limit meat, poultry, and seafood portions.

Vietnamese: Vietnamese food is one of the world's oldest and most exquisite cuisines. Its subtle flavors and textures blend the Far East with French cooking for a marvelous dining experience. And many of the dishes are low in fat.

✔ Quick Tip

Many ethnic cuisines offer lots of low fat, low calorie choices. So, if you want to eat healthy and still have lots of different choices, take a taste adventure with ethnic foods. Here's a sample of healthy food choices (lower in calories and fat) and terms to look for when making your selection:

Chinese

• Steamed

• Jum (poached)

• Kow (roasted)

• Shu (barbecued)

• Steamed rice

• Dishes without monosodium glutamate (MSG) added

Italian

• Red sauces

• Primavera (no cream)

• Piccata (lemon)

• Sun-dried tomatoes

• Crushed tomatoes

• Lightly sautéed

• Grilled

Mexican

• Spicy chicken

• Rice and black beans

• Salsa or Picante

• Soft corn tortillas

Source: "Eating Healthy With Ethnic Food," an undated *Tipsheet* produced by the National Heart, Lung, and Blood Institute in cooperation with the National Institute of Diabetes and Digestive and Kidney Diseases, December 2004.

Chapter 9

Healthy Eating For Teen Vegetarians

Is A Vegetarian Diet Right For Me?

For much of the world, vegetarianism is largely a matter of economics—meat costs a lot more than, say, beans or rice. As such, meat becomes a special-occasion dish (if it's eaten at all). Even where meat is more plentiful, it's still used in moderation, often providing a side note to a meal rather than taking center stage.

In countries like the United States where meat is not as expensive, though, people choose to be vegetarians for reasons other than economics. Parental preferences, religious beliefs, lifestyle factors, and health issues are among the most common reasons for choosing to be a vegetarian. Many people choose a vegetarian diet out of concern over animal rights or the environment. And lots of people have more than one reason for choosing vegetarianism.

Vegetarian And Semi-Vegetarian Diets

Different people follow different forms of vegetarianism. A true vegetarian eats no meat at all, including chicken and fish. A lacto-ovo vegetarian eats dairy products and eggs, but excludes meat, fish, and poultry. It follows, then, that a lacto vegetarian eats dairy products but not eggs, whereas an ovo vegetarian eats eggs but not dairy products.

A stricter form of vegetarianism is a vegan (pronounced: vee-gun or vee-jan) diet. Not only are eggs and dairy products excluded from a vegan diet, so are animal products like honey and gelatin. There are a surprising number of foods that you'd think might be vegetarian but aren't—foods like gelatin, which are made using meat byproducts; cheese, which is made using an animal-based product called rennet, and sauces such as Worcestershire sauce. Vegans avoid all these foods.

Some macrobiotic diets fall into the vegan category. Macrobiotic diets restrict not only animal products but also refined and processed foods, foods with preservatives, and foods that contain caffeine or other stimulants.

Following a macrobiotic or vegan diet could lead to nutritional deficiencies in teens, who need to be sure their diets include enough nutrients to fuel growth, particularly protein and calcium. If you're interested in following a vegan or macrobiotic diet it's a good idea to talk to a registered dietitian. He or she can help you design meal plans that include adequate vitamins and minerals.

Some people consider themselves semi-vegetarians and eat fish and maybe a small amount of poultry as part of a diet that's primarily made up of vegetables, fruits, grains, legumes, seeds, and nuts. A pesci-vegetarian eats fish, but not poultry.

Are These Diets OK For Teens?

In the past, choosing not to eat meat or animal-based foods was considered unusual in the United States. Times and attitudes have changed dramatically, however. Vegetarians are still a minority in the United States, but a large and growing one. The American Dietetic Association (ADA) has officially endorsed vegetarianism, stating "appropriately planned vegetarian diets are healthful, are nutritionally adequate, and provide health benefits in the prevention and treatment of certain diseases."

So what does this mean for you? If you're already a vegetarian, or are thinking of becoming one, it means that you're in good company. There are more choices in the supermarket than ever before, and an increasing number of restaurants and schools are providing vegetarian options—way beyond a basic peanut butter and jelly sandwich.

If you're choosing a vegetarian diet, the most important thing you can do is to educate yourself. That's why the ADA says that a vegetarian diet needs to be "appropriately planned." Simply dropping certain foods from your diet isn't the way to go if you're interested in maintaining good health, a high energy level, and strong muscles and bones.

Vegetarians have to be careful to include the following key nutrients because they may be lacking in a vegetarian diet: iron, calcium, protein, vitamins D and B_{12}, and zinc. If meat, fish, dairy products, and/or eggs are not going to be part of your diet, you'll need to know how to get enough of these nutrients, or you may need to take a daily multiple vitamin and mineral supplement.

Here are some suggestions:

Iron: Sea vegetables like nori, wakame, and dulse are very high in iron. Less exotic but still good options are iron-fortified breakfast cereals, legumes (chickpeas, lentils, and baked beans), soybeans and tofu, dried fruit (raisins and figs), pumpkin seeds, broccoli, and blackstrap molasses. Eating these foods with a food high in vitamin C (citrus fruits and juices, tomatoes, and broccoli) will help you to better absorb the iron. Girls need to be particularly concerned about getting adequate iron because some iron is lost during menstruation. Some girls who are vegetarians may not get adequate iron from vegetable sources and require a daily supplement. Check with your doctor about your own iron needs.

Calcium: Milk and yogurt are tops if you're eating dairy products; otherwise, tofu, fortified soy milk, calcium-fortified orange juice, green leafy vegetables, and dried figs are excellent choices. Remember that as a teen you're building up your bones for the rest of your life. Because women have a greater risk for getting osteoporosis (weak bones) as adults, it's particularly important for them to make sure they get enough calcium. Again, taking a supplement may be necessary to ensure this.

♣ It's A Fact!!
What Vegetarian Teens Need Every Day

Legumes, Eggs, Soy-Based Meat Substitutes, And Nuts/Seeds

- Servings: 2–3

- Serving Size:

    - ½ c. cooked dry beans, peas, or lentils

    - 3 oz. soy-based meat substitute

    - ¼ c. tofu or tempeh

    - 1 egg or 2 egg whites

    - 2 T. nuts, seeds, peanut butter, other nut butter, or seed butter

Nutrition Tip: Select tofu set with calcium sulfate for a calcium bonus: ½ cup can have as much calcium as 1 cup of milk

Milk Or Milk Substitute

- Servings: 4

- Serving Size:

    - 1 c. milk or yogurt

    - 1 c. calcium- and vitamin D-fortified soy milk or soy yogurt

    - 1 ½ oz. cheese or soy cheese

Nutrition Tip: Protect your bones: Calcium-fortified juice, cereals, and calcium-rich plant foods like collard greens and tofu with calcium sulfate can also help meet calcium needs.

Grains

- Servings: 8–11

- Serving Size:

    - 1 slice bread

    - ½ c. pasta or rice

    - 1 oz. ready-to-eat cereal

Nutrition Tip: Check the label: Look for 100% whole grain breads and fortified cereals. Whole grains provide fiber, vitamins, minerals, and protein.

Vegetables

- Servings: 4–5
- Serving Size:
  - ¾ c. juice
  - 1 c. raw, leafy greens
  - ½ c. chopped cooked vegetables

Nutrition Tip: Eat plenty of nutrient-rich dark green, deep red, and yellow-orange vegetables for vitamins A and C.

Fruits

- Servings: 3–4
- Serving Size:
  - ¾ c. juice
  - ¼ c. dried fruit
  - ½ c. fresh or canned
  - 1 medium-size piece

Nutrition Tip: Vitamin C-rich foods like strawberries and orange juice boosts iron absorption from iron-rich foods like legumes and iron-fortified cereals

Added Fats And Sugars

- Servings: As needed for extra calories

Nutrition Tip: Tannins in tea and coffee reduce iron absorption, so avoid overdoing these beverages.

Notes

*Most teenage girls need the lower number of servings; boys and very active girls need the higher number.

This information was prepared with the assistance of the Vegetarian Nutrition Practice Group, American Dietetic Association.

Source: From "What Vegetarian Teens Need Every Day," *Nutrition and Your Child Newsletter,* Winter 2000. © 2000 USDA/ARS (U.S. Department of Agriculture/Agricultural Research Service) Children's Nutrition Research Center at Baylor College of Medicine; reprinted with permission.

Vitamin D: Cow's milk and sunshine are tops on the list for this vitamin, which you need to get calcium into your bones. Vegans can try fortified soy milk and fortified breakfast cereals, but they may need a supplement that includes vitamin D, especially during the winter months. Everyone should have some exposure to the sun to help the body produce vitamin D.

Protein: Some people believe that vegetarians must combine incomplete plant proteins in one meal—like red beans and rice—to make the type of complete proteins found in meat. We now know that it's not that complicated. Current recommendations are that vegetarians eat a wide variety of foods during the course of a day. Eggs and dairy products are good sources of protein, but also try nuts, peanut butter, tofu, beans, seeds, soy milk, grains, cereals, and vegetables to get all the protein your body needs.

Vitamin B$_{12}$: B$_{12}$ is an essential vitamin found only in animal products, including eggs and dairy. Fortified soy milk and fortified breakfast cereals

♣ It's A Fact!!
Nutrients To Focus On For Vegetarians

- Protein has many important functions in the body and is essential for growth and maintenance. Protein needs can easily be met by eating a variety of plant-based foods. Combining different protein sources in the same meal is not necessary. Sources of protein for vegetarians include beans, nuts, nut butters, peas, and soy products (tofu, tempeh, veggie burgers). Milk products and eggs are also good protein sources for lacto-ovo vegetarians.

- Iron functions primarily as a carrier of oxygen in the blood. Iron sources for vegetarians include iron-fortified breakfast cereals, spinach, kidney beans, black-eyed peas, lentils, turnip greens, molasses, whole wheat breads, peas, and some dried fruits (dried apricots, prunes, raisins).

- Calcium is used for building bones and teeth and in maintaining bone strength. Sources of calcium for vegetarians include fortified breakfast also have this important vitamin. It's hard to get enough vitamin B$_{12}$ in your diet if you are vegan, so a supplement may be needed.

Zinc: If you're not eating dairy foods, make sure fortified cereals, dried beans, nuts, and soy products like tofu and tempeh are part of your diet so you can meet your daily requirement for this important mineral.

In addition to vitamins and minerals, vegetarians need to keep an eye on their total intake of calories and fat. Vegetarian diets tend to be high in fiber and low in fat and calories. That may be good for people who need to lose weight or lower their cholesterol but it can be a problem for kids and teens who are still growing and people who are already at a healthy weight. Diets that are high in fiber tend to be more filling, and as a result strict vegetarians may feel full before they've eaten enough calories to keep their bodies healthy and strong. It's a good idea to let your doctor know that you're a vegetarian so that he or she can keep on eye on your growth and make sure you're still getting adequate amounts of calories and fat.

cereals, soy products (tofu, soy-based beverages), calcium-fortified orange juice, and some dark green leafy vegetables (collard greens, turnip greens, bok choy, mustard greens). Milk products are excellent calcium sources for lacto vegetarians.

• Zinc is necessary for many biochemical reactions and also helps the immune system function properly. Sources of zinc for vegetarians include many types of beans (white beans, kidney beans, and chickpeas), zinc-fortified breakfast cereals, wheat germ, and pumpkin seeds. Milk products are a zinc source for lacto vegetarians.

• Vitamin B$_{12}$ is found in animal products and some fortified foods. Sources of vitamin B$_{12}$ for vegetarians include milk products, eggs, and foods that have been fortified with vitamin B$_{12}$. These include breakfast cereals, soy-based beverages, veggie burgers, and nutritional yeast.

Source: Excerpted from "Vegetarian Diets," U.S. Department of Agriculture (MyPyramid.gov), 2005.

✔ Quick Tip

• Build meals around protein sources that are naturally low in fat, such as beans, lentils, and rice. Don't overload meals with high-fat cheeses to replace the meat.

• Calcium-fortified soy-based beverages can provide calcium in amounts similar to milk. They are usually low in fat and do not contain cholesterol.

• Many foods that typically contain meat or poultry can be made vegetarian. This can increase vegetable intake and cut saturated fat and cholesterol intake. Consider:

  • pasta primavera or pasta with marinara or pesto sauce

  • veggie pizza

  • vegetable lasagna

  • tofu-vegetable stir fry

  • vegetable lo mein

  • vegetable kabobs

  • bean burritos or tacos

• A variety of vegetarian products look (and may taste) like their non-vegetarian counterparts, but are usually lower in saturated fat and contain no cholesterol.

  • For breakfast, try soy-based sausage patties or links.

Getting Some Guidance

When Danielle's mom knew that she was serious about becoming a vegetarian, she made an appointment for Danielle to talk with a registered dietitian. The dietitian and Danielle went over lists of foods and recipe ideas that would give her the nutrients she needs. They discussed ways to prevent conditions such as iron-deficiency anemia that Danielle might be at an increased risk of developing. And whenever Danielle sees her family doctor, the doctor reminds her to eat many different kinds of foods each day and to get enough protein and iron.

- Rather than hamburgers, try veggie burgers. A variety of kinds are available, made with soy beans, vegetables, and/or rice.

- Add vegetarian meat substitutes to soups and stews to boost protein without adding saturated fat or cholesterol. These include tempeh (cultured soybeans with a chewy texture), tofu, or wheat gluten (seitan).

- For barbecues, try veggie or garden burgers, soy hot dogs, marinated tofu or tempeh, and veggie kabobs.

- Make bean burgers, lentil burgers, or pita halves with falafel (spicy ground chick pea patties).

- Some restaurants offer soy options (texturized vegetable protein) as a substitute for meat, and soy cheese as a substitute for regular cheese.

- Most restaurants can accommodate vegetarian modifications to menu items by substituting meatless sauces, omitting meat from stir-fries, and adding vegetables or pasta in place of meat. These substitutions are more likely to be available at restaurants that make food to order.

- Many Asian and Indian restaurants offer a varied selection of vegetarian dishes.

Source: Excerpted from "Vegetarian Diets," U.S. Department of Agriculture (MyPyramid.gov), 2005.

Danielle also tries to remember to take a daily standard multivitamin, just in case she's missed getting enough vitamins or minerals that day.

Tips For Eating Out

Danielle admits that eating out can be difficult sometimes, but because she does eat fish, she can usually find something suitable on a restaurant menu. If not, she opts for salad and an appetizer or two. Even fast food places sometimes have vegetarian choices, such as bean tacos and burritos, veggie burgers made from soybeans, and soy cheese pizza.

Because both she and her sister are vegetarians, Danielle's family rarely eats red meat anymore. Her mom serves salmon frequently, and Danielle eats a lot of pasta, along with plenty of vegetables, grains, and fruits. Danielle is also psyched about some of the vegetarian products now available in the grocery store. The veggie burgers, hot dogs, and chicken substitutes taste very much like the real thing. She especially likes the ground soy "beef" that makes a great stand-in for ground beef in foods like tacos and spaghetti sauce.

Remember that it's important to eat a wide variety of foods, and to try out new foods, too—regardless of whether you choose a vegetarian way of life.

☞ Remember!!

Vegetarian diets can meet all the recommendations for nutrients. The key is to consume a variety of foods and the right amount of foods to meet your calorie needs. Follow the food group recommendations for your age, sex, and activity level to get the right amount of food and the variety of foods needed for nutrient adequacy. Nutrients that vegetarians may need to focus on include protein, iron, calcium, zinc, and vitamin B_{12}.

Source: Excerpted from "Vegetarian Diets," U.S. Department of Agriculture (MyPyramid.gov), 2005.

Chapter 10

Eating In The School Cafeteria

School Cafeteria—How To Make Healthy Choices

Most school calendars are about 180 days long. That's a lot of school lunches. Cafeteria food may not seem awesome—not like home cooking—but it's actually gotten a lot healthier in recent years. News that children in the United States are becoming increasingly overweight has pushed many schools to make their cafeteria food healthier. A lot of schools still serve fast food, though. But with a little thought and planning, you can eat healthy meals at school every day.

One way to make sure your meal is healthy is to pack it at home. That way, you can make sure to get enough from different sections of the food guide pyramid. For example, you can have a turkey, low-fat cheese, lettuce, and tomato sandwich on whole wheat bread with mustard; an apple, orange, or pear; a small salad; and a carton of non-fat milk. For dessert, try low-fat pudding or yogurt with low-fat dry cereal or granola, or even a couple of fig bars. Overall, that's a pretty healthy meal, even with dessert. Here are some tips in packing:

• Keep hot foods hot and cold foods cold by using insulated containers.

About This Chapter: From "School Cafeteria—How To Make Healthy Choices," Girl Power! U.S. Department of Health and Human Services (www.girlpower.gov), updated 2004.

- Pack lunch the night before to avoid the morning rush.

- Make sure to throw out leftovers that may spoil (meat, cheese, egg, milk, foods with mayonnaise) and clean the containers thoroughly.

When you don't have time to pack a lunch, eating cafeteria food is okay, too. Just take a minute to think about what you're eating. Vending machine snacks, soda, and fast food may sound tasty and quick, but they should be eaten on occasion, not as everyday meals. Ask your school food service director or administrator to provide healthy choices in vending machines and school stores. Ask them to make it easier for you to make healthy choices everywhere food is sold or provided at school.

Here are some things to keep in mind when choosing a cafeteria meal:

✔ Quick Tip
Packing A Safe School Lunch

How often do you pack a lunch to take to school with you?

If you take a lunch to school, it is important to know what to do to keep from getting sick.

Some foods need special attention, like milk, meats, and cheeses. These foods can make you sick if food poisoning bacteria is allowed to grow on them.

A bacteria is a one-celled organism that can only be seen with a microscope. Some types of bacteria on food can make you sick, so it is important to know what to do. If you eat foods that have these bacteria on them, you could get food poisoning. Food poisoning will give you a stomach ache, but it can be very serious.

How To Make Sure Your Lunch Is Safe

- Put something cold in the lunch box. A fun trick is to freeze a juice box overnight and put that in your lunch box right next to your sandwich. That way, your sandwich will not get too warm and you still have a cold drink at lunchtime. If you do not take a juice box, a small, plastic refrigerator dish filled with water and put into the freezer the night before will do the trick.

- You can have fried chicken, if there aren't better options, but a way to cut down on the fat is to take off the skin.

- Vegetable soup and a salad with some whole-grain bread is a filling and healthy option.

- Fruit, low-fat granola, and low-fat yogurt is a good choice if you're not starving, but still want a good lunch.

- Choose non-fat or low-fat milk instead of whole milk.

- Fruit, frozen yogurt, or frozen fruit pops are good dessert options.

Keeping to a healthy eating pattern while you're at school takes a little more thought and work, but it's worth it to stay on track. You'll have more energy and be more alert during afternoon classes.

- Freeze your sandwiches. This works better with coarse-textured breads that won't get soggy when they thaw. The sandwich will be thawed by the time you eat lunch, and it keeps everything else in the lunch box cold. (If you like lettuce, tomato, and mayonnaise on your sandwich, pack those separately. They do not freeze well, and you may not like the taste when they thaw.)

- Use a thermos to keep milk or juice cold until lunchtime. Some juices do not even need to be refrigerated.

- Keep your lunch in the coolest place possible. If you have a refrigerator at school, put your lunch in there. If not, keep it out of the sun and away from the heat.

Every day, you can practice these food safety tips and you can feel a lot healthier because of it.

Source: "Packing a Safe School Lunch," reprinted with permission from the Michigan Department of Agriculture. Copyright © 2004 State of Michigan.

♣ It's A Fact!!

• 19.7% of schools usually give students less than 20 minutes to eat lunch once they are seated.

• 26.4% of schools begin serving lunch before 11:00 am, and 4.5% of schools begin serving lunch before 10:30 am. In 12.9% of schools, lunch is served until after 1:00 p.m., and in 2.2% of schools, lunch is served until after 1:30 p.m.

Source: From "Fact Sheet: Food Service," School Health Policies and Programs Study (SHPPS 2000), Centers for Disease Control and Prevention.

Chapter 11

Plan For Snacking

For many of today's active and time-strapped teens, eating healthy may be a priority, but who really has the time? Between after-school activities, sports, homework, and active social lives, many teens don't have time to sit down for a balanced meal with the family. Instead they grab something quick for refueling, like potato chips or a candy bar. Snacks keep teens going when they are dragging—but nutritious snacks can keep them going longer.

Smart Snacking

Snacks can be an important part of a healthy diet. Well-chosen, balanced, and moderate-sized snacks can help teens manage weight, hunger, health, and energy. Since most adolescents don't eat perfectly balanced meals, snacks can help them meet their recommended daily guidelines for fruits, vegetables, protein, dairy, and grain intake. Snacking can be a great way to get all the vitamins and nutrients a growing body needs, especially calcium. And speaking of growing bodies, teens going through growth spurts require more calories. You may have already noticed that you sometimes eat like you can never get enough. This is perfectly normal as you go through puberty.

About This Chapter: Reprinted with permission from "Smart Snacking For Teens," part of the Tips to Grow By© series produced as a public service by Akron Children's Hospital. Copyright © 2005 Akron Children's Hospital. All rights reserved. For additional information, visit http://www.akronchildrens.org/tips/.

Keep snacks on hand that contain complex carbohydrates—like whole wheat bagels, graham crackers, or unsweetened cereal—and foods that contain protein—such as low-fat yogurt, hard-boiled eggs, and skim milk. These will help keep your energy level consistent throughout the day. Include some fruit, pretzels, or low-fat granola bars in your school bag so you have a nutritious snack available before sports practice.

To start the day off right make sure you eat breakfast. It increases metabolism and energy, allowing your brain to function more effectively. This means better school performance, better athletic performance, and more calories burned. If you just can't sit down for breakfast, take nuts or a banana to eat on the bus.

Snacks On The Go

Stock your refrigerator and cupboards with ready-to-go snack fixings like these:

- **Refrigerator snacks:** Yogurt, cottage cheese, hummus, pita, low-fat cheese, lean deli meats, fruit juice, milk, and ready-to-eat fruits and vegetables are some great ideas.

✔ Quick Tip

It's easy to make tasty, healthy snacks. Each of these snacks counts toward servings from two or three food groups. They're ranked from super-easy to prepare to takes-some-effort.

Ultra-Easy, No Fuss

- Reduced fat yogurt topped with a favorite fruit.
- Baked tortilla chips with salsa.
- Baby carrots.

Easy, Minor Preparation

- Ice cream sandwich made with oatmeal cookies.
- Microwaved chicken noodle soup mixed with corn or other vegetables.
- Peanut butter sandwich made with banana slices.

A Little More Effort

- Fruit smoothie made with ice cream, fruit, and reduced fat milk.
- Ham and lettuce, rolled up in a soft tortilla.
- Microwaved potato topped with reduced fat cheese.

Source: "Snack Attack," Bodywise, www.girl power.gov, U.S. Department of Health and Human Services, 2004.

- **Shelf snacks:** Make sure you are prepared for the munchies by stashing nutritious snacks in your locker: pretzels, whole-grain cereal, cans of water-packed tuna, peanut butter, boxes of raisins, baked tortilla chips, instant oatmeal, dried fruit, single serving fruit cups or applesauce, or whole-wheat crackers.

- **Microwave snacks:** Make an instant pizza by topping a bagel or English muffin with tomato sauce and cheese. Make a hot bean dip with refried beans, salsa, and mild green chilies, and serve with baked tortillas.

✔ **Quick Tip**
Microwave Safety

- Reheat hot dogs until they are hot and steaming. Pierce hot dogs with a fork before putting them into the microwave oven to keep them from exploding.

- Foods and liquids are heated unevenly in the microwave, so stir or rotate food midway through cooking. If you don't, you'll have cold spots where harmful bacteria can survive.

- Cover a dish of food for microwaving with a lid or plastic wrap and wrap loose to let steam escape. The moist heat will help destroy harmful bacteria.

- To prevent burns, carefully remove food from the microwave oven. Use potholders and uncover foods away from your face so steam can escape.

- Do not use plastic containers such as margarine tubs or other one-time use containers in the microwave. They can warp or melt, possibly causing harmful chemicals to get in the food.

- Do not use metal or aluminum foil containers in the microwave. They can get too hot and burn. Use only glass and other containers labeled "made for microwave use."

- Throw away leftovers (and any perishable food) that stays out longer than two hours—or one hour if it's over 90°F. When in doubt, throw it out.

Source: Excerpted from "Home Alone? After School Snacks and Food Safety USDA Quiz for Parents and Kids," Food Safety and Inspection Service, U.S. Department of Agriculture, September 2004.

- **Sweet snacks:** Try these goodies: pudding, oatmeal-raisin cookies, fig bars, graham crackers, hot chocolate, frozen yogurt, dried fruit, raisin toast, vanilla wafers, frozen juice bars, smoothies, or a fruit flavored bagel.

- **Other snack ideas:** For long car rides take along canned or boxed 100 percent juice, crackers and cheese, pretzels, air-popped or microwave popcorn, fresh fruit, dried fruit, raisin-nut mixes, or sunflower seeds.

Read The Food Labels

Make it a point to read the nutrition facts label that appears on most processed or prepared foods. These labels provide valuable information on serving size, total calories, calories from carbohydrates, protein, and fat and other nutritional information. In addition, these labels list their primary ingredients in descending order. Try to choose snacks that don't have sugar, salt, or oil listed as their prime

♣ **It's A Fact!!**
These days, many kids don't just open a bag of chips—some make cookies from scratch; others use a microwave to heat up instant noodles or soup. Sound safe? Not if the cookie maker tastes the raw homemade cookie dough because that could lead to *Salmonella* poisoning and sometimes hospitalization. And heating soup in the microwave isn't safe if the cook isn't tall enough to reach the microwave and spills hot soup on himself. That's a major cause of serious burns in children.

Before you take over in the kitchen, USDA advises you to take a little quiz:

Quiz: True Or False

1. Put backpacks on the floor, not the counter.

2. Washing your hands with warm water and soap washes bacteria down the drain.

3. You need to wash fruits and vegetables under cold running water before eating.

4. Cooked foods should not be put on the same plate that held raw meat or poultry (unless the plate has been thoroughly washed.).

5. Lunch meat or deli meat does not need to be refrigerated until the package is opened.

6. Don't leave leftovers on the counter for more than two hours.

7. Always wash your hands after touching raw meat or poultry.

8. Eating homemade cookie dough is not safe because it may contain raw eggs.

(Answers: 1, 2, 3, 4–True. 5–False. 6,7,8–True.)

Source: Excerpted from "Home Alone? After School Snacks and Food Safety USDA Quiz for Parents and Kids," Food Safety and Inspection Service, U.S. Department of Agriculture, September 2004.

ingredients. Many food manufacturers are now labeling their products with words like "all natural" and "pure." This doesn't necessarily mean that the foods are nutritious. A food may contain all natural ingredients but may still be high in fat. A good example is granola. Although granola may be a good source of certain vitamins and nutrients, it also contains a large amount of fat. If you are a granola fan, look for the low-fat variety.

When choosing snack foods, you may occasionally prefer eating a smaller amount of the full-fat version of a snack food rather than a larger portion of something with reduced fat. For instance, if a serving of potato chips is 1 ounce (28 grams), there may be 16 chips per serving for the full-fat version and 30 for the fat-free version. Consider keeping single serving bags of chips on hand so you can fulfill your craving without going overboard.

If you know certain snacks will "call your name" from the cupboard, and you won't be able to control yourself, ask your parents not to buy them. You're better off having to make a special trip to the ice cream parlor or frozen yogurt stand for a single serving of a favorite treat than keeping a half gallon container in your freezer.

Snack Strategies

Going without food for long periods between meals, eating large meals at the end of the day when activity levels are low, and skipping meals can increase impulsive binging. Instead try these tips:

- Make snacks part of your day's food pyramid choices. Rather than thinking of them as "extras," choose snacks that contribute food-group servings for your recommended daily allowances. Choose fruits, vegetables, milk, or whole grains.

- Snack only when hungry. Skip the urge to nibble when bored, frustrated, or stressed. "Nourish" stress or boredom with a walk or a good book instead of a cookie.

- Match snack calories to your activity level. A physically active person can consume more substantial snacks—with more calories—than someone who never exercises. Snack portions should be smaller than meal portions. Snacks shouldn't "fill you up" but rather help you to be "not hungry."

- Snack consciously. Snacking absent-mindedly while doing other things, like watching TV, leads to overeating.

- Plan ahead. Keep a variety of tasty, nutritious, ready-to-eat snacks on hand at home, at school, or wherever you need a light bite to take the edge off hunger. That way you won't be limited to snacks from vending machines, fast-food restaurants, or convenience stores.

Avoid the rut of selecting the same snack all the time. Rotate snack choices among the food groups. Eat snacks to meet a physical need. Avoid eating snacks out of boredom, frustration, or loneliness. Instead try some physical activity.

> ✔ **Quick Tip**
>
> **Recipe Idea:** In the summer when fresh fruit is abundant, fruit smoothies are a great idea for a snack or a quick breakfast. Get creative and add any or all the fruits you love.
>
> *Magnificent Mixed Berry Smoothie*
>
> Ingredients
>
> ¼ cup orange juice
>
> ½ cup plain, non-fat yogurt
>
> ¼ cup washed, stemmed strawberries
>
> ¼ cup washed, stemmed blackberries
>
> ¼ cup washed, stemmed blueberries
>
> Preparation
>
> Place all ingredients in a blender. Blend on high speed until smooth.
>
> Source: © 2005 Akron Children's Hospital.

Evenings can be a tempting time for indulging in fatty, sugary snacks. Don't ignore these cravings—if you're hungry, your body is probably telling you that it needs nutrients. The trick is to pick the right snacks to fill the hunger gap. Pay attention to the hidden fats in many snack foods such as cake, biscuits, and chips. Select snacks that have a limited amount of refined or concentrated sugars. Try to limit sweets, chocolate, ice cream, and cookies, etc. Snacks should be packed with nutrients rather than empty calories.

☞ Remember!!

Snacks are not intended to replace meals, but to supplement them.

Source: © 2005 Akron Children's Hospital.

Part Two

Nutrients, Foods, And Food Groups

Chapter 12

Vitamins: Vital For Good Health

Vitamin A And Carotenoids

Vitamin A: What is it?

Vitamin A is a family of fat-soluble compounds that play an important role in vision, bone growth, reproduction, cell division, and cell differentiation (in which a cell becomes part of the brain, muscle, lungs, etc.). Vitamin A helps regulate the immune system, which helps prevent or fight off infections by making white blood cells that destroy harmful bacteria and viruses. Vitamin A also may help lymphocytes, a type of white blood cell, fight infections more effectively.

Vitamin A promotes healthy surface linings of the eyes and the respiratory, urinary, and intestinal tracts. When those linings break down, it becomes easier for bacteria to enter the body and cause infection. Vitamin A also helps maintain the integrity of skin and mucous membranes, which also function as a barrier to bacteria and viruses.

This chapter includes excerpts from the following *Dietary Supplement Fact Sheets*, produced by the Office of Dietary Supplements, National Institutes of Health: "Vitamin A and Carotenoids," June 2005, "Vitamin B6," March 2005, "Vitamin B12," March 2005, "Folate," August 2004, "Vitamin D," May 2004, and "Vitamin E," October 2004. Text under the heading "Vitamin C" is from "Ascorbic Acid (Vitamin C) (Systemic)," reprinted with permission. USP DI® is a registered trademark used herein under license. Originally created and edited by the United States Pharmacopeia until January 1, 2004, and now entirely edited and maintained by Thomson Healthcare, Inc. Klasko RK (ed): *USP DI® Vol II Advice for the Patient®*, (accessed 7/13/2005), Copyright 2005.

Retinol is one of the most active, or usable, forms of vitamin A, and is found in animal foods such as liver and whole milk and in some fortified food products. Retinol is also called preformed vitamin A. It can be converted to retinal and retinoic acid, other active forms of the vitamin A family.

What foods provide vitamin A?

Retinol is found in animal foods such as whole eggs, milk, and liver. Most fat-free milk and dried nonfat milk solids sold in the United States are fortified with vitamin A to replace the amount lost when the fat is removed. Fortified foods such as fortified breakfast cereals also provide vitamin A. Provitamin A carotenoids are abundant in darkly colored fruits and vegetables. The 2000 National Health and Nutrition Examination Survey (NHANES) indicated that major dietary contributors of retinol are milk, margarine, eggs, beef liver, and fortified ready-to-eat cereals, whereas major contributors of provitamin A carotenoids are carrots, cantaloupes, sweet potatoes, and spinach.

Table 12.1. Recommended Dietary Allowances (RDAs) For Vitamin A For Children And Adults (excluding pregnant and lactating women)

Age (years)	Children (mcg RAE*)	Males (mcg RAE*)	Females (mcg RAE*)
1–3	300 (1,000 IU)		
4–8	400 (1,320 IU)		
9–13	600 (2,000 IU)		
14–18		900 (3,000 IU)	700 (2,310 IU)
19+		900 (3,000 IU)	700 (2,310 IU)

*Retinol Activity Equivalents

Vitamin B$_6$

Vitamin B$_6$: What is it?

Vitamin B$_6$ is a water-soluble vitamin that exists in three major chemical forms: pyridoxine, pyridoxal, and pyridoxamine. It performs a wide variety of functions in your body and is essential for your good health. For example, vitamin B$_6$ is needed for more than 100 enzymes involved in protein metabolism. It is also essential for red blood cell metabolism. The nervous and immune systems need vitamin B$_6$ to function efficiently, and it is also needed for the conversion of tryptophan (an amino acid) to niacin (a vitamin).

♣ It's A Fact!!

Retinoids are compounds that are chemically similar to vitamin A. Over the past 15 years, synthetic retinoids have been prescribed for acne, psoriasis, and other skin disorders. Isotretinoin (Roaccutane® or Accutane®) is considered an effective anti-acne therapy. At very high doses, however, it can be toxic, which is why this medication is usually saved for the most severe forms of acne. The most serious consequence of this medication is birth defects. It is extremely important for sexually active females who may become pregnant and who take these medications to use an effective method of birth control. Women of childbearing age who take these medications are advised to undergo monthly pregnancy tests to make sure they are not pregnant.

Source: Office of Dietary Supplements, National Institutes of Health, June 2005.

Hemoglobin within red blood cells carries oxygen to tissues. Your body needs vitamin B$_6$ to make hemoglobin. Vitamin B$_6$ also helps increase the amount of oxygen carried by hemoglobin. A vitamin B$_6$ deficiency can result in a form of anemia that is similar to iron deficiency anemia.

Vitamin B$_6$ also helps maintain your blood glucose (sugar) within a normal range. When caloric intake is low your body needs vitamin B$_6$ to help convert stored carbohydrate or other nutrients to glucose to maintain normal blood sugar levels. While a shortage of vitamin B$_6$ will limit these functions, supplements of this vitamin do not enhance them in well-nourished individuals.

✎ What's It Mean?

Adequate Intakes (AI): A recommended average daily nutrient intake level based on observed or experimentally determined approximations or estimates of mean nutrient intake by a group (or groups) of apparently healthy people. The AI is used when the Estimated Average Requirement cannot be determined.

Dietary Reference Intakes (DRIs): A set of nutrient-based reference values that expand upon and replace the former Recommended Dietary Allowances (RDAs) in the United States and the Recommended Nutrient Intakes (RNIs) in Canada. They are actually a set of four reference values: Estimated Average Requirements (EARs), RDAs, AIs, and Tolerable Upper Intake Levels (ULs).

Estimated Average Requirements: EAR is the average daily nutrient intake level estimated to meet the requirement of half the healthy individuals in a particular life stage and gender group.

Micronutrient: Vitamins and minerals that are required in the human diet in very small amounts.

Recommended Dietary Allowance (RDA): The dietary intake level that is sufficient to meet the nutrient requirement of nearly all (97 to 98 percent) healthy individuals in a particular life stage and gender group.

Tolerable Upper Intake Level (UL): The highest average daily nutrient intake level likely to pose no risk of adverse health affects for nearly all individuals in a particular life stage and gender group. As intake increases above the UL, the potential risk of adverse health affects increases.

Source: Excerpted from "Appendix C: Glossary of Terms," *Dietary Guidelines for Americans 2005*, U.S. Department of Agriculture, 2005.

What foods provide vitamin B$_6$?

Vitamin B$_6$ is found in a wide variety of foods including fortified cereals, beans, meat, poultry, fish, and some fruits and vegetables.

Who may need extra vitamin B₆ to prevent a deficiency?

Asthmatic children treated with the medicine theophylline may need to take a vitamin B₆ supplement. Theophylline decreases body stores of vitamin B₆, and theophylline-induced seizures have been linked to low body stores of the vitamin. A physician should be consulted about the need for a vitamin B₆ supplement when theophylline is prescribed.

Individuals with a poor quality diet or an inadequate B₆ intake for an extended period may also benefit from taking a vitamin B₆ supplement if they are unable to increase their dietary intake of vitamin B₆. Alcoholics and older adults are more likely to have inadequate vitamin B₆ intakes than other segments of the population because they may have limited variety in their diet. Alcohol also promotes the destruction and loss of vitamin B₆ from the body.

What is the health risk of too much vitamin B₆?

Too much vitamin B₆ can result in nerve damage to the arms and legs. This neuropathy is usually related to high intake of vitamin B₆ from supplements and is reversible when supplementation is stopped.

Table 12.2. The 1998 RDAs For Vitamin B₆ For Adults, In Milligrams (excluding pregnant and lactating women)

Life-Stage	Men	Women
Ages 19–50	1.3 mg	1.3 mg
Ages 51+	1.7 mg	1.5 mg

Results of two national surveys, the National Health and Nutrition Examination Survey (NHANES III 1988–94) and the Continuing Survey of Food Intakes by Individuals (1994–96 CSFII), indicated that diets of most Americans meet current intake recommendations for vitamin B₆.

Vitamin B_{12}

What is vitamin B_{12}?

Vitamin B_{12} is also called cobalamin because it contains the metal cobalt. This vitamin helps maintain healthy nerve cells and red blood cells. It is also needed to help make DNA, the genetic material in all cells.

Vitamin B_{12} is bound to the protein in food. Hydrochloric acid in the stomach releases B_{12} from proteins in foods during digestion. Once released, vitamin B_{12} combines with a substance called gastric intrinsic factor (IF). This complex can then be absorbed by the intestinal tract.

What foods provide vitamin B_{12}?

Vitamin B_{12} is naturally found in animal foods including fish, meat, poultry, eggs, milk, and milk products. Fortified breakfast cereals are a particularly valuable source of vitamin B_{12} for vegetarians.

Table 12.3. Recommended Dietary Allowances (RDA) For Vitamin B_{12} For Children And Adults (excluding pregnant and lactating women)

Age (years)	Males and Females (ig/day)
1–3	0.9
4–8	1.2
9–13	1.8
14–18	2.4
19 and older	2.4

When is a deficiency of vitamin B_{12} likely to occur?

Most children and adults in the United States consume recommended amounts of vitamin B_{12}. A deficiency may still occur as a result of an inability to absorb B_{12} from food and in strict vegetarians who do not consume any animal foods.

Folate

Folate: What is it?

Folate is a water-soluble B vitamin that occurs naturally in food. Folic acid is the synthetic form of folate that is found in supplements and added to fortified foods.

Folate gets its name from the Latin word "folium" for leaf. A key observation of researcher Lucy Wills nearly 70 years ago led to the identification of folate as the nutrient needed to prevent the anemia of pregnancy. Dr. Wills demonstrated that the anemia could be corrected by a yeast extract. Folate was identified as the corrective substance in yeast extract in the late 1930s, and was extracted from spinach leaves in 1941.

Folate helps produce and maintain new cells. This is especially important during periods of rapid cell division and growth such as infancy and pregnancy. Folate is needed to make DNA and RNA, the building blocks of cells. It also helps prevent changes to DNA that may lead to cancer. Both adults and children need folate to make normal red blood cells and prevent anemia. Folate is also essential for the metabolism of homocysteine and helps maintain normal levels of this amino acid.

What foods provide folate?

Leafy green vegetables (like spinach and turnip greens), fruits (like citrus fruits and juices), and dried beans and peas are all natural sources of folate.

In 1996, the Food and Drug Administration (FDA) published regulations requiring the addition of folic acid to enriched breads, cereals, flours, corn meals, pastas, rice, and other grain products. Since cereals and grains are widely consumed in the U.S., these products have become a very important contributor of folic acid to the American diet.

Do girls and women of childbearing age and pregnant women have a special need for folate?

Folic acid is very important for all women who may become pregnant. Adequate folate intake during the periconceptual period (the time just before and

Table 12.4. Recommended Dietary Allowances For Folate For Children And Adults (excluding pregnant and lactating women)

Age (years)	Males and Females (ìg/day)
1–3	150
4–8	200
9–13	300
14–18	400
19+	400

just after a woman becomes pregnant) protects against neural tube defects. Neural tube defects result in malformations of the spine (spina bifida), skull, and brain (anencephaly). The risk of neural tube defects is significantly reduced when supplemental folic acid is consumed in addition to a healthful diet prior to and during the first month following conception. Since January 1, 1998, when the folate food fortification program took effect, data suggest that there has been a significant reduction in neural tube birth defects. Women who could become pregnant are advised to eat foods fortified with folic acid or take a folic acid supplement in addition to eating folate-rich foods to reduce the risk of some serious birth defects. For this population, researchers recommend a daily intake of 400 μg of synthetic folic acid per day from fortified foods and/or dietary supplements.

Vitamin C

Description

Ascorbic acid, also known as vitamin C, is necessary for wound healing. It is needed for many functions in the body, including helping the body use carbohydrates, fats, and protein. Vitamin C also strengthens blood vessel walls.

Lack of vitamin C can lead to a condition called scurvy, which causes muscle weakness, swollen and bleeding gums, loss of teeth, and bleeding under the skin, as well as tiredness and depression. Wounds also do not heal easily. Your health care professional may treat scurvy by prescribing vitamin C for you.

Some conditions may increase your need for vitamin C. These include the following:

- AIDS (acquired immune deficiency syndrome)

- Alcoholism

- Burns

- Cancer

- Diarrhea (prolonged)

- Fever (prolonged)

- Infection (prolonged)

- Intestinal diseases

- Overactive thyroid (hyperthyroidism)

- Stomach ulcer

- Stress (continuing)

- Surgical removal of stomach

- Tuberculosis

Also, the following groups of people may have a deficiency of vitamin C:

- Infants receiving unfortified formulas

- Smokers

- Patients using an artificial kidney (on hemodialysis)

- Patients who undergo surgery

- Individuals who are exposed to long periods of cold temperatures

Increased need for vitamin C should be determined by your health care professional.

Vitamin C may be used for other conditions as determined by your health care professional.

Claims that vitamin C is effective for preventing senility and the common cold, and for treating asthma, some mental problems, cancer, hardening of the arteries, allergies, eye ulcers, blood clots, gum disease, and pressure sores have not been proven. Although vitamin C is being used to reduce the risk of cardiovascular disease and certain types of cancer, there is not enough information to show that these uses are effective.

Injectable vitamin C is given by or under the supervision of a health care professional. Other forms of vitamin C are available without a prescription.

Importance Of Diet

For good health, it is important that you eat a balanced and varied diet. Follow carefully any diet program your health care professional may recommend. For your specific dietary vitamin and/or mineral needs, ask your health care professional for a list of appropriate foods. If you think that you are not getting enough vitamins and/or minerals in your diet, you may choose to take a dietary supplement. Vitamin C is found in various foods, including citrus fruits (oranges, lemons, grapefruit), green vegetables (peppers, broccoli, cabbage), tomatoes, and potatoes. It is best to eat fresh fruits and vegetables whenever possible since they contain the most vitamins. Food processing may destroy some of the vitamins. For example, exposure to air, drying, salting, or cooking (especially in copper pots), mincing of fresh vegetables, or mashing potatoes may reduce the amount of vitamin C in foods. Freezing does not usually cause loss of vitamin C unless foods are stored for a very long time.

Vitamins alone will not take the place of a good diet and will not provide energy. Your body also needs other substances found in food such as protein, minerals, carbohydrates, and fat. Vitamins themselves often cannot work without the presence of other foods.

The daily amount of vitamin C needed is defined in several different ways.

For U.S.

- Recommended dietary allowances (RDAs) are the amount of vitamins and minerals needed to provide for adequate nutrition in most healthy persons. RDAs for a given nutrient may vary depending on a person's age, sex, and physical condition (for example, pregnancy).

- Daily values (DVs) are used on food and dietary supplement labels to indicate the percent of the recommended daily amount of each nutrient that a serving provides. DV replaces the previous designation of United States recommended daily allowances (RDAs).

For Canada

Recommended nutrient intakes (RNIs) are used to determine the amounts of vitamins, minerals, and protein needed to provide adequate nutrition and lessen the risk of chronic disease.

✤ **It's A Fact!!**

What vitamin do you associate with oranges and other citrus fruits? Vitamin C is correct! Citrus fruits are rich in this vitamin, but did you know that strawberries, mangoes, red peppers, and tomatoes are also sources of vitamin C? Vitamin C helps heal cuts and wounds and also keeps your gums healthy.

Source: Excerpted from "Fabulous Fruits... Versatile Vegetables," U.S. Department of Agriculture, No. HG 267-4, June 2003.

Table 12.5. Normal Daily Recommended Intakes For Vitamin C

Persons	U.S. (mg)	Canada (mg)
Infants and children birth to 3 years of age	30–40	20
4 to 6 years of age	45	25
7 to 10 years of age	45	25
Adolescent and adult males	50–60	25–40
Adolescent and adult females	50–60	25–30
Pregnant females	70	30–40
Breast-feeding females	90–95	55
Smokers	100	45–60

Vitamin D

What is vitamin D?

Vitamin D is a fat soluble vitamin that is found in food and can also be made in your body after exposure to ultraviolet (UV) rays from the sun. Sunshine is a significant source of vitamin D because UV rays from sunlight trigger vitamin D synthesis in the skin.

Vitamin D exists in several forms, each with a different level of activity. Calciferol is the most active form of vitamin D. Other forms are relatively inactive in the body. The liver and kidney help convert vitamin D to its active hormone form. Once vitamin D is produced in the skin or consumed in food, it requires chemical conversion in the liver and kidney to form 1,25 dihydroxyvitamin D, the physiologically active form of vitamin D. Active vitamin D functions as a hormone because it sends a message to the intestines to increase the absorption of calcium and phosphorus.

The major biologic function of vitamin D is to maintain normal blood levels of calcium and phosphorus. By promoting calcium absorption, vitamin D helps to form and maintain strong bones. Vitamin D also works in concert with a number of other vitamins, minerals, and hormones to promote bone mineralization. Without vitamin D, bones can become thin, brittle, or misshapen. Vitamin D sufficiency prevents rickets in children and osteomalacia in adults, two forms of skeletal diseases that weaken bones.

Research also suggests that vitamin D may help maintain a healthy immune system and help regulate cell growth and differentiation, the process that determines what a cell is to become.

What are the sources of vitamin D?

Food Sources: Fortified foods are common sources of vitamin D. In the 1930s, rickets was a major public health problem in the United States (U.S.). A milk fortification program was implemented to combat rickets, and it nearly eliminated this disorder in the U.S.

Although milk is fortified with vitamin D, dairy products made from milk, such as cheese and ice creams, are generally not fortified with vitamin D and contain only small amounts. Some ready-to-eat breakfast cereals may be fortified with vitamin D, often at a level of 10% to 15% of the daily value. There are only a few commonly consumed foods that are good sources of vitamin D.

Sun Exposure: Sun exposure is perhaps the most important source of vitamin D because exposure to sunlight provides most humans with their vitamin D requirement. UV rays from the sun trigger vitamin D synthesis in skin. Season, geographic latitude, time of day, cloud cover, smog, and sunscreen affect UV ray exposure and vitamin D synthesis. For example, sunlight exposure from November through February in Boston is insufficient to produce significant vitamin D synthesis in the skin. Complete cloud cover halves the energy of UV rays, and shade reduces it by 60%. Industrial pollution, which increases shade, also decreases sun exposure and may contribute to the development of rickets in individuals with insufficient dietary intake of vitamin D. Sunscreens with a sun protection factor (SPF) of 8 or greater will block UV rays that produce vitamin D, but it is still important to routinely use sunscreen to help prevent skin cancer and other negative consequences of excessive sun exposure. An initial exposure to sunlight (10–15 minutes) allows adequate time for vitamin D synthesis and should be followed by application of a sunscreen with an SPF of at least 15 to protect the skin. Ten to fifteen minutes of sun exposure at least two times per week to the face, arms, hands, or back without sunscreen is usually sufficient to provide adequate vitamin D. It is very important for individuals with limited sun exposure to include good sources of vitamin D in their diet.

Who may need extra vitamin D to prevent a deficiency?

It can be difficult to obtain enough vitamin D from natural food sources. For many people, consuming vitamin D fortified foods and adequate sunlight exposure are essential for maintaining a healthy vitamin D status. In some groups, dietary supplements may be needed to meet the daily need for vitamin D.

Infants Who Are Exclusively Breastfed: In infants, vitamin D requirements cannot be met by human (breast) milk alone. Sunlight is a potential source of vitamin D for infants, but the American Academy of Pediatrics (AAP) advises that infants be kept out of direct sunlight and wear protective clothing and sunscreen when exposed to sunlight. The American Academy of Pediatrics (AAP) recommends a daily supplement of 200 IU vitamin D for breastfed infants beginning within the first two months of life unless they are weaned to receive at least 500 ml (about 2 cups) per day of vitamin D-fortified formula.

Persons With Limited Sun Exposure: Homebound individuals, people living in northern latitudes such as in New England and Alaska, women who wear robes and head coverings for religious reasons, and individuals working in occupations that prevent sun exposure are unlikely to obtain much vitamin D from sunlight. It is important for people with limited sun exposure to consume recommended amounts of vitamin D in their diets or consider vitamin D supplementation. Children and adolescents who are not routinely exposed to sunlight and do not consume at least two, 8-fluid ounce servings of vitamin D-fortified milk per day are also at higher risk of vitamin D deficiency and may need a dietary supplement containing 200 IU vitamin D.

Older Adults: Americans age 50 and older are believed to be at increased risk of developing vitamin D deficiency. As people age, skin cannot synthesize vitamin D as efficiently and the kidney is less able to convert vitamin D to its active hormone form. It is estimated that as many as 30% to 40% of older adults with hip fractures are vitamin D insufficient. Therefore, older adults may benefit from supplemental vitamin D.

Persons With Greater Skin Melanin Content: Melanin is the pigment that gives skin its color. Greater amounts of melanin result in darker skin. The high melanin content in darker skin reduces the skin's ability to produce vitamin D from sunlight. It is very important for African Americans and other populations with dark-pigmented skin to consume recommended amounts of vitamin D. Some studies suggest that older adults, especially women, in these groups are at even higher risk of vitamin D deficiency. Individuals with darkly pigmented skin who are unable to get adequate sun exposure and/or consume recommended amounts of vitamin D may benefit from a vitamin D supplement.

Persons With Fat Malabsorption: As a fat soluble vitamin, vitamin D requires some dietary fat for absorption. Individuals who have a reduced ability to absorb dietary fat may require vitamin D supplements. Symptoms of fat malabsorption include diarrhea and oily stools.

What are the health risks of too much vitamin D?

Vitamin D toxicity can cause nausea, vomiting, poor appetite, constipation, weakness, and weight loss. It can also raise blood levels of calcium, causing mental status changes such as confusion. High blood levels of calcium also can cause heart rhythm abnormalities. Calcinosis, the deposition of calcium and phosphate in the body's soft tissues such as the kidney, can also be caused by vitamin D toxicity.

Sun exposure is unlikely to result in vitamin D toxicity. Diet is also unlikely to cause vitamin D toxicity, unless large amounts of cod liver oil are consumed. Vitamin D toxicity is much more likely to occur from high intakes of vitamin D in supplements. The Food and Nutrition Board of the Institute of Medicine has set the tolerable upper intake level (UL) for vitamin D at 25 µg (1,000 IU) for infants up to 12 months of age and 50 µg (2,000 IU) for children, adults, pregnant, and lactating women. Long-term intakes above the UL increase the risk of adverse health effects.

Table 12.6. Adequate Intake For Vitamin D (excluding pregnant and lactating women)

Age	Children (µg/day)	Men (µg/day)	Women (µg/day)
Birth to 13 years	5 (=200 IU)		
14 to 18 years		5 (=200 IU)	5 (=200 IU)
19 to 50 years		5 (=200 IU)	5 (=200 IU)
51 to 70 years		10 (=400 IU)	10 (=400 IU)
71+ years		15 (=600 IU)	15 (=600 IU)

Vitamin E

Vitamin E: What is it?

Vitamin E is a fat-soluble vitamin that exists in eight different forms. Each form has its own biological activity, which is the measure of potency or functional use in the body. Alpha-tocopherol is the name of the most active form of vitamin E in humans. It is also a powerful biological antioxidant. Vitamin E in supplements is usually sold as alpha-tocopheryl acetate, a form that protects its ability to function as an antioxidant. The synthetic form is labeled "D, L" while the natural form is labeled "D". The synthetic form is only half as active as the natural form.

Antioxidants such as vitamin E act to protect your cells against the effects of free radicals, which are potentially damaging byproducts of energy metabolism. Free radicals can damage cells and may contribute to the development of cardiovascular disease and cancer. Studies are underway to determine whether vitamin E, through its ability to limit production of free radicals, might help prevent or delay the development of those chronic diseases. Vitamin E has also been shown to play a role in immune function, in DNA repair, and other metabolic processes.

What foods provide vitamin E?

Vegetable oils, nuts, green leafy vegetables, and fortified cereals are common food sources of vitamin E in the United States.

Table 12.7. Recommended Dietary Allowances For Vitamin E For Children And Adults (excluding pregnant and lactating women)

Age (years)	Children (mg/day)	Men (mg/day)	Women (mg/day)
1–3	6 mg (=9 IU)		
4–8	7 mg (=10.5 IU)		
9–13		11 mg (=16.5 IU)	11 mg (=16.5 IU)
14 +		15 mg (=22.5 IU)	15 mg (=22.5 IU)

Chapter 13

Minerals: An Overview

Calcium

Calcium: What is it?

Calcium, the most abundant mineral in the human body, has several important functions. More than 99% of total body calcium is stored in the bones and teeth where it functions to support their structure. The remaining 1% is found throughout the body in blood, muscle, and the fluid between cells. Calcium is needed for muscle contraction, blood vessel contraction and expansion, the secretion of hormones and enzymes, and sending messages through the nervous system. A constant level of calcium is maintained in body fluid and tissues so that these vital body processes function efficiently.

Bone undergoes continuous remodeling, with constant resorption (breakdown of bone) and deposition of calcium into newly deposited bone (bone

About This Chapter: This chapter includes excerpts from the following *Dietary Supplement Fact Sheets*, produced by the Office of Dietary Supplements, National Institutes of Health: "Calcium," April 2005, "Iron," July 2004, "Magnesium," January 2005, "Selenium," August 2004, and "Zinc," December 2002. Text under the heading "Sodium," is reprinted with permission from "Sodium Savvy," by Catherine A. Broihier, University of Iowa Hospitals and Clinics Dietary Department, © 2003 by the author and University of Iowa Hospitals. Copyright protected material used with permission of the author and the University of Iowa's Virtual Hospital © 2003, www.vh.org. Text under the heading "Potassium," is reprinted with permission from "Potassium Recommendations Fact Sheet," © 2004 National Diary Council (www.nationaldiarycouncil.org).

formation). The balance between bone resorption and deposition changes as people age. During childhood there is a higher amount of bone formation and less breakdown. In early and middle adulthood, these processes are relatively equal. In aging adults, particularly among postmenopausal women, bone breakdown exceeds its formation, resulting in bone loss, which increases the risk for osteoporosis (a disorder characterized by porous, weak bones).

What is the recommended intake for calcium?

For calcium, the recommended intake is listed as an Adequate Intake (AI), which is a recommended average intake level based on observed or experimentally determined levels. Table 13.1 contains the current recommendations for calcium for infants, children, and adults.

There is a widespread concern that Americans are not meeting the recommended intake for calcium.

What foods provide calcium?

In the United States, milk, yogurt, and cheese are the major contributors of calcium in the typical diet. The inadequate intake of dairy foods may explain why some Americans are deficient in calcium since dairy foods are the major source of calcium in the diet.

Although dairy products are the main source of calcium in the U.S. diet, other foods also contribute to overall calcium intake. Individuals with lactose intolerance (those who experience symptoms such as bloating and diarrhea because they cannot completely digest the milk sugar lactose) and those who are vegan (people who consume no animal products) tend to avoid or completely eliminate

Table 13.1. Recommended Adequate Intake for Calcium (excluding pregnant and lactating women).

Male and Female Age	Calcium (mg*/day)
0 to 6 months	210
7 to 12 months	270
1 to 3 years	500
4 to 8 years	800
9 to 13 years	1300
14 to 18 years	1300
19 to 50 years	1000
51+ years	1200

*mg = milligrams

dairy products from their diets. Thus, it is important for these individuals to meet their calcium needs with alternative calcium sources. Foods such as Chinese cabbage, kale, and broccoli are other alternative calcium sources. Although most grains are not high in calcium (unless fortified), they do contribute calcium to the diet because they are consumed frequently. Additionally, there are several calcium-fortified food sources presently available, including fruit juices, fruit drinks, tofu, and cereals.

Who may need extra calcium to prevent a deficiency?

Amenorrheic Women and the Female Athlete Triad: Amenorrhea is the condition when menstrual periods stop or fail to begin The condition "female athlete triad" refers to the combination of disordered eating, amenorrhea, and osteoporosis. Exercise-induced amenorrhea has been shown to result in decreases in bone mass. In female athletes, low bone mineral density, menstrual irregularities, dietary factors, and a history of prior stress fractures are associated with an increased risk of future stress fractures.

Lactose Intolerant Individuals: Lactose maldigestion describes the inability of an individual to completely digest lactose, the naturally occurring sugar in milk. Lactose intolerance refers to the symptoms that occur when the amount of lactose exceeds the ability of an individual's digestive tract to break down lactose. In the U.S., approximately 25% of all adults have a limited ability to digest lactose. Lactose maldigestion varies by ethnicity, with a prevalence of 85% in Asians, 50% in African Americans, and 10% in Caucasians. If an individual chooses to avoid dairy products, it is important for them to include non-dairy sources of calcium in their daily diet or consider taking a calcium supplement to help meet their recommended calcium needs.

Vegetarians: There are several types of vegetarian eating practices. Individuals may choose to include some animal products (ovo-vegetarian, lacto-vegetarian, lacto-ovo vegetarian, pesco-vegetarian) or no animal products (vegan) in their diet. Vegans may be at increased risk for inadequate intake of calcium because of their lack of consumption of dairy products. Therefore, it is important for vegans to include adequate amounts of non-dairy sources of calcium in their daily diet or consider taking a calcium supplement to meet their recommended calcium intake.

> **✔ Quick Tip**
>
> The following are strategies and tips to help you meet your calcium needs each day:
>
> * Use low-fat or fat-free milk instead of water in recipes such as pancakes, mashed potatoes, pudding, and instant, hot breakfast cereals.
>
> * Blend a fruit smoothie made with low-fat or fat-free yogurt for a great breakfast.
>
> * Sprinkle grated low-fat or fat-free cheese on salad, soup or pasta.
>
> * Choose low-fat or fat-free milk instead of carbonated soft drinks.
>
> * Serve raw fruits and vegetables with a low-fat or fat-free yogurt based dip.
>
> * Create a vegetable stir-fry and toss in diced calcium-set tofu.
>
> * Enjoy a parfait with fruit and low-fat or fat-free yogurt.
>
> * Complement your diet with calcium-fortified foods such as certain cereals, orange juice, and soy beverages.
>
> Source: "Calcium," Office of Dietary Supplements, April 2005.

Post-Menopausal Women: Menopause often leads to increases in bone loss with the most rapid rates of bone loss occurring during the first five years after menopause. Drops in estrogen production after menopause result in increased bone resorption, and decreased calcium absorption.

Is there a health risk of too much calcium?

While low intakes of calcium can result in deficiency and undesirable health conditions, excessively high intakes of calcium can also have adverse effects. Adverse conditions associated with high calcium intakes are hypercalcemia (elevated levels of calcium in the blood), impaired kidney function, and decreased absorption of other minerals. Hypercalcemia can also result from excess intake of vitamin D, such as from supplement overuse at levels of 50,000 IU or higher. However, hypercalcemia from diet and supplements is very rare. Most cases of hypercalcemia occur as a result of malignancy (cancer)—especially in the advanced stages.

Iron

Iron: What is it?

Iron, one of the most abundant metals on Earth, is essential to most life forms and to normal human physiology. Iron is an integral part of many proteins and enzymes that maintain good health. In humans, iron is an essential component of proteins involved in oxygen transport. It is also essential for the regulation of cell growth and differentiation. A deficiency of iron limits oxygen delivery to cells, resulting in fatigue, poor work performance, and decreased immunity. On the other hand, excess amounts of iron can result in toxicity and even death.

Almost two-thirds of iron in the body is found in hemoglobin, the protein in red blood cells that carries oxygen to tissues. Smaller amounts of iron are found in myoglobin, a protein that helps supply oxygen to muscle, and in enzymes that assist biochemical reactions. Iron is also found in proteins that store iron for future needs and that transport iron in blood. Iron stores are regulated by intestinal iron absorption.

What foods provide iron?

There are two forms of dietary iron: heme and nonheme. Heme iron is derived from hemoglobin, the protein in red blood cells that delivers oxygen to cells. Heme iron is found in animal foods that originally contained hemoglobin, such as red meats, fish, and poultry. Iron in plant foods, such as lentils and beans, is arranged in a chemical structure called nonheme iron. This is the form of iron added to iron-enriched and iron-fortified foods. Heme iron is absorbed better than nonheme iron, but most dietary iron is nonheme iron.

When can iron deficiency occur?

The World Health Organization considers iron deficiency the number one nutritional disorder in the world. As many as 80% of the world's population may be iron deficient, while 30% may have iron deficiency anemia.

Iron deficiency anemia can be associated with low dietary intake of iron, inadequate absorption of iron, or excessive blood loss. Women of childbearing age, pregnant women, preterm and low birth weight infants, older infants and toddlers, and teenage girls are at greatest risk of developing iron deficiency anemia because they have the greatest need for iron. Women with heavy menstrual losses can lose a significant amount of iron and are at considerable risk for iron deficiency. Adult men and post-menopausal women lose very little iron and have a low risk of iron deficiency.

Individuals with kidney failure, especially those being treated with dialysis, are at high risk for developing iron deficiency anemia. This is because their kidneys cannot create enough erythropoietin, a hormone needed to make red blood cells. Both iron and erythropoietin can be lost during kidney dialysis. Individuals who receive routine dialysis treatments usually need extra iron and synthetic erythropoietin to prevent iron deficiency.

♣ **It's A Fact!!**

Teenage girls must be sure get enough iron (to replace what you lose each month). Include meats, fortified breakfast cereals, and dried fruits in your diet. Eat foods high in vitamin C at the same time and you'll improve iron absorption. Folic acid is also important, and is found in oranges, whole grains, dark green leafy vegetables, nuts, legumes, and fortified cereals.

Source: Excerpted from "Nutrition Tips for Teens," © 2003 Munson Healthcare. All rights reserved. Reprinted with permission.

Eating nonnutritive substances (such as dirt and clay) often referred to as pica or geophagia, is sometimes seen in persons with iron deficiency. There is disagreement about the cause of this association. Some researchers believe that these eating abnormalities may result in an iron deficiency. Other researchers believe that iron deficiency may somehow increase the likelihood of these eating problems.

What are some facts about iron supplements?

Supplemental iron is available in two forms: ferrous and ferric. Ferrous iron salts (ferrous fumarate, ferrous sulfate, and ferrous gluconate) are the best absorbed forms of iron supplements. Elemental iron is the amount of iron in a supplement that is available for absorption.

The amount of iron absorbed decreases with increasing doses. For this reason, it is recommended that most people take their prescribed daily iron supplement in two or three equally spaced doses. For adults who are not pregnant, the Centers for Disease Control and Prevention (CDC) recommends taking 50 mg to 60 mg of oral elemental iron (the approximate amount of elemental iron in one 300 mg tablet of ferrous sulfate) twice daily for three months for the therapeutic treatment of iron deficiency anemia. However, physicians evaluate each person individually and prescribe according to individual needs.

Who should be cautious about taking iron supplements?

Iron deficiency is uncommon among adult men and postmenopausal women. Because of their greater risk of iron overload, these individuals should only take iron supplements when prescribed by a physician. Iron overload is a condition in which excess iron is found in the blood and stored in organs such as the liver and heart. Iron overload is associated with several genetic diseases, including hemochromatosis—which affects approximately 1 in 250 individuals of northern European descent. Individuals with hemochromatosis absorb iron very efficiently, which can result in a build up of excess iron and can cause organ damage such as cirrhosis of the liver and heart failure. Hemochromatosis is often not diagnosed until excess iron stores have damaged an organ. Iron supplementation may accelerate the effects of hemochromatosis, an important reason why adult men and postmenopausal women who are not iron deficient should avoid iron supplements. Individuals with blood disorders that require frequent blood transfusions are also at risk of iron overload and are usually advised to avoid iron supplements.

Table 13.2. Recommended Dietary Allowances for Iron for Infants (7 to 12 months), Children, and Adults (excluding pregnant and lactating women).

Age	Males (mg/day)	Females (mg/day)
7 to 12 months	11	11
1 to 3 years	7	7
4 to 8 years	10	10
9 to 13 years	8	8
14 to 18 years	11	15
19 to 50 years	8	18
51+ years	8	8

What is the risk of iron toxicity?

There is considerable potential for iron toxicity because very little iron is excreted from the body. Thus, iron can accumulate in body tissues and organs when normal storage sites are full. For example, people with hemochromatosis are at risk of developing iron toxicity because of their high iron stores.

In children, death has occurred from ingesting 200 mg of iron. It is important to keep iron supplements tightly capped and away from children's reach. Any time excessive iron intake is suspected, immediately call your physician or Poison Control Center, or visit your local emergency room. Doses of iron prescribed for iron deficiency anemia in adults are associated with constipation, nausea, vomiting, and diarrhea, especially when the supplements are taken on an empty stomach.

Magnesium

Magnesium: What is it?

Magnesium is the fourth most abundant mineral in the body and is essential to good health. Approximately 50% of total body magnesium is found in bone. The other half is found predominantly inside cells of body tissues and organs. Only 1% of magnesium is found in blood, but the body works very hard to keep blood levels of magnesium constant.

Magnesium is needed for more than 300 biochemical reactions in the body. It helps maintain normal muscle and nerve function, keeps heart rhythm steady, supports a healthy immune system, and keeps bones strong.

Table 13.3. Recommended Dietary Allowances for Magnesium For Children And Adults (excluding pregnant and lactating women).

Age (years)	Male (mg/day)	Female (mg/day)
1–3	80	80
4–8	130	130
9–13	240	240
14–18	410	360
19–30	400	310
31+	420	320

Magnesium also helps regulate blood sugar levels, promotes normal blood pressure, and is known to be involved in energy metabolism and protein synthesis. There is an increased interest in the role of magnesium in preventing and managing disorders such as hypertension (high blood pressure), cardiovascular disease, and diabetes. Dietary magnesium is absorbed in the small intestines. Magnesium is excreted through the kidneys.

What foods provide magnesium?

Green vegetables such as spinach are good sources of magnesium because the center of the chlorophyll molecule (which gives green vegetables their color) contains magnesium. Some legumes (beans and peas), nuts and seeds, and whole, unrefined grains are also good sources of magnesium. Refined grains are generally low in magnesium. When white flour is refined and processed, the magnesium-rich germ and bran are removed. Bread made from whole grain wheat flour provides more magnesium than bread made from white refined flour. Tap water can be a source of magnesium, but the amount varies according to the water supply. Water that naturally contains more minerals is described as "hard". "Hard" water contains more magnesium than "soft" water.

Eating a wide variety of legumes, nuts, whole grains, and vegetables will help you meet your daily dietary need for magnesium.

What is the health risk of too much magnesium?

Dietary magnesium does not pose a health risk, however pharmacologic doses of magnesium in supplements can promote adverse effects such as diarrhea and abdominal cramping. Risk of magnesium toxicity increases with kidney failure—when the kidney loses the ability to remove excess magnesium. Very large doses of magnesium-containing laxatives and antacids also have been associated with magnesium toxicity. For example, a case of hypermagnesemia after unsupervised intake of aluminum magnesia oral suspension occurred after a 16-year-old girl decided to take the antacid every two hours rather than four times per day, as prescribed. Three days later, she became unresponsive and demonstrated loss of deep tendon reflex. Doctors were unable to determine her exact magnesium intake, but the young lady presented with blood levels of magnesium five times higher than normal. Therefore, it is important for medical professionals to be aware of the use of any magnesium-containing laxatives or antacids. Signs of excess magnesium can be similar to magnesium deficiency and include changes in mental status, nausea, diarrhea, appetite loss, muscle weakness, difficulty breathing, extremely low blood pressure, and irregular heartbeat.

Potassium

What is potassium's function?

Potassium is a mineral that helps regulate fluids and mineral balance and is needed for muscle contractions and transmission of nerve impulses. It also helps regulate blood pressure; an important role considering one in five Americans is living with hypertension.

Potassium plays such an important role in blood pressure regulation and stroke prevention that the Food and Drug Administration has approved the use of the health claim "diets containing foods that are good sources of potassium and low in sodium may reduce the risk of high blood pressure and stroke," for foods that are naturally low in sodium, fat, and cholesterol, and provide at least 350 mg of potassium per serving, such as fat free milk and some yogurts.

Table 13.4. Dietary Reference Intake For Potassium For Children And Adults (excluding pregnant and lactating women)

Males and Females	Adequate Intake, mg/d
1–3 years	3500
4–8 years	3800
9–18 years	4500
19–50 years	4700
>50 years	4700

How much potassium is needed?

Until recently no official recommendation for potassium intake existed, although many health professionals recommended 2 grams a day. But in February of 2004, after an extensive review of scientific literature, the Institute of Medicine set the adequate intake of potassium for adults at 4.7 grams a day—more than double previous estimates. However, more than 90% of American children and adults are not meeting these recommendations.

What are the effects of potassium deficiency?

Potassium deficiency can result in high blood pressure, stroke, congestive heart failure, cardiac arrhythmias, weakness, depression, and glucose intolerance, as well as increased risk of kidney stones, and increased bone turnover.

What foods provide potassium?

Milk provides most of the potassium in the American diet. An 8-ounce serving of milk provides about 350–400 mg of potassium. Three to four servings of milk a day provides 1050–1600 mg of potassium, up to a third of the potassium recommendation. Other common sources of potassium include: potato (with skin), yogurt, pasta sauce, bananas, almonds, oranges, and cottage cheese.

Selenium

What is selenium?

Selenium is a trace mineral that is essential to good health but required only in small amounts. Selenium is incorporated into proteins to make selenoproteins, which are important antioxidant enzymes. The antioxidant properties of selenoproteins help prevent cellular damage from free radicals. Free radicals are natural by-products of oxygen metabolism that may contribute to the development of chronic diseases such as cancer and heart disease. Other selenoproteins help regulate thyroid function and play a role in the immune system.

Table 13.5. Recommended Dietary Allowances (RDA) for Selenium For Children And Adults (excluding pregnant and lactating women).

Age (years)	Males and Females (µg/day)
1–3	20
4–8	30
9–13	40
14–18	55
19+	55

What foods provide selenium?

Plant foods are the major dietary sources of selenium in most countries throughout the world. The content of selenium in food depends on the selenium content of the soil where plants are grown or animals are raised. For example, researchers know that soils in the high plains of northern Nebraska and the Dakotas have very high levels of selenium. People living in those regions generally have the highest selenium intakes in the United States. In the U.S., food distribution patterns across the country help prevent people living in low-selenium geographic areas from having low dietary selenium intakes. Soils in some parts of China and Russia have very low amounts of selenium. Selenium deficiency is often reported in those regions because most food in those areas is grown and eaten locally.

Selenium also can be found in some meats and seafood. Animals that eat grains or plants that were grown in selenium-rich soil have higher levels of selenium in their muscle. In the U.S., meats and bread are common sources of dietary selenium. Some nuts are also sources of selenium.

Selenium content of foods can vary. For example, Brazil nuts may contain as much as 544 micrograms of selenium per ounce. They also may contain far less selenium. It is wise to eat Brazil nuts only occasionally because of their unusually high intake of selenium.

What is the health risk of too much selenium?

High blood levels of selenium (greater than 100 μg/dL) can result in a condition called selenosis. Symptoms of selenosis include gastrointestinal upsets, hair loss, white blotchy nails, garlic breath odor, fatigue, irritability, and mild nerve damage.

Selenium toxicity is rare in the U.S. The few reported cases have been associated with industrial accidents and a manufacturing error that led to an excessively high dose of selenium in a supplement.

Sodium

Did you know that the average American consumes about 3½ pounds of sodium in one year? That is almost ten times more than the amount required by the human body. If you are concerned about the amount of sodium in your diet, read on.

Sodium in the diet, mainly in the form of salt, is also known as sodium chloride (NaCl). Salt is a mixture of 40% sodium and 60% chloride; therefore, the words "sodium" and "salt" are not synonymous. A food product may contain little salt and still contain sources of sodium.

The human body requires about 500 mg of sodium per day, while the average American usually ingests between 2,300–6,900 mg each day. The Estimated Safe and Adequate Daily Intake (ESADDI) for sodium was determined by the Committee on Dietary Allowance and the Food and Nutrition Board to be approximately 1,100–3,300 mg per day.

For most individuals, reducing dietary sodium levels to the ESADDI range simply means decreasing the amount of salt used in cooking and at the table. For example, one might omit salt in cooking, and only add salt at the table after tasting the food. Not adding any salt would be even more effective. If further sodium control is desired, one must start reading labels and become familiar with the new reduced sodium foods.

There are numerous products entering the market that can be used to help decrease the amount of sodium in one's diet. Canned soups, some snack foods, and canned vegetables are currently available in low sodium variations. When reading labels, however, be aware of the number of servings per unit. Some can be misleading if manufacturers have made the serving sizes smaller so that the amount of sodium per serving is lower.

Salt substitution can be useful, but be sure to read the labels. True salt substitutes, such as Morton's Salt Substitute, contain no sodium and are usually made from potassium chloride. Some products, such as Lite Salt, are not true substitutes because they contain both sodium chloride and potassium chloride; and therefore, are not free of sodium. One of the best sodium substitutes can be a spice mixture suited to your own taste.

There are other sources of sodium that aren't as obvious as the foods we eat. Softened water, bottled waters, medications, and chewing tobacco are sources of hidden sodium.

Reducing the sodium content of one's diet can be achieved in a variety of ways, and the method is not as crucial as is actually doing it. Be aware of the amount of salt added in cooking and at the table, and consciously try to limit it. Small changes can significantly reduce sodium intake. Also, with the new lower sodium foods on the market, reducing sodium can be easier and tastier than ever.

Zinc

Zinc: What is it?

Zinc is an essential mineral that is found in almost every cell. It stimulates the activity of approximately 100 enzymes, which are substances that promote biochemical reactions in your body. Zinc supports a healthy immune system, is needed for wound healing, helps maintain your sense of taste and smell, and is needed for DNA synthesis. Zinc also supports normal growth and development during pregnancy, childhood, and adolescence.

What foods provide zinc?

Zinc is found in a wide variety of foods. Oysters contain more zinc per serving than any other food, but red meat and poultry provide the majority of zinc in the American diet. Other good food sources include beans, nuts, certain seafood, whole grains, fortified breakfast cereals, and dairy products. Zinc absorption is greater from a diet high in animal protein than a diet rich in plant proteins. Phytates, which are found in whole grain breads, cereals, legumes, and other products, can decrease zinc absorption.

Table 13.6. Recommended Dietary Allowances for Zinc for Infants over 7 Months, Children, and Adults (excluding pregnant and lactating women)

Age	Infants and Children
7 months to 3 years	3 mg
4 to 8 years	5 mg
9 to 13 years	8 mg

Age (years)	Males	Females
14 to 18	11 mg	9 mg
19+	11 mg	8 mg

Results of two national surveys, the National Health and Nutrition Examination Survey (NHANES III 1988–91) and the Continuing Survey of Food Intakes of Individuals (1994 CSFII) indicated that most infants, children, and adults consume recommended amounts of zinc.

Chapter 14

Calcium: A Special Concern For Teens

Why Calcium?

Bones are living structures that need the mineral calcium to help them develop and stay strong. Most of the calcium in our bodies—99 percent of it—is found in our bones. Without enough calcium, bones can become fragile and break easily with very little stress. Because many children and teens aren't getting the calcium they need, the number of broken and fractured bones continues to increase. Other effects of too little calcium, like osteoporosis, don't show up until we are adults, but these problems start by not getting enough calcium as children and teens.

Eating and drinking lots of foods with calcium during childhood can help build a "bone bank" to store calcium for later in life. As adults, this stored calcium can help keep bones strong. Our bodies continually re-move and replace small amounts of calcium from our bones. If your body removes more calcium than it replaces, your bones will become weaker

About This Chapter: This chapter begins with "Why Calcium?" National Institute of Child Health and Human Development (www.nichd.nih.gov), 2005; "Issues Affecting Consumption" is excerpted and reprinted with permission from "Dairy/Calcium Coun-seling Resource," © 2005 National Dairy Council (the complete text of this document including references and additional material is available online at www.national diarycouncil.org); "Calcium-Cool Cuisine," is from a fact sheet produced by the Centers for Disease Control and Prevention (CDC), September 2001.

and have a greater chance of breaking. But by getting the recommended amount of calcium, you can help your bones stay strong.

Calcium also keeps teeth and gums healthy throughout our lives by helping baby teeth and adult teeth develop properly and to remain strong and resist tooth decay. Calcium is also important for preventing gum disease.

♣ It's A Fact!!
Osteoporosis Prevention Starts Early

Most people think osteoporosis is a disease of the elderly. People lose bone mass as they age. Bone growth during childhood and adolescence is just as important in developing osteoporosis. That's what experts said at the National Institutes of Health (NIH) conference on Osteoporosis Prevention, Diagnosis and Therapy in March 2000. (Primary sponsors were the National Institute of Arthritis and Musculoskeletal and Skin Diseases and the NIH Office of Medical Applications of Research.)

Bones grow in size and strength during childhood. The bone mass you reach while young helps determine your skeletal health for the rest of your life. The more bone mass you have after adolescence, the more protection you have against losing bone density later.

Childhood is critical for developing lifestyle habits that support good bone health. Cigarette smoking could start in childhood. It has a harmful effect on reaching peak bone mass.

Good nutrition is vital for normal growth. Like all tissues, bone needs a balanced diet, enough calories, and appropriate nutrients. But not everyone follows a diet that is best for bone health. For example, the Institute of Medicine recommends calcium intake for children ages 9 to 17 of 1,300 mg/day (800 mg/day for children ages 3 to 8). Only about 25 percent of boys and 10 percent of girls ages 9 to 17 have a diet that meets these recommendations.

Calcium is the most important nutrient for reaching peak bone mass. It prevents and treats osteoporosis. The body requires vitamin D to absorb calcium effectively. Most infants and young children in the United States get enough vitamin D from fortified milk. But adolescents don't consume as many dairy products. They may not get adequate levels of vitamin D. Dieting and fasting to be thin may harm nutrition and bone health. Teens who diet may need to take calcium and vitamin D supplements.

Issues Affecting Consumption

There are several barriers undermining consumption of milk and milk products that may cause calcium consumption to lag far behind dietary recommendations for this nutrient. Factors influencing dietary behavior are complex and include physiological and sociodemographic factors, as well as

Risk Factors And Prevention

Several groups of children and adolescents may be at risk for poor bone health. They include the following:

- Premature and low birthweight infants who have lower-than-expected bone mass in the first few months of life

- Children who take medications such as systemic or inhaled steroids to treat chronic inflammatory or respiratory diseases such as asthma

- Children who have cystic fibrosis, celiac disease, and inflammatory bowel disease because these conditions make it difficult for the body to absorb nutrients appropriately

- Adolescent girls who have minimal, delayed, or irregular menstrual cycles because of strenuous athletic training, emotional stress, or low body weight

- Children with cerebral palsy and other conditions causing limited weight bearing, especially when children are taking chronic medications for seizure control

Many more studies are needed on ways to maximize peak bone mass in girls and boys. Parents and children alike can benefit from following these suggestions:

- Make sure you get enough calcium and vitamin D throughout your life.

- Exercise regularly, using resistance and high-impact activities.

- Eat a healthy diet and follow a healthy lifestyle.

Source: "Osteoporosis Prevention Starts Early," © 2004 American Academy of Orthopaedic Surgeons. Reprinted with permission from *Your Orthopaedic Connection*, the patient education website of the American Academy of Orthopaedic Surgeons located at http://orthoinfo.aaos.org.

lifestyle choices, knowledge, and attitudes. The following are examples of these factors:

Taste: Taste is an important factor influencing food choices, including milk and other dairy products. People who enjoy the taste of dairy foods are more likely to consume these foods more often and, as such, have higher calcium intakes. According to a study of factors affecting teenagers' intake of milk and milk products, teens who enjoyed the taste consumed these foods more often and consequently were more likely to have higher calcium intakes. In this study, 79% of the teens' calcium intake came from the milk group such as cheese, yogurt, frozen yogurt, cottage cheese, and ice cream. Children's taste preference for flavored milk (for example, chocolate) increases their consumption of milk and their calcium intake.

> **✔ Quick Tip**
>
> While most experts agree that calcium should be obtained from natural dietary sources whenever possible, calcium supplements can be given to teens who don't get enough through their foods. For best absorption, no more than 500 mg of calcium supplements should be taken at any one time.
>
> Source: From "Why Calcium?" National Institute of Child Health and Human Development, 2005.

Body Weight Concerns: The misperception that milk and other dairy foods are fattening, coupled with strong societal pressures to be thin, prevents many people, especially teenage girls and adult women, from consuming calcium-rich milk and milk products that would contribute the amount of calcium needed for optimal bone health. According to a study of over 34,000 Minnesota students in grades 7 through 12, dieting and dissatisfaction with body weight are strongly linked to low intake of dairy foods.

The American Academy of Pediatrics (AAP), in its report on calcium requirements of children, acknowledges that preoccupation with being thin, especially among teenage girls, and the misperception that all dairy foods are fattening, is contributing to low calcium intakes in this age group.

Research demonstrates that young girls and adults can increase their calcium intake to recommended levels with foods from the milk group without excessive fat or calorie intake, weight gain, or adversely affecting blood lipid [fat] levels. Furthermore, emerging scientific research findings indicate that increasing calcium intake, especially from calcium-rich dairy foods, may help control body fat and encourage weight loss on a reduced calorie diet.

Lactose Maldigestion: Some people who have lactose maldigestion (a reduced ability to digest lactose), or believe that they have lactose intolerance, avoid milk and milk products. However, research indicates that many individuals who are lactose maldigesters can consume the amount of lactose in one cup of milk with breakfast or two cups of milk with meals—one cup with breakfast and one with dinner—without symptoms. Aged cheeses are well tolerated by lactose-intolerant individuals since they contain less lactose than milk. And yogurt with "live active cultures" is well tolerated since the active bacteria cultures "autodigest" ingested lactose within the intestinal tract. Gradually increasing intake of lactose-containing foods improves tolerance to lactose. Other options include lactose-reduced milk or lactase tablets with milk. Many individuals attribute gastrointestinal symptoms to lactose intolerance when in fact the symptoms may be due to other causes. Lactose intolerance is reportedly high among African Americans and many of the chronic diseases (for example, hypertension) for which African Americans are at disproportionately high risk may be exacerbated by their low intake of dairy foods. A consensus statement of the National Medical Association recognizes that African Americans would greatly benefit from improved intake of calcium by consuming 3–4 servings of dairy products daily.

Image: For teens in particular, milk-drinking is linked to images of home and family, which may be at odds with teens' need for peer approval and independence. As children get older, drinking milk, especially at school, is often not considered to be "cool." However, if a teen's peers drink milk, he/she is also likely to consume this beverage. Substituting soft drinks for milk compromises calcium intake. One study of 460 ninth and tenth grade students linked increased intake of soft drinks with a higher risk for fractures.

Family Influence: Parents, particularly mothers, can influence their children's milk intake. In the early years, moms encourage their children to consume milk and make it readily available. However, as children enter the pre-teen years (9–12), parents' influence starts to wane. This, coupled with

Table 14.1. Sources of Calcium: Dairy Foods

Serving Size	Food Item	Calcium (mg)	% Daily Value
1 cup	Plain yogurt, fat-free	450	45%
2 oz.	American cheese	350	35%
½ cup	Ricotta cheese, part skim	340	34%
1 cup	Yogurt with fruit (low-fat or fat-free)	315	31%
8 oz.	Milk (fat-free, low fat or whole)	300	30%
6-8 nachos	Nachos with cheese	272	25%
1 slice	Cheese pizza	220	22%
1 oz.	Cheddar cheese	204	20%
½ cup	Macaroni and cheese	180	18%
1 cup	Cottage cheese	138	10%
½ cup	Ice cream, soft serve	118	10%

Calcium content in many foods varies depending on ingredients. Check your food labels to get exact content.

Source of data: Bowes and Church's. *Food Values of Portions Commonly Used*, revised by Jean A.T. Pennington, Lippincot: Raven Publishers, 1998.

Source of table: From "Why Calcium?" National Institute of Child Health and Human Development.

Table 14.2. Sources of Calcium: Non-Diary

Serving Size	Food Item	Calcium (mg)	% Daily Value
Vegetables			
1 oz.	Cooked dried white beans	161	15%
½ cup	Spinach	122	10%
½ cup	Turnip greens	99	8%
½ cup	Soybeans, cooked	90	8%
1 cup	Broccoli, cooked or fresh	90	8%
½ cup	Bok choy, cooked or fresh	80	8%
1 cup	Garbanzo beans	80	8%
½ cup	Kale, cooked	45	4%
Grains and Nuts			
3	Corn tortillas (lime-treated)	132	10%
1 oz.	Dry roasted almonds	80	8%
1 slice	Bread, white or whole wheat	30	2%
Other Foods Naturally Containing Calcium			
10	Dried figs	269	25%
6 oz.	Small taco	221	20%
2 burritos	Burrito with beans and cheese	214	20%
3 oz.	Salmon, canned with bones	180	15%
Fortified Foods (foods with calcium added)			
½ cup	Frozen yogurt, fat-free, calcium added	450	45%
8 fluid oz.	Calcium fortified orange juice	300	30%
1 cup	Soy milk, calcium added	250–300	25–30%
½ cup	Tofu made with calcium	260	25%

Other foods with calcium added include many cereals, breads, and soy products. Check the packages and food labels to see if calcium has been added.

Source of data: Bowes and Church's. *Food Values of Portions Commonly Used*, revised by Jean A.T. Pennington, Lippincot: Raven Publishers, 1998.

Source of table: From "Why Calcium? Sources of Calcium," National Institute of Child Health and Human Development, 2005.

other factors such as pre-teens' and teens' growing independence with their choices, contributes to decreased milk consumption. Intake of soft drinks was negatively associated with milk and calcium intake.

Cultural Influence: Cultural factors can influence intake of calcium-rich foods such as milk and other dairy foods. One study found that white girls are more likely to prefer the taste of milk than either Asian or Hispanic girls. Also, white girls liked milk served cold, whereas Asian girls preferred milk warm and sweetened in combination with other beverages such as tea. Hispanic girls preferred milk in the form of shakes, puddings, and flan. African Americans' low intake of dairy foods, especially milk and yogurt, is related to culturally determined food preferences. Compared to the general population, African Americans are less likely to consume milk "as a glass" or with meals.

Eating Away from Home and Participating in School Nutrition Programs: Eating away from home, especially at fast food establishments, can jeopardize calcium intake. A study of more than 6,000 children and teens aged 4 to 19 years found that on a typical day 30% of them reported consuming fast foods. Fast food intake is associated with a low intake of milk and a high intake of soft drinks, which can compromise calcium intake. With the exception of foods served as part of the school

♣ It's A Fact!!

How much calcium do children and teens get every day on average?

According to the National Health and Nutrition Examination Survey (NHANES), many kids and teens are not getting enough calcium. The following percentages show how many children and teens get enough calcium every day, on average:

• Females 2–8 years: 79% get enough calcium

• Females 9–19 years: 19% get enough calcium

• Males 2–8 years: 89% get enough calcium

• Males 9–19 years: 52% get enough calcium

Source: From "Why Calcium? Getting Enough Calcium," National Institute of Child Health and Human Development, 2005.

nutrition programs, the calcium density of restaurant or fast foods is lower than that of home foods. In contrast to eating away from home, consuming family meals, and participating in school nutrition programs (school breakfast and lunch), improves intake of calcium or calcium-rich foods such as dairy foods. When the nutrient contributions of five meal components of school lunch were examined, milk contributed the most calcium and protein per 100 calories and per penny. Encouraging children to improve their food choices when eating away from home and to consume more meals at home may improve their overall nutrient intakes, including their calcium and dairy intakes.

Calcium-Cool Cuisine

Breakfast Ideas: Start your day with these treats to get an energy boost and give your bones more power.

- Munch on a bowl of cereal with added calcium, fat-free or low-fat milk, and fresh fruit.

- Top a whole wheat English muffin with your favorite melted low-fat cheese.

- Make waffles or pancakes for the whole family. Be sure to make them with milk or top them with fat-free or low-fat yogurt, and enjoy a glass of fat-free or low-fat milk with them.

- Enjoy a glass of fruit juice—the kind with added calcium.

- Make a breakfast banana split. Top a sliced banana with a small container of low-fat or fat-free fruit yogurt, a sprinkle of frosted cereal, and pieces of your favorite fruit.

- Fruit adds a flavorful punch to foods like cereal, smoothies, and yogurt. Although it's generally not high in calcium, fruit has lots vitamins and minerals.

Bus Stop Eats: Munch these convenient treats when you're running to catch the bus.

- A cereal bar with added calcium.

- A whole wheat English muffin, spread with low-fat ricotta cheese and topped with tomato or salsa.

- Add a handful of almonds to dried fruit and toss it in a zipped plastic bag. (Keep a couple of bags on hand for those super-busy days.)

Scrumptious Lunches and Snacks: Spice up lunch or snack time with these fun foods with calcium.

- Try a soy beverage with added calcium. (Believe it or not, these cool treats can help you get the calcium you need.)

- Top a fruit salad with fat-free or low-fat yogurt and almonds. (Who would guess that almonds can deliver calcium?)

- Add almonds or low-fat cheddar cheese cubes to a snack of apple slices.

- Warm up with a bowl of tomato or mushroom soup made with fat-free or low-fat milk.

- Make some pudding with fat-free or low-fat milk.

- Steam chopped broccoli and top it with low-fat ranch dressing.

- Add almonds and fruit to a bowl of low-fat cottage cheese.

Slumber Party Treats: With your best pal or ten friends, enjoy these bone-healthy foods between the gossip and videos.

- Top baked tortilla chips with low-fat cheddar cheese and heat until melted. This slumber party sensation will keep your pals coming back for more.

- Mix up bowls of your favorite pudding made with low-fat or fat-free milk.

- Combine chopped collards and low-fat cheese in a bowl, heat until bubbly. Eat with crackers, toasted bread, or practically anything you can dip.

- Top whole wheat English muffins with your favorite veggies and low-fat cheeses. Toast in the oven for a treat your friends will love.

- Serve up tortillas, grated low-fat cheese, lettuce, tomatoes, and salsa—for a south-of-the-border treat.

- Melt low-fat cheese on a whole-wheat pita. Add apple slices.

- Set up a baked potato bar. Let your guests get calcium from toppings like broccoli, grated low-fat cheese, or plain yogurt (fat-free or low-fat).

- Sip mugs of hot chocolate made with fat-free or low-fat milk.

- Scoop up fat-free or low-fat frozen yogurt. Top with sprinkles or fruit.

- Make a frozen treat by pouring fat-free or low-fat drinkable yogurt into a paper cup. Add a stick and freeze. Then, peel the cup, and enjoy.

- Wash it all down with a glass of fat-free or low-fat milk (with chocolate or strawberry flavor to make it extra yummy). Lactose-free milk or a soy beverage with added calcium works, too.

Wrap It Up: Wraps are the most portable meals ever. Just fill a tortilla with your favorite sandwich ingredients, and in a jif you'll have a tasty, on-the-go meal. Wrap up your favorite fillings. Be sure to include ingredients like these:

- All kinds of low-fat cheeses

- Low-fat cottage cheese

- An ounce of slivered almonds

- Tofu (look for calcium sulfate on the ingredient list)

Slammin' Smoothies: Chat with your friends over these yummy bone-healthy treats. Toss all ingredients in a blender and mix up a smooth snack. Remember to get your parents' OK.

- *Sunshine Smoothie:* 1 cup of orange juice with added calcium, fat-free or low-fat milk, ice cubes, and a handful of fruit.

- *Very Berry Smoothie:* 1 cup of fat-free or low-fat milk, a handful of fresh or frozen blueberries, and a dash of honey. Toss in some ice cubes to make it extra thick.

- *Fruit Smash Smoothie:* 1 cup of fat-free or low-fat milk, a bunch of frozen strawberries, apricots, bananas, and fresh raspberries. Toss in some ice cubes to make it extra thick.

- *Vanilla Smoothie:* 1 cup of orange juice with added calcium, a handful of strawberries, a banana, and 1 cup of fat-free or low-fat vanilla yogurt.

Delicious Dinners: Create these dinners at home (with your parents' OK) to help your family build powerful bones.

- Create an Italian feast by combining low-fat cottage and mozzarella cheeses, garlic, and basil with cooked pasta and covering it with your favorite sauce. Bake for 20 minutes.

- Make a sesame stir-fry sensation by combining pieces of tofu (look for calcium sulfate on the ingredient list), chicken, or shrimp with your favorite calcium-containing vegetables, like bok choy and broccoli, in a skillet and cook. Then, sprinkle on some yummy sesame seeds.

- Cheesy rice and broccoli makes a great dinner or side dish. Just combine cooked rice, broccoli, and low-fat cheddar cheese for a dinnertime treat.

Stop for a Snack: If you're out to shop till you drop, make sure you fuel up with these calcium-cool treats.

- Grab a piece of cheese or veggie pizza in the food court, some low-fat frozen yogurt with sprinkles, or a shake from the closest yogurt stand.

- Sit and chat with your friends over a smoothie made with low-fat or fat-free milk, yogurt, and your favorite fruits.

Calcium Cool at School: At lunchtime or after school, pick (or pack) these foods with calcium to help build powerful bones.

- Bring a cereal bar or bottle of juice with added calcium to boost your body into after-school sports practice mode.

- At lunch, try a carton of plain or chocolate low-fat or fat-free milk or orange juice with added calcium.

- Whether you pack your lunch or buy it at school, be sure to look for these foods to help build your bones while you build your mind:

  - Cubes of low-fat or fat-free cheese

  - Low-fat yogurt (fruit or plain)

  - Fruit juice with added calcium

  - Pudding made with low-fat or fat-free milk

- Low-fat or fat-free cottage cheese (sprinkle with almonds for added calcium)

- A sandwich made with low-fat cheese and your favorite veggies

- One cup rice beverage with added calcium

- A slice of cheese pizza

What's on the Menu? Order one of these delicious menu items with calcium when you're out on the town.

- Eating out? Don't worry. Plenty of restaurants have calcium cool menu items such as: grilled cheese; a slice of cheese pizza; stir fry made with bok choy, kale, or broccoli; macaroni and cheese; low-fat or fat-free ice cream or frozen yogurt; and pudding made with fat-free or low-fat milk.

- Be your own chef. Check out salad bars and buffets to find fun foods with calcium like broccoli, macaroni and cheese, low-fat cottage cheese, pudding, collards or kale, and low-fat frozen yogurt.

Pack Your Picnic: Don't forget to fill your basket with some of these calcium-cool favorites.

- On the hiking trail, snack on almonds and fruit juice with added calcium to keep you climbing to the top. For a picnic lunch, munch on low-fat American cheese sandwiches, low-fat yogurt, pudding packs, or broccoli.

- Plan a perfect picnic by packing pitas (Say *that* three times fast). Along with low-fat cheese or tofu (look for calcium sulfate on the ingredient list), fill your pita with apples, turkey, or vegetables.

Holiday Season Ideas: Try these suggestions to add calcium to your special parties.

- You're planning an awesome Halloween bash, but you don't want your guests chowing down on candy all night. Use a pumpkin, bat, ghost, or other ghoulish cookie cutter to cut shapes out of soft flour or corn tortillas and bake until they get crispy. Top with low-fat cheese for a calcium kick and serve up this frightful treat that's sure to please any ghost or ghoul.

• Give your New Year's Eve a little punch—add some orange juice with added calcium to lemon lime soda or ginger ale. Slice oranges and drop them in, too, for a creative calcium celebration.

Chapter 15

Dietary Supplements

Dietary Supplements—More Than Vitamins

Today's dietary supplements are not only vitamins and minerals. They also include other less familiar substances, such as herbals, botanicals, amino acids, and enzymes. Dietary supplements come in a variety of forms, such as tablets, capsules, powders, energy bars, or drinks.

If you do not consume a variety of foods, as recommended in the Food Guide Pyramid and *Dietary Guidelines for Americans*, some supplements may help ensure that you get adequate amounts of essential nutrients or help promote optimal health and performance. However, dietary supplements are not intended to treat, diagnose, mitigate, prevent, or cure diseases; therefore, manufacturers may not make such claims. In some cases, dietary supplements may have unwanted effects, especially if taken before surgery or with other dietary supplements or medicines, or if you have certain health conditions.

Unlike drugs, but like conventional foods, dietary supplements are not approved by the Food and Drug Administration (FDA) for safety and effectiveness. It is the responsibility of dietary supplement manufacturers/

About This Chapter: From "What Dietary Supplements Are You Taking," Center for Food Safety and Applied Nutrition, U.S. Food and Drug Administration, December 2004.

distributors to ensure that their products are safe and that their label claims are accurate and truthful. Once a product enters the marketplace, FDA has the authority to take action against any dietary supplement product that presents a significant or unreasonable risk of illness or injury.

Scientific evidence supporting the benefits of some dietary supplements (for example, vitamins and minerals) is well established for certain health conditions, but others need further study. Whatever your choice, supplements should not replace prescribed medications or the variety of foods important to a healthful diet.

How can I recognize a dietary supplement?

At times, it can be confusing to tell the difference between a dietary supplement, a food, or an over-the-counter (OTC) medicine. An easy way to recognize a dietary supplement is to look for the Supplement Facts Panel on the product.

What are the potential risks of using dietary supplements?

Although certain products may be helpful to some people, there may be circumstances when these products can pose unexpected risks. Many supplements contain active ingredients that can have strong effects in the body. Taking a combination of supplements, using these products together with medicine, or substituting them in place of prescribed medicines could lead to harmful, even life-threatening results. Also, some supplements can have unwanted effects before, during, and after surgery. It is important to let your doctor and other health professionals know about the vitamins, minerals, botanicals, and other products you are taking, especially before surgery.

Here a few examples of dietary supplements believed to interact with specific drugs:

- **Calcium and heart medicine** (for example, Digoxin), thiazide diuretics (Thiazide), and aluminum and magnesium-containing antacids.

- **Magnesium** and thiazide and loop diuretics (such as Lasix®, etc.), some cancer drugs (for example, Cisplatin, etc.), and magnesium-containing antacids.

- **Vitamin K** and a blood thinner (for example, Coumadin).

- **St. John's Wort** and selective serotonin reuptake inhibitor (SSRI) drugs (such as anti-depressant drugs) and birth control pills.

What should I know before using dietary supplements?

Be savvy! Follow the following tips before buying a dietary supplement:

- **Remember:** Safety first. Some supplement ingredients, including nutrients and plant components, can be toxic based on their activity in your body. Do not substitute a dietary supplement for a prescription medicine or therapy.

- **Think twice about chasing the latest headline.** Sound health advice is generally based on research over time, not a single study touted by the media. Be wary of results claiming a "quick fix" that depart from scientific research and established dietary guidance.

- **Learn to Spot False Claims. Remember:** "If something sounds too good to be true, it probably is." Some examples of false claims on product labels include the following:

  - Quick and effective "cure-all."

  - Can treat or cure disease.

  - "Totally safe," "all natural," and has "definitely no side effects."

  - Limited availability, "no-risk, money-back guarantees," or requires advance payment.

- **More may not be better.** Some products can be harmful when consumed in high amounts, for a long time, or in combination with certain other substances.

> **✔ Quick Tip**
>
> More is not better when it comes to vitamins and minerals. Overdoing some nutrients can crowd out others. Taking vitamin and mineral supplements to ensure meeting the 100% Recommended Daily Intake is fine, but supplements cannot replace a healthy diet of varied foods. Many healthy substances in foods are not contained in supplements. So, still pay attention to your food choices.
>
> Source: Excerpted from "Nutrition Tips for Teens," © 2003 Munson Healthcare. All rights reserved. Reprinted with permission.

☞ **Remember!!**

- Do not self diagnose any health condition. Work with your health care providers to determine how best to achieve optimal health.

- Check with your health care providers before taking a supplement, especially when combining or substituting them with other foods or medicine.

- Some supplements can help you meet your daily requirements for certain nutrients, but others may cause health problems.

- Dietary supplements are not intended to treat, diagnose, mitigate, prevent, or cure disease, or to replace the variety of foods important to a healthful diet.

Source: FDA, 2004.

- **The term "natural" doesn't always mean safe.** Do not assume that this term ensures wholesomeness or safety. For some supplements, "natural" ingredients may interact with medicines, be dangerous for people with certain health conditions, or be harmful in high doses. For example, tea made from peppermint leaves is generally considered safe to drink, but peppermint oil (extracted from the leaves) is much more concentrated and can be toxic if used incorrectly.

- **Is the product worth the money?** Resist the pressure to buy a product or treatment "on the spot." Some supplement products may be expensive or may not provide the benefit you expect. For example, excessive amounts of water-soluble vitamins, like vitamin C and B vitamins, are not used by the body and are eliminated in the urine.

Examples Of Products Marketed As Dietary Supplements

Because many products are marketed as dietary supplements, it is important to remember that supplements include vitamins and minerals, as well as botanicals and other substances. The list below (Adapted from *A Healthcare Professional's Guide to Evaluating Dietary Supplements*, the American Dietetic Association and American Pharmaceutical Association Special Report, 2000) gives some examples of products you may see sold as dietary supplements. It is not possible to list them all here. The examples provided do not represent an endorsement or approval by any agency or organization that contributed to this material.

Vitamins, Minerals, And Nutrients

- Multiple Vitamin/Mineral
- Vitamin B Complex
- Vitamin C
- Vitamin D
- Vitamin E
- Beta-Carotene
- Calcium
- Omega-3 Fatty Acids
- Folic Acid
- Zinc
- Iron

Botanicals And Other Substances

- Acidophilus
- Black Cohosh
- Ginger
- Evening Primrose Oil
- Echinacea
- Fiber
- Garlic
- Ginkgo Biloba
- Fish Oil
- Glucosamine and/or Chondroitin Sulfate
- St. John's Wort
- Saw Palmetto

✔ Quick Tip
To Report An Illness Or Injury
Associated With A Dietary Supplement

FDA can be contacted to report general complaints or concerns about food products, including dietary supplements. You may telephone or write to FDA.

If you think you have suffered a serious harmful effect or illness from a dietary supplement, your health care provider can report this by calling FDA's MedWatch hotline at 800-FDA-1088 or using the website http://www.fda.gov/medwatch/report/hcp.htm. The MedWatch program allows health care providers to report problems possibly caused by FDA-regulated products such as drugs, medical devices, medical foods and dietary supplements. The identity of the patient is kept confidential.

Consumers may also report an adverse event or illness they believe to be related to the use of a dietary supplement by calling FDA at 800-FDA-1088 or using the website http://www.fda.gov/medwatch/report/consumer/consumer.htm. FDA would like to know when a product causes a problem even if you are unsure the product caused the problem or even if you do not visit a doctor or clinic.

Source: "Adverse Event Reporting," Center for Food Safety and Applied Nutrition, U.S. Food and Drug Administration, 2002.

Chapter 16

Why Is It Important To Eat Grains?

Eating grains, especially whole grains, provides health benefits. People who eat whole grains as part of a healthy diet have a reduced risk of some chronic diseases. Grains provide many nutrients that are vital for the health and maintenance of our bodies.

Health Benefits

- Consuming foods rich in fiber, such as whole grains, as part of a healthy diet, reduces the risk of coronary heart disease.

- Consuming foods rich in fiber, such as whole grains, as part of a healthy diet, may reduce constipation.

- Eating at least three ounce equivalents a day of whole grains may help with weight management.

- Eating grains fortified with folate before and during pregnancy helps prevent neural tube defects during fetal development.

Nutrients

- Grains are important sources of many nutrients, including dietary fiber, several B vitamins (thiamin, riboflavin, niacin, and folate), and minerals (iron, magnesium, and selenium).

About This Chapter: Excerpted from "Inside the Pyramid: Grains," U.S. Department of Agriculture (MyPyramid.gov), 2005.

- Dietary fiber from whole grains, as part of an overall healthy diet, helps reduce blood cholesterol levels and may lower risk of heart disease. Fiber is important for proper bowel function. It helps reduce constipation and diverticulosis. Fiber-containing foods such as whole grains help provide a feeling of fullness with fewer calories. Whole grains are good sources of dietary fiber; most refined (processed) grains contain little fiber.

- B vitamins (thiamin, riboflavin, niacin, and folate)play a key role in metabolism—they help the body release energy from protein, fat, and carbohydrates. B vitamins are also essential for a healthy nervous system. Many refined grains are enriched with these B vitamins.

- Folate (folic acid), another B vitamin, helps the body form red blood cells. Women of childbearing age who may become pregnant and those in the first trimester of pregnancy should consume adequate folate, including folic acid from fortified foods or supplements. This reduces the risk of neural tube defects, spina bifida, and anencephaly during fetal development.

- Iron is used to carry oxygen in the blood. Many teenage girls and women in their childbearing years have iron-deficiency anemia. They should eat foods high in heme-iron (meats) or eat other iron containing foods along with foods rich in vitamin C, which can improve absorption of non-heme iron. Whole and enriched refined grain products are major sources of non-heme iron in American diets.

- Whole grains are sources of magnesium and selenium. Magnesium is a mineral used in building bones and releasing energy from muscles. Selenium protects cells from oxidation. It is also important for a healthy immune system.

Foods In The Grain Group

Any food made from wheat, rice, oats, cornmeal, barley or another cereal grain is a grain product. Bread, pasta, oatmeal, breakfast cereals, tortillas, and grits are examples of grain products.

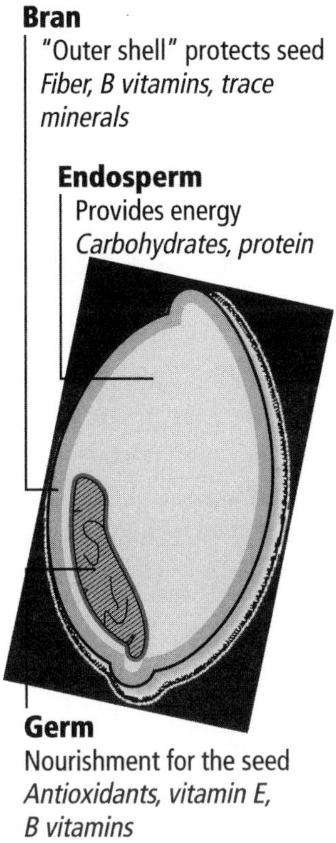

Bran
"Outer shell" protects seed
Fiber, B vitamins, trace minerals

Endosperm
Provides energy
Carbohydrates, protein

Germ
Nourishment for the seed
Antioxidants, vitamin E, B vitamins

Figure 16.1. Whole grain kernel (Source: "Get on the Grain Train," U.S. Department of Agriculture, May 2002).

Grains are divided into two subgroups, whole grains and refined grains.

Whole grains contain the entire grain kernel—the bran, germ, and endosperm. Examples include the following:

• whole-wheat flour

• bulgur (cracked wheat)

• oatmeal

• whole cornmeal

• brown rice

Refined grains have been milled, a process that removes the bran and germ. This is done to give grains a finer texture and improve their shelf life, but it also removes dietary fiber, iron, and many B vitamins. Some examples of refined grain products include the following:

• white flour

• degermed cornmeal

• white bread

• white rice

✤ It's A Fact!!
How many grain foods are needed daily?

The amount of grains you need to eat depends on your age, sex, and level of physical activity. Most Americans consume enough grains, but few are whole grains. At least ½ of all the grains eaten should be whole grains.

Source: U.S. Department of Agriculture
(MyPyramid.gov), 2005.

Most refined grains are enriched. This means certain B vitamins (thiamin, riboflavin, niacin, folic acid) and iron are added back after processing. Fiber is not added back to enriched grains. Check the ingredient list on refined grain products to make sure that the word "enriched" is included in the grain name. Some food products are made from mixtures of whole grains and refined grains.

Some commonly eaten grain products are as follows:

Whole Grains

- brown rice

- buckwheat

- bulgur (cracked wheat)

- oatmeal

- popcorn

- Ready-to-eat breakfast cereals:
  - whole wheat cereal flakes
  - muesli

- whole grain barley

- whole grain cornmeal

- whole rye

- whole wheat bread

- whole wheat crackers

- whole wheat pasta

✔ Quick Tip
Tips To Help You Eat Whole Grains

At Meals

- To eat more whole grains, substitute a whole-grain product for a refined product—such as eating whole-wheat bread instead of white bread or brown rice instead of white rice. It's important to substitute the whole-grain product for the refined one, rather than adding the whole-grain product.

- For a change, try brown rice or whole-wheat pasta. Try brown rice stuffing in baked green peppers or tomatoes and whole-wheat macaroni in macaroni and cheese.

- Use whole grains in mixed dishes, such as barley in vegetable soup or stews and bulgur wheat in casserole or stir-fries.

- Create a whole grain pilaf with a mixture of barley, wild rice, brown rice, broth and spices. For a special touch, stir in toasted nuts or chopped dried fruit.

- Experiment by substituting whole wheat or oat flour for up to half of the flour in pancake, waffle, muffin or other flour-based recipes. They may need a bit more leavening.

- Use whole-grain bread or cracker crumbs in meatloaf.

- Try rolled oats or a crushed, unsweetened whole grain cereal as breading for baked chicken, fish, veal cutlets, or eggplant parmesan.

- Try an unsweetened, whole grain ready-to-eat cereal as croutons in salad or in place of crackers with soup.

- Freeze leftover cooked brown rice, bulgur, or barley. Heat and serve it later as a quick side dish.

As Snacks

- Snack on ready-to-eat, whole grain cereals such as toasted oat cereal.

- Add whole-grain flour or oatmeal when making cookies or other baked treats.

- Try a whole-grain snack chip, such as baked tortilla chips.

- Popcorn, a whole grain, can be a healthy snack with little or no added salt and butter.

Source: U.S. Department of Agriculture (MyPyramid.gov), 2005.

- whole wheat sandwich buns and rolls

- whole wheat tortillas

- wild rice

- Less common whole grains:

- amaranth

- millet

- quinoa

- sorghum

- triticale

Refined Grains

- cornbread*

- corn tortillas*

- couscous*

- crackers*

- flour tortillas*

- grits

- noodles*

- Pasta*

- spaghetti

- macaroni

- pitas*

- pretzels

- Ready-to-eat breakfast cereals

- corn flakes

- white bread

- white sandwich buns and rolls

- white rice

*Most of these products are made from refined grains. Some are made from whole grains. Check the ingredient list for the words "whole grain" or "whole wheat" to decide if they are made from a whole grain. Some foods are made from a mixture of whole and refined grains.

Some grain products contain significant amounts of bran. Bran provides fiber, which is important for health. However, products with added bran or bran alone (for example, oat bran) are not necessarily whole grain products.

> ✔ **Quick Tip**
> **Make Half Your Grains Whole**
>
> Eat at least 3 ounces of whole-grain cereals, breads, crackers, rice, or pasta every day. One ounce is about 1 slice of bread, 1 cup of breakfast cereal, or ½ cup of cooked rice or pasta. Look to see that grains such as wheat, rice, oats, or corn are referred to as "whole" in the list of ingredients.
>
> Source: Excerpted from "Finding Your Way to a Healthier You," U.S. Department of Agriculture, Home and Garden Bulletin No. 232-CP, 2005.

What To Look For On The Food Label

Choose foods that name one of the following whole-grain ingredients first on the label's ingredient list:

- "brown rice"
- "bulgur"
- "graham flour"

> ♣ **It's A Fact!!**
> **What counts as an ounce equivalent of grains?**
>
> In general, 1 slice of bread, 1 cup of ready-to-eat cereal, or ½ cup of cooked rice, cooked pasta, or cooked cereal can be considered as 1 ounce equivalent from the grains group.
>
> Source: U.S. Department of Agriculture (MyPyramid.gov), 2005.

- "oatmeal"
- "whole-grain corn"
- "whole oats"
- "whole rye"
- "whole wheat"
- "wild rice"

Foods labeled with the words "multi-grain," "stone-ground," "100% wheat," "cracked wheat," "seven-grain," or "bran" are usually not whole-grain products.

Color is not an indication of a whole grain. Bread can be brown because of molasses or other added ingredients. Read the ingredient list to see if it is a whole grain.

✔ **Quick Tip**

Fiber keeps your intestinal walls and their contents healthy. Fiber is the part of food you do not digest, so it passes through your intestines. How many grams of fiber do you need each day? Add your age plus five, up to 25 grams a day. Foods high in fiber include fruits, vegetables, legumes, and whole grains, such as oatmeal, graham crackers, higher fiber cereals, whole wheat bread, and whole grain crackers.

Source: Excerpted from "Nutrition Tips for Teens," © 2003 Munson Healthcare. All rights reserved. Reprinted with permission.

Use the Nutrition Facts label and choose products with a higher % Daily Value (%DV) for fiber—the %DV for fiber is a good clue to the amount of whole grain in the product.

Chapter 17

Why Is It Important To Eat Vegetables?

Eating vegetables provides health benefits—people who eat more fruits and vegetables as part of an overall healthy diet are likely to have a reduced risk of some chronic diseases. Vegetables provide nutrients vital for health and maintenance of your body.

Health Benefits

- Eating a diet rich in fruits and vegetables as part of an overall healthy diet may reduce risk for stroke and perhaps other cardiovascular diseases.

- Eating a diet rich in fruits and vegetables as part of an overall healthy diet may reduce risk for type 2 diabetes.

- Eating a diet rich in fruits and vegetables as part of an overall healthy diet may protect against certain cancers, such as mouth, stomach, and colon-rectum cancer.

- Diets rich in foods containing fiber, such as fruits and vegetables, may reduce the risk of coronary heart disease.

- Eating fruits and vegetables rich in potassium as part of an overall

About This Chapter: Excerpted from "Inside the Pyramid: Vegetables," U.S. Department of Agriculture (MyPyramid.gov), 2005.

healthy diet may reduce the risk of developing kidney stones and may help to decrease bone loss.

- Eating foods such as vegetables that are low in calories per cup instead of some other higher-calorie food may be useful in helping to lower calorie intake.

Nutrients

- Most vegetables are naturally low in fat and calories. None have cholesterol. (Sauces or seasonings may add fat, calories, or cholesterol.)

- Vegetables are important sources of many nutrients, including potassium, dietary fiber, folate (folic acid), vitamin A, vitamin E, and vitamin C.

- Diets rich in potassium may help to maintain healthy blood pressure. Vegetable sources of potassium include sweet potatoes, white potatoes, white beans, tomato products (paste, sauce, and juice), beet greens, soybeans, lima beans, winter squash, spinach, lentils, kidney beans, and split peas.

- Dietary fiber from vegetables, as part of an overall healthy diet, helps reduce blood cholesterol levels and may lower risk of heart disease. Fiber is important for proper bowel function. It helps reduce constipation and diverticulosis. Fiber-containing foods such as vegetables help provide a feeling of fullness with fewer calories.

- Folate (folic acid) helps the body form red blood cells. Women of childbearing age who may become pregnant and those in the first trimester of pregnancy should consume adequate folate, including folic acid from fortified foods or supplements. This reduces the risk of neural tube defects, spina bifida, and anencephaly during fetal development.

- Vitamin A keeps eyes and skin healthy and helps to protect against infections.

- Vitamin E helps protect vitamin A and essential fatty acids from cell oxidation.

- Vitamin C helps heal cuts and wounds and keeps teeth and gums healthy. Vitamin C aids in iron absorption.

Foods In The Vegetable Group

Any vegetable or 100% vegetable juice counts as a member of the vegetable group. Vegetables may be raw or cooked; fresh, frozen, canned, or dried/dehydrated; and may be whole, cut-up, or mashed.

Vegetables are organized into five subgroups, based on their nutrient content. Some commonly eaten vegetables in each subgroup are as follows:

Dark Green Vegetables

- bok choy
- broccoli
- collard greens
- dark green leafy lettuce
- kale
- mesclun
- mustard greens
- romaine lettuce
- spinach
- turnip greens
- watercress

Orange Vegetables

- acorn squash
- butternut squash
- carrots
- Hubbard squash
- pumpkin
- sweet potatoes

♣ It's A Fact!!

Phytochemicals are natural substances found only in plants. Hundreds of thousands have been identified. As plants grow, their phytochemicals fight off bacteria, virus, and fungus. When we eat plants (fruits, veggies, whole grains, nuts, seeds, legumes) they help protect our bodies as well, including keeping our blood vessels healthier and lowering our risk of cancer.

Source: Excerpted from "Nutrition Tips for Teens," © 2003 Munson Healthcare. All rights reserved. Reprinted with permission.

Dry Beans And Peas

- black beans
- garbanzo beans (chickpeas)
- lentils
- navy beans
- soy beans
- tofu (bean curd made from soybeans)
- black-eyed peas
- kidney beans
- lima beans (mature)
- pinto beans
- split peas
- white beans

Starchy Vegetables

- corn
- lima beans (green)
- green peas
- potatoes

Other Vegetables

- artichokes
- bean sprouts
- Brussels sprouts
- cauliflower
- cucumbers
- green beans
- iceberg (head) lettuce
- okra
- parsnips
- tomato juice
- turnips
- zucchini
- asparagus
- beets
- cabbage
- celery
- eggplant
- green or red peppers
- mushrooms
- onions
- tomatoes
- vegetable juice
- wax beans

♣ It's A Fact!!
What counts as a cup of vegetables?

In general, 1 cup of raw or cooked vegetables or vegetable juice, or 2 cups of raw leafy greens can be considered as 1 cup from the vegetable group.

Source: U.S. Department of Agriculture (MyPyramid.gov), 2005.

Tips To Help You Eat Vegetables

General

- Buy fresh vegetables in season. They cost less and are likely to be at their peak flavor.

- Stock up on frozen vegetables for quick and easy cooking in the microwave.

- Buy vegetables that are easy to prepare. Pick up pre-washed bags of salad greens and add baby carrots or grape tomatoes for a salad in minutes. Buy packages of such as baby carrots or celery sticks for quick snacks.

- Use a microwave to quickly "zap" vegetables. White or sweet potatoes can be baked quickly this way.

- Vary your veggie choices to keep meals interesting.

- Try crunchy vegetables, raw or lightly steamed.

Best Nutritional Value

- Select vegetables with more potassium often, such as sweet potatoes, white potatoes, white beans, tomato products (paste, sauce, and juice), beet greens, soybeans, lima beans, winter squash, spinach, lentils, kidney beans, and split peas.

- Sauces or seasonings can add calories, fat, and sodium to vegetables. Use the Nutrition Facts label to compare the calories and % Daily Value for fat and sodium in plain and seasoned vegetables.

- Prepare more foods from fresh ingredients to lower sodium intake. Most sodium in the food supply comes from packaged or processed foods.

- Buy canned vegetables labeled "no salt added." If you want to add a little salt it will likely be less than the amount in the regular canned product.

Meals

- Plan some meals around a vegetable main dish, such as a vegetable stir-fry or soup. Then add other foods to complement it.

- Try a main dish salad for lunch. Go light on the salad dressing.

- Include a green salad with your dinner every night.

- Shred carrots or zucchini into meatloaf, casseroles, quick breads, and muffins.

♣ It's A Fact!!

More Color More Health

Nutrition research shows that colorful vegetables and fruit contain essential vitamins, minerals, fiber, and phytochemicals that your body needs to promote health and help you feel great. Here are the specifics.

Reds: When you add deep reds or bright pinks to your daily diet, you are also adding a powerful antioxidant called lycopene. Lycopene is found in tomatoes, red and pink grapefruit, watermelon, papaya and guava. Diets rich in lycopene are being studied for their ability to fight heart disease and some cancers.

Greens: Do you know why this color is so essential to your diet? Not only do green vegetables look great and taste wonderful, but they are rich in the phytochemicals that keep you healthy. For example, the carotenoids lutein and zeaxanthin that are found in spinach, collards, kale and broccoli have antioxidant properties and are being studied for their ability to protect your eyes by keeping your retina strong. Also, research is being done on cruciferous vegetables like cabbage, Brussels sprouts, cauliflower, kale, and turnips to see if they may reduce the risk of cancerous tumors. Greens are also loaded with essential vitamins (folate), minerals, and fiber.

Oranges/Yellows: Orange, the color of a blazing sun, is a must have in your daily diet. Orange vegetables and fruits like sweet potatoes, mangos, carrots, and apricots, contain beta-carotene. This carotenoid is a natural antioxidant that is being studied for its role in enhancing the immune system. In addition to being touted as a powerful health-protector, the orange group is rich in Vitamin C. Folate, most often found in leafy greens, is also found in orange fruits and vegetables, and is a B vitamin that may help prevent some birth defects and reduce your risk of heart disease. With a chemical make-up this good, make the orange group always a part of your five to nine a day.

- Include chopped vegetables in pasta sauce or lasagna.

- Order a veggie pizza with toppings like mushrooms, green peppers, and onions, and ask for extra veggies.

- Use pureed, cooked vegetables such as potatoes to thicken stews, soups and gravies. These add flavor, nutrients, and texture.

- Grill vegetable kabobs as part of a barbecue meal. Try tomatoes, mushrooms, green peppers, and onions.

Bright yellows have many of the same perks as the orange groups: high in essential vitamins and carotenoids. Pineapple, for example, is rich with Vitamin C, manganese, and the natural enzyme, bromelain. Additionally, corn and pears are high in fiber. Yellow fruits and vegetables belong to many different families, but they all share the common bond of being health enhancing with great taste. Go for the gold!

Blues/Purples: Blues and purples not only add beautiful shades of tranquility and richness to your plate, they add health-enhancing flavonoids, phytochemicals, and antioxidants. Anthocyanins, a phytochemical, are pigments responsible for the blue color in vegetables and fruits, and are being studied for their role in the body's defense of harmful carcinogens. Blueberries, in particular, are rich in Vitamin C and folic acid and high in fiber and potassium.

Whites: Vegetables from the onion family, which include garlic, chives, scallions, leeks, and any variety of onion, contain the phytochemical allicin. Research is being conducted on the following:

- Allicin to learn how it may help lower cholesterol and blood pressure and increase the body's ability to fight infections.

- Indoles and sulfaforaphanes, phytochemicals in cruciferous vegetables like cauliflower, for how they may inhibit cancer growth.

- Polyphenols, another important phytochemical in pears and green grapes for how they may reduce the risk of certain cancers.

Source: Centers for Disease Control and Prevention, June 2005.

Make Vegetables More Appealing

- Many vegetables taste great with a dip or dressing. Try a low-fat salad dressing with raw broccoli, red and green peppers, celery sticks or cauliflower.

- Add color to salads by adding baby carrots, shredded red cabbage, or spinach leaves. Include in-season vegetables for variety through the year.

- Include cooked dry beans or peas in flavorful mixed dishes, such as chili or minestrone soup.

- Decorate plates or serving dishes with vegetable slices.

- Keep a bowl of cut-up vegetables in a see-through container in the refrigerator. Carrot and celery sticks are traditional, but consider broccoli floretes, cucumber slices, or red or green pepper strips.

♣ **It's A Fact!!**
Are there nutritional differences between fresh foods and canned foods?

The heating process during canning destroys from one-third to one-half of vitamins A and C, riboflavin, and thiamin. For every year the food is stored, canned food loses an additional 5 to 20% of these vitamins. However, the amounts of other vitamins are only slightly lower in canned food than in fresh food.

Most produce will begin to lose some of its nutrients when harvested. When produce is handled properly and canned quickly after harvest, it can be more nutritious than fresh produce sold in stores.

When refrigerated, fresh produce will lose half or more of some of its vitamins within one to two weeks. If it's not kept chilled or preserved, nearly half of the vitamins may be lost within a few days of harvesting. For optimum nutrition, it is generally recommended that a person eat a variety of foods.

Source: Excerpted from *FDA/CFSAN Food Safety A to Z Reference Guide*, U.S. Food and Drug Administration (FDA), September 2001.

Chapter 18

Why Is It Important To Eat Fruit?

Eating fruit provides health benefits—people who eat more fruits and vegetables as part of an overall healthy diet are likely to have a reduced risk of some chronic diseases. Fruits provide nutrients vital for health and maintenance of your body.

Health Benefits

* Eating a diet rich in fruits and vegetables as part of an overall healthy diet may reduce risk for stroke and perhaps other cardiovascular diseases.

* Eating a diet rich in fruits and vegetables as part of an overall healthy diet may reduce risk for type 2 diabetes.

* Eating a diet rich in fruits and vegetables as part of an overall healthy diet may protect against certain cancers, such as mouth, stomach, and colon-rectum cancer.

* Diets rich in foods containing fiber, such as fruits and vegetables, may reduce the risk of coronary heart disease.

* Eating fruits and vegetables rich in potassium as part of an overall healthy diet may reduce the risk of developing kidney stones and may help to decrease bone loss.

About This Chapter: Excerpted from "Inside the Pyramid: Fruits," U.S. Department of Agriculture (MyPyramid.gov), 2005.

- Eating foods such as fruits that are low in calories per cup instead of some other higher-calorie food may be useful in helping to lower calorie intake.

Nutrients

- Most fruits are naturally low in fat, sodium, and calories. None have cholesterol.

- Fruits are important sources of many nutrients, including potassium, dietary fiber, vitamin C, and folate (folic acid).

- Diets rich in potassium may help to maintain healthy blood pressure. Fruit sources of potassium include bananas, prunes and prune juice, dried peaches and apricots, cantaloupe, honeydew melon, and orange juice.

> ✔ **Quick Tip**
> **Focus On Fruits**
>
> Eat a variety of fruits—whether fresh, frozen, canned, or dried—rather than fruit juice for most of your fruit choices. For a 2,000-calorie diet, you will need 2 cups of fruit each day (for example, 1 small banana, 1 large orange, and ¼ cup of dried apricots or peaches).
>
> Source: Excerpted from "Finding Your Way to a Healthier You," U.S. Department of Agriculture, Home and Garden Bulletin No. 232-CP, 2005.

- Dietary fiber from fruits, as part of an overall healthy diet, helps reduce blood cholesterol levels and may lower risk of heart disease. Fiber is important for proper bowel function. It helps reduce constipation and diverticulosis. Fiber-containing foods such as fruits help provide a feeling of fullness with fewer calories. Whole or cut-up fruits are sources of dietary fiber; fruit juices contain little or no fiber.

- Vitamin C is important for growth and repair of all body tissues, helps heal cuts and wounds, and keeps teeth and gums healthy.

- Folate (folic acid) helps the body form red blood cells. Women of childbearing age who may become pregnant and those in the first trimester of pregnancy should consume adequate folate, including folic acid from fortified foods or supplements. This reduces the risk of neural tube defects, spina bifida, and anencephaly during fetal development.

Tips To Help You Eat Fruits

General

- Keep a bowl of whole fruit on the table, counter, or in the refrigerator.

- Refrigerate cut-up fruit to store for later.

- Buy fresh fruits in season when they may be less expensive and at their peak flavor.

- Buy fruits that are dried, frozen, and canned (in water or juice) as well as fresh, so that you always have a supply on hand.

- Consider convenience when shopping. Buy pre-cut packages of fruit (such as melon or pineapple chunks) for a healthy snack in seconds. Choose packaged fruits that do not have added sugars.

Best Nutritional Value

- Make most of your choices whole or cut-up fruit rather than juice, for the benefits dietary fiber provides.

- Select fruits with more potassium often, such as bananas, prunes and prune juice, dried peaches and apricots, cantaloupe, honeydew melon, and orange juice.

- When choosing canned fruits, select fruit canned in 100% fruit juice or water rather than syrup.

- Vary your fruit choices. Fruits differ in nutrient content.

Meals

- At breakfast, top your cereal with bananas or peaches; add blueberries to pancakes; drink 100% orange or grapefruit juice. Or, try a fruit mixed with low-fat or fat-free yogurt.

- At lunch, pack a tangerine, banana, or grapes to eat, or choose fruits from a salad bar. Individual containers of fruits like peaches or applesauce are easy and convenient.

- At dinner, add crushed pineapple to coleslaw, or include mandarin oranges or grapes in a tossed salad.

- Make a Waldorf salad, with apples, celery, walnuts, and dressing.

- Try meat dishes that incorporate fruit, such as chicken with apricots or mango chutney.

- Add fruit like pineapple or peaches to kabobs as part of a barbecue meal.

- For dessert, have baked apples, pears, or a fruit salad.

♣ It's A Fact!!
What foods are in the fruit group?

Any fruit or 100% fruit juice counts as part of the fruit group. Fruits may be fresh, canned, frozen, or dried, and may be whole, cut-up, or pureed. Some commonly eaten fruits are as follows:

- Apples
- Apricots
- Avocado
- Bananas
- Berries:
    - strawberries
    - blueberries
    - raspberries
    - cherries
- Grapefruit
- Grapes
- Kiwi fruit
- Lemons
- Limes
- Mangoes
- Melons:
    - cantaloupe
    - honeydew
    - watermelon
- Mixed fruits:
    - fruit cocktail
- Nectarines
- Oranges
- Peaches
- Pears
- Papaya
- Pineapple
- Plums
- Prunes
- Raisins
- Tangerines
- 100% Fruit juice:
    - orange
    - apple
    - grape
    - grapefruit

Source: U.S. Department of Agriculture (MyPyramid.gov), 2005.

Snacks

- Cut-up fruit makes a great snack. Either cut them yourself, or buy pre-cut packages of fruit pieces like pineapples or melons. Or, try whole fresh berries or grapes.

- Dried fruits also make a great snack. They are easy to carry and store well. Because they are dried, ¼ cup is equivalent to ½ cup of other fruits.

- Keep a package of dried fruit in your desk or bag. Some fruits that are available dried include apricots, apples, pineapple, bananas, cherries, figs, dates, cranberries, blueberries, prunes (dried plums), and raisins (dried grapes).

- As a snack, spread peanut butter on apple slices or top frozen yogurt with berries or slices of kiwi fruit.

- Frozen juice bars (100% juice) make healthy alternatives to high-fat snacks.

✤ It's A Fact!!

Does freezing affect the level of nutrients contained in foods?

Fortunately, the freezing process itself does not reduce nutrients, and, for meat and poultry products, there is little change in protein value during freezing.

Source: Excerpted from *FDA/CFSAN Food Safety A to Z Reference Guide*, U.S. Food and Drug Administration (FDA), September 2001.

Make Fruit More Appealing

- Many fruits taste great with a dip or dressing. Try low-fat yogurt or pudding as a dip for fruits like strawberries or melons.

- Make a fruit smoothie by blending fat-free or low-fat milk or yogurt with fresh or frozen fruit. Try bananas, peaches, strawberries, or other berries.

- Try applesauce as a fat-free substitute for some of the oil when baking cakes.

- Try different textures of fruits. For example, apples are crunchy, bananas are smooth and creamy, and oranges are juicy.

- For fresh fruit salads, mix apples, bananas, or pears with acidic fruits like oranges, pineapple, or lemon juice to keep them from turning brown.

Chapter 19

Food From The Meat And Beans Group Is Essential For Health

Make Lean Or Low-Fat Choices From The Meat And Beans Group

Foods in the meat, poultry, fish, eggs, nuts, and seed group provide nutrients that are vital for health and maintenance of your body. However, choosing foods from this group that are high in saturated fat and cholesterol may have health implications.

Nutrients

• Meat, poultry, fish, dry beans and peas, eggs, nuts, and seeds supply many nutrients. These include protein, B vitamins (niacin, thiamin, riboflavin, and B_6), vitamin E, iron, zinc, and magnesium.

• Proteins function as building blocks for bones, muscles, cartilage, skin, and blood. They are also building blocks for enzymes, hormones, and vitamins. Proteins are one of three nutrients that provide calories (the others are fat and carbohydrates).

About This Chapter: From "Inside the Pyramid," U.S. Department of Agriculture (www.mypyramid.gov), 2005.

- B vitamins found in this food group serve a variety of functions in the body. They help the body release energy, play a vital role in the function of the nervous system, aid in the formation of red blood cells, and help build tissues.

- Vitamin E is an anti-oxidant that helps protect vitamin A and essential fatty acids from cell oxidation.

- Iron is used to carry oxygen in the blood. Many teenage girls and women in their child-bearing years have iron-deficiency anemia. They should eat foods high in heme-iron (meats) or eat other non-heme iron containing foods along with a food rich in vitamin C, which can improve absorption of non-heme iron.

- Magnesium is used in building bones and in releasing energy from muscles.

- Zinc is necessary for biochemical reactions and helps the immune system function properly.

♣ **It's A Fact!!**

What foods are included in the meat, poultry, fish, dry beans, eggs, and nuts (meat and beans) group?

All foods made from meat, poultry, fish, dry beans, or peas, eggs, nuts, and seeds are considered part of this group. Dry beans and peas are part of this group as well as the vegetable group.

Most meat and poultry choices should be lean or low-fat. Fish, nuts, and seeds contain healthy oils, so choose these foods frequently instead of meat or poultry.

Source: U.S. Department of Agriculture (MyPyramid.gov), 2005.

Health Implications

- Diets that are high in saturated fats raise "bad" cholesterol levels in the blood. The "bad" cholesterol is called LDL (low-density lipoprotein) cholesterol. High LDL cholesterol, in turn, increases the risk for coronary heart disease. Some food choices in this group are high in saturated fat. These include fatty cuts of beef, pork, and lamb; regular (75% to 85% lean) ground beef; regular sausages, hot dogs, and bacon; some luncheon meats such as regular bologna and salami; and some poultry such as duck. To help keep blood cholesterol levels healthy, limit the amount of these foods you eat.

- Diets that are high in cholesterol can raise LDL cholesterol levels in the blood. Cholesterol is only found in foods from animal sources. Some foods from this group are high in cholesterol. These include egg yolks (egg whites are cholesterol-free) and organ meats such as liver and giblets. To help keep blood cholesterol levels healthy, limit the amount of these foods you eat.

- A high intake of fats makes it difficult to avoid consuming more calories than are needed.

Why Is It Important To Include Fish, Nuts, And Seeds?

- Many people do not make varied choices from this food group, selecting meat or poultry everyday as their main dishes. Varying choices and including fish, nuts, and seeds in meals can boost intake of monounsaturated fatty acids (MUFAs) and polyunsaturated fatty acids (PUFAs). Most fat in the diet should come from MUFAs and PUFAs. Some of the PUFAs are essential for health—the body cannot create them from other fats.

- Some fish (such as salmon, trout, and herring) are high in a type of PUFA called "omega-3 fatty acids." The omega-3 fatty acids in fish are commonly called "EPA" and "DHA." There is some limited evidence that suggests eating fish rich in EPA and DHA may reduce the risk for mortality from cardiovascular disease. (EPA is eicosapentaenoic acid and DHA is docosahexaenoic acid.)

• Some nuts and seeds (flax, walnuts) are excellent sources of essential fatty acids, and some (sunflower seeds, almonds, hazelnuts) are good sources of vitamin E.

Make Wise Choices From The Meat And Beans Group

Go Lean With Protein

• Start with a lean choice:

  • The leanest beef cuts include round steaks and roasts (round eye, top round, bottom round, round tip), top loin, top sirloin, and chuck shoulder and arm roasts.

  • The leanest pork choices include pork loin, tenderloin, center loin, and ham.

  • Choose extra lean ground beef. The label should say at least "90% lean." You may be able to find ground beef that is 93% or 95% lean.

  • Buy skinless chicken parts, or take off the skin before cooking.

✔ **Quick Tip**
Selection Tips

• Choose lean or low-fat meat and poultry. If higher fat choices are made, such as regular ground beef (75 to 80% lean) or chicken with skin, the fat in the product counts as part of the discretionary calorie allowance.

• If solid fat is added in cooking, such as frying chicken in shortening or frying eggs in butter or stick margarine, this also counts as part of the discretionary calorie allowance.

• Select fish rich in omega-3 fatty acids, such as salmon, trout, and herring, more often.

• Liver and other organ meats are high in cholesterol. Egg yolks are also high in cholesterol, but egg whites are cholesterol-free.

- Boneless skinless chicken breasts and turkey cutlets are the leanest poultry choices.

- Choose lean turkey, roast beef, ham, or low-fat luncheon meats for sandwiches instead of luncheon meats with more fat, such as regular bologna or salami.

- Keep it lean:

  - Trim away all of the visible fat from meats and poultry before cooking.

  - Broil, grill, roast, poach, or boil meat, poultry, or fish instead of frying.

  - Drain off any fat that appears during cooking.

  - Skip or limit the breading on meat, poultry, or fish. Breading adds fat and calories. It will also cause the food to soak up more fat during frying.

  - Prepare dry beans and peas without added fats.

  - Choose and prepare foods without high fat sauces or gravies.

- Processed meats such as ham, sausage, frankfurters, and luncheon or deli meats have added sodium. Check the ingredient and Nutrition Facts label to help limit sodium intake. Fresh chicken, turkey, and pork that have been enhanced with a salt-containing solution also have added sodium. Check the product label for statements such as "self-basting" or "contains up to __% of __", which mean that a sodium-containing solution has been added to the product.

- Sunflower seeds, almonds, and hazelnuts (filberts) are the richest sources of vitamin E in this food group. To help meet vitamin E recommendations, make these your nut and seed choices more often.

Source: U.S. Department of Agriculture (MyPyramid.gov), 2005.

Vary Your Protein Choices

- Choose fish more often for lunch or dinner. Look for fish rich in omega-3 fatty acids, such as salmon, trout, and herring. Here are some ideas:

  - Salmon steak or filet

  - Salmon loaf

  - Grilled or baked trout

- Choose dry beans or peas as a main dish or part of a meal often. Here are some choices:

  - Chili with kidney or pinto beans

  - Stir-fried tofu

  - Split pea, lentil, minestrone, or white bean soups

  - Baked beans

  - Black bean enchiladas

  - Garbanzo or kidney beans on a chef's salad

  - Rice and beans

  - Veggie burgers or garden burgers

  - Hummus (chickpeas) spread on pita bread

- Choose nuts as a snack, on salads, or in main dishes. Use nuts to replace meat or poultry, not in addition to these items:

  - Use pine nuts in pesto sauce for pasta.

  - Add slivered almonds to steamed vegetables.

  - Add toasted peanuts or cashews to a vegetable stir fry instead of meat.

  - Sprinkle a few nuts on top of low-fat ice cream or frozen yogurt.

  - Add walnuts or pecans to a green salad instead of cheese or meat.

♣ **It's A Fact!!**

Vegetarian Choices In The Meat And Beans Group

- Vegetarians get enough protein from this group as long as the variety and amounts of foods selected are adequate.

- Protein sources from the Meat and Beans group for vegetarians include eggs (for ovo-vegetarians), beans, nuts, nut butters, peas, and soy products (tofu, tempeh, veggie burgers).

Source: U.S. Department of Agriculture (MyPyramid.gov), 2005.

What To Look For On The Food Label

• Check the Nutrition Facts label for the saturated fat, trans fat, cholesterol, and sodium content of packaged foods.

  • Processed meats such as hams, sausages, frankfurters, and lun-
    cheon or deli meats have added sodium. Check the ingredient
    and Nutrition Facts label to help limit sodium intake.

  • Fresh chicken, turkey, and pork that have been enhanced with a
    salt-containing solution also have added sodium. Check the prod-
    uct label for statements such as "self-basting" or "contains up to
    __% of __."

  • Lower fat versions of many processed meats are available. Look
    on the Nutrition Facts label to choose products with less fat and
    saturated fat.

Keep It Safe To Eat

• Separate raw, cooked and ready-to-eat foods.

• Do not wash or rinse meat or poultry.

• Wash cutting boards, knives, utensils and counter tops in hot soapy
  water after preparing each food item and before going on to the
  next one.

• Store raw meat, poultry and seafood on the bottom shelf of the refrigerator so juices don't drip onto other foods.

• Cook foods to a safe temperature to kill microorganisms. Use a meat
  thermometer, which measures the internal temperature of cooked
  meat and poultry, to make sure that the meat is cooked all the way
  through.

• Chill (refrigerate) perishable food promptly and defrost foods properly. Refrigerate or freeze perishables, prepared food and leftovers within
  two hours.

• Plan ahead to defrost foods. Never defrost food on the kitchen counter
  at room temperature. Thaw food by placing it in the refrigerator,

submerging air-tight packaged food in cold tap water, or defrosting on a plate in the microwave.

- Avoid raw or partially cooked eggs or foods containing raw eggs and raw or undercooked meat and poultry.

✎ What's It Mean?

Adzuki Beans are small, with a vivid red color, solid flavor and texture. Originally from Asia, its name means "little bean" in Japanese. Its red coloring—red being the most important color in Eastern celebrations—means that it is greatly used in festive or special meals.

Large Lima Bean are large and flat with a greenish-white color. It has a buttery flavor and creamy texture. This bean is named after Lima, Peru, and is extremely popular in the Americas, both in its natural state and dried.

Pink Beans have beautiful pink color and is very popular in the countries of the Caribbean. Pink beans are of medium size (similar to the Great Northern and the Pinto) and have a refined texture and delicate flavor.

Green Baby Lima Beans come from Peru and are very popular in the Americas. The baby variety is much loved in Japan for making desserts from bean paste known as "an." These are medium-sized flat beans with a greenish white color, buttery flavor, and creamy texture.

Small Red Beans are particularly popular in the Caribbean region, where they are normally eaten with rice. Dark red in color, small red beans are also smoother in taste and texture than the dark red kidney bean.

Dark Red Kidney Beans are large and kidney-shaped with a deep glossy red color. They have a solid flavor and texture. These beans are produced mainly in the northern U.S.A. and owes its popularity in America and Europe to its large size, bright color and solid texture.

Black Beans are sweet tasting with an almost mushroom-like flavor and soft floury texture. These beans are medium sized, oval, with a matt black color. They are the most popular beans in the Costa Rica and Cuba.

Light Red Kidney Beans have a solid texture and flavor. They are characterized by their large, kidney-shape with a pink color. This bean is popular in the Caribbean region as well as in Portugal and Spain for its similarity to the canela bean.

- Women who may become pregnant, pregnant women, nursing mothers, and young children should avoid some types of fish and eat types lower in mercury. Go to www.cfsan.fda.gov/~dms/admehg3.html or call 1-888-SAFEFOOD for more information.

Navy Beans are small, white and oval with a refined texture and delicate flavor. These are the beans used for the famous Boston and English baked beans. Because their skin and fine texture do not break up on cooking. These beans were named for their part of the U.S. Navy diet during the second half of the 19th century.

Cranberry Beans are known for their creamy texture with a flavor similar to chestnuts. Cranberry beans are rounded with red specks, which disappear on cooking. These beans are a favorite in northern Italy and Spain. You can find them fresh in their pods in Autumn. They also freeze well.

Black-eyed Beans have a scented aroma, creamy texture and distinctive flavor. These beans are characterized by their kidney shaped, white skin with a small black eye and very fine wrinkles. Originally from Africa, it is one of the most widely dispersed beans in the world. Black-eyed peas are really a type of pea, which gives it its distinctive flavor and rapid cooking potential, with no pre-soaking needed.

Pinto Beans are the most widely produced bean in the United States and is one of the most popular in the Americas. It also contains the most fiber of all beans. Characteristically known by their medium size oval shape, with speckled reddish brown over a pale pink base and solid texture and flavor.

Great Northern Beans are a North American bean, which is popular in France for making cassoulet (a white bean casserole) and in the whole Mediterranean where many beans of a similar appearance are cultivated. These beans have a delicate flavor, thin skin, and are flat, kidney shaped, medium-sized white beans.

Garbanzo Beans or chickpeas are the most widely consumed legume in the world. Originating in the Middle East, they have a firm texture with a flavor somewhere between chestnuts and walnuts. Garbanzo beans are usually pale yellow in color. In India there are red, black, and brown chickpeas.

Source: Excerpted from "5 A Day: Vegetable of the Month: Beans," Centers for Disease Control and Prevention, June 2005.

Ounce Equivalents In The Meat And Beans Group

In general, 1 ounce of meat, poultry, or fish, ¼ cup cooked dry beans, 1 egg, 1 tablespoon of peanut butter, or ½ ounce of nuts or seeds can be considered as 1 ounce equivalent from the meat and beans group.

These amounts that count as 1 ounce equivalent in the meat and beans group towards your daily recommended intake:

Meats:

- 1 ounce cooked lean beef, lean pork, or ham

Poultry:

- 1 ounce cooked chicken or turkey, without skin
- 1 sandwich slice of turkey (4 ½ x 2 ½ x 1/8")

Fish:

- 1 ounce cooked fish or shell fish

Eggs:

- 1 egg

Nuts and seeds:

- ½ ounce of nuts (12 almonds, 24 pistachios, 7 walnut halves)
- ½ ounce of seeds (pumpkin, sunflower or squash seeds, hulled, roasted)
- 1 Tablespoon of peanut butter or almond butter

Dry beans and peas:

- ¼ cup of cooked dry beans (such as black, kidney, pinto, or white beans)
- ¼ cup of cooked dry peas (such as chickpeas, cow peas, lentils, or split peas)
- ¼ cup of baked beans, refried beans
- ¼ cup (about 2 ounces) of tofu
- 1 oz. tempeh, cooked
- ¼ cup roasted soybeans 1 falafel patty (2 ¼", 4 oz)
- 2 Tbsp. hummus

Chapter 20

Soy Foods And Health

Vegetarians and health enthusiasts have known for years that foods rich in soy protein offer a good alternative to meat, poultry, and other animal-based products. As consumers have pursued healthier lifestyles in recent years, consumption of soy foods has risen steadily, bolstered by scientific studies showing health benefits from these products.

Scientists agree that foods rich in soy protein can have considerable value to heart health, a fact backed by dozens of controlled clinical studies. A year-long review of the available human studies in 1999 prompted the U.S. Food and Drug Administration (FDA) to allow a health claim on food labels stating that a daily diet containing 25 grams of soy protein, also low in saturated fat and cholesterol, may reduce the risk of heart disease.

"Soy by itself is not a magic food," says Christine Lewis, acting director of the Center for Food Safety and Applied Nutrition's Office of Nutritional Products, Labeling and Dietary Supplements. "But rather it is an example of the different kinds of foods that together in a complete diet can have a positive effect on health."

About This Chapter: Excerpted from "Soy: Health Claims for Soy Protein, Questions About Other Components," by John Henkel, *FDA Consumer magazine*, May-June 2000.

Soy Benefits

Soy protein products can be good substitutes for animal products because, unlike some other beans, soy offers a "complete" protein profile. Soybeans contain all the amino acids essential to human nutrition, which must be supplied in the diet because they cannot be synthesized by the human body. Soy protein products can replace animal-based foods—which also have complete proteins but tend to contain more fat, especially saturated fat—without requiring major adjustments elsewhere in the diet.

While foreign cultures, especially Asians, have used soy extensively for centuries, mainstream America has been slow to move dietary soy beyond a niche market status. In the United States, soybean is a huge cash crop, but the product is used largely as livestock feed.

With the increased emphasis on healthy diets, that may be changing. Sales of soy products are up and are projected to increase, due in part, say industry officials, to the FDA-approved health claim. "We've seen this before with other claims FDA has approved," says Brian Sansoni, senior manager for public policy at the Grocery Manufacturers of America. "It brings attention to products; there are newspaper and TV stories and information on the internet."

To qualify for the health claim, foods must contain at least 6.25 grams of soy protein per serving and fit other criteria, such as being low in fat, cholesterol, and sodium. The claim is similar to others the agency has approved in recent years to indicate heart benefits, including claims for the cholesterol-lowering effects of soluble fiber in oat bran and psyllium seeds.

FDA determined that diets with four daily soy servings can reduce levels of low-density lipoproteins (LDLs), the so-called "bad cholesterol" that builds up in blood vessels, by as much as 10 percent. This number is significant because heart experts generally agree that a 1 percent drop in total cholesterol can equal a 2 percent drop in heart disease risk. Heart disease kills more Americans than any other illness. Disorders of the heart and blood vessels, including stroke, cause nearly 1 million deaths yearly.

Studies also hint that soy may have benefits beyond fostering a healthy heart. At the Third International Symposium on the Role of Soy in Preventing and Treating Chronic Disease, held in late 1999, researchers presented data linking soy consumption to a reduced risk of several illnesses. Disorders as diverse as osteoporosis, prostate cancer, and colon cancer are under investigation.

✎ What's It Mean?

Miso is a fermented soybean paste used for seasoning and in soup stock.

Soy flour is created by grinding roasted soybeans into a fine powder. The flour adds protein to baked goods, and, because it adds moisture, it can be used as an egg substitute in these products. It also can be found in cereals, pancake mixes, frozen desserts, and other common foods.

Soymilk, the name some marketers use for a soy beverage, is produced by grinding dehulled soybeans and mixing them with water to form a milk-like liquid. It can be consumed as a beverage or used in recipes as a substitute for cow's milk. Soymilk, sometimes fortified with calcium, comes plain or in flavors such as vanilla, chocolate, and coffee. For lactose-intolerant individuals, it can be a good replacement for dairy products.

Tempeh is made from whole, cooked soybeans formed into a chewy cake and used as a meat substitute.

Textured soy protein is made from defatted soy flour, which is compressed and dehydrated. It can be used as a meat substitute or as filler in dishes such as meatloaf.

Tofu is made from cooked puréed soybeans processed into a custard-like cake. It has a neutral flavor and can be stir-fried, mixed into "smoothies," or blended into a cream cheese texture for use in dips or as a cheese substitute. It comes in firm, soft, and silken textures.

Adding Soy Protein To The Diet

For consumers interested in increasing soy protein consumption to help reduce their risk of heart disease, health experts say they need not completely eliminate animal-based products such as meat, poultry, and dairy foods to reap soy's benefits. While soy protein's direct effects on cholesterol levels are well documented, replacing some animal protein with soy protein is a valuable way to lower fat intake. "If individuals begin to substitute soy products, for example, soy burgers, for foods high in saturated fat, such as hamburgers, there would be the added advantage of replacing saturated fat and cholesterol [in] the diet," says Alice Lichtenstein, D.Sc., professor of nutrition at Tufts University. Whole soy foods also are a good source of fiber, B vitamins, calcium, and omega-3 essential fatty acids, all important food components.

The American Heart Association recommends that soy products be used in a diet that includes fruits, vegetables, whole grains, low-fat dairy products, poultry, fish, and lean meats. The AHA also emphasizes that a diet to effectively lower cholesterol should consist of no more than 30 percent of total daily calories from fat and no more than 10 percent of calories from saturated fat.

Nowadays, a huge variety of soy foods is on shelves not only in health food stores, but increasingly in mainstream grocery stores. As the number of soy-based products grows, it becomes increasingly easy for consumers to add enough soy to their daily diets to meet the 25-gram amount that FDA says is beneficial to heart health. According to soybean industry figures, the numbers add up quickly when you look at the protein contained in typical soy foods. For example:

- Four ounces of firm tofu contains 13 grams of soy protein.

- One soy "sausage" link provides 6 grams of protein.

- One soy "burger" includes 10 to 12 grams of protein.

- An 8-ounce glass of plain soymilk contains 10 grams of protein.

- One soy protein bar delivers 14 grams of protein.

- One-half cup of tempeh provides 19.5 grams of protein.

- And a quarter cup of roasted soy nuts contains 19 grams of soy protein.

Though some consumers may try soy products here and there, it takes a sustained effort to eat enough to reach the beneficial daily intake. This is especially true for those who have elevated cholesterol levels. "Dietary interventions that can lower cholesterol are important tools for physicians," says Antonio Gotto, M.D., professor of medicine at Cornell University, "particularly since diet is usually prescribed before medication and is continued after drug therapy is begun." He emphasizes that in order to succeed, such diets must have enough variety that patients don't get bored and lapse back into old eating habits. He says his experience with patients suggests that it's important to learn how to "sneak" soy into the diet painlessly.

"People think it's challenging to get a high concentration of soy into your diet," says chef and cookbook author Dana Jacobi. "But it's actually easy to consume 25 grams [of soy protein], once you realize what a wide range of soy products is available." For those new to soy, she recommends what she calls "good-tasting" soy foods such as smoothies, muffins made with soy flour, protein bars, and soy nuts.

The American Dietetic Association recommends introducing soy slowly by adding small amounts to the daily diet or mixing into existing foods. Then, once the taste and texture have become familiar, add more.

Because some soy products have a mild or even neutral flavor, it's possible to add soy to dishes and barely know it's there. Soy flour can be used to thicken sauces and gravies. Soymilk can be added to baked goods and desserts. And tofu takes on the flavor of whatever it is cooked in, making it suitable for stews and stir-fries. "Cook it with strong flavors such as garlic, crushed red pepper, or ginger," says Amy Lanou, a New York-based nutritionist. "One of my favorites is tofu sautéed with a spicy barbecue sauce." She also suggests commercial forms of baked tofu, which she says has a "cheese-like texture and a mild, but delicious, flavor." For soy "newbies," she also recommends trying a high-quality restaurant that really knows how to prepare soy dishes—just to see how professionals handle soy.

Soy chefs and nutritionists suggest the following further possibilities for adding soy to the diet:

- Include soy-based beverages, muffins, sausages, yogurt, or cream cheese at breakfast.

- Use soy deli meats, soy nut butter (similar to peanut butter), or soy cheese to make sandwiches.

- Top pizzas with soy cheese, pepperoni, sausages, or "crumbles" (similar to ground beef).

- Grill soy hot dogs, burgers, marinated tempeh, and baked tofu.

- Cube and stir fry tofu or tempeh and add to a salad.

- Pour soymilk on cereal and use it in cooking or to make "smoothies."

- Order soy-based dishes such as spicy bean curd and miso soup at Asian restaurants.

- Eat roasted soy nuts or a soy protein bar for a snack.

Chapter 21

Health Benefits Of Dairy Products

Health Benefits And Nutrients

Consuming milk and milk products provides health benefits—people who have a diet rich in milk and milk products can reduce the risk of low bone mass throughout the life cycle. Foods in the milk group provide nutrients that are vital for health and maintenance of your body. These nutrients include calcium, potassium, vitamin D, and protein.

Nutrients

• Calcium is used for building bones and teeth and in maintaining bone mass. Milk products are the primary source of calcium in American diets. Diets that provide 3 cups or the equivalent of milk products per day can improve bone mass.

• Diets rich in potassium may help to maintain healthy blood pressure. Milk products, especially yogurt and fluid milk, provide potassium.

• Vitamin D functions in the body to maintain proper levels of calcium and phosphorous, thereby helping to build and maintain bones. Milk that is fortified with vitamin D is a good source of this nutrient. Other

About This Chapter: Excerpted from "Inside the Pyramid: Milk," U.S. Department of Agriculture (MyPyramid.gov), 2005.

sources include vitamin D-fortified yogurt and vitamin D-fortified ready-to-eat breakfast cereals.

- Milk products that are consumed in their low-fat or fat-free forms provide little or no solid fat.

Make Fat-Free Or Low-Fat Choices From The Milk Group

Choosing foods from the milk group that are high in saturated fats and cholesterol can have health implications. Diets high in saturated fats raise "bad" cholesterol levels in the blood. The "bad" cholesterol is called LDL (low-density lipoprotein) cholesterol. High LDL cholesterol, in turn, increases the risk for coronary heart disease. Many cheeses, whole milk, and products made from them are high in saturated fat. To help keep blood cholesterol levels healthy, limit the amount of these foods you eat. In addition, a high intake of fats makes it difficult to avoid consuming more calories than are needed.

Foods Included In The Milk, Yogurt, And Cheese (Milk) Group

All fluid milk products and many foods made from milk are considered part of this food group. Foods made from milk that retain their calcium content are part of the group, while foods made from milk that have little to no calcium, such as cream cheese, cream, and butter, are not. Most milk group choices should be fat-free or low-fat.

♣ It's A Fact!!

- Diets rich in milk and milk products help build and maintain bone mass throughout the lifecycle. This may reduce the risk of osteoporosis.

- The intake of milk products is especially important to bone health during childhood and adolescence, when bone mass is being built.

- Diets that include milk products tend to have a higher overall nutritional quality.

Some commonly eaten choices in the milk, yogurt, and cheese group include the following:

Milk*

- all fluid milk:
  - fat-free (skim)
  - low fat (1%)
  - reduced fat (2%)
  - whole milk
- flavored milks:
  - chocolate
  - strawberry
- lactose reduced milks
- lactose free milks

Milk-Based Desserts*

- puddings made with milk
- ice milk
- frozen yogurt
- ice cream

Cheese*

- hard natural cheeses:
  - cheddar
  - mozzarella
  - Swiss
  - parmesan
- soft cheeses
  - ricotta
  - cottage cheese
- processed cheeses
  - American

Yogurt*

- all yogurt
- fat-free
- low fat
- reduced fat
- whole milk yogurt

*Selection Tips

Choose fat-free or low-fat milk, yogurt, and cheese. If you choose milk or yogurt that is not fat-free, or cheese that is not low-fat, the fat in the product counts as part of the discretionary calorie allowance.

If sweetened milk products are chosen (flavored milk, yogurt, drinkable yogurt, desserts), the added sugars also count as part of the discretionary calorie allowance.

For those who are lactose intolerant, lactose-free and lower-lactose products are available. These include hard cheeses and yogurt. Also, enzyme preparations can be added to milk to lower the lactose content. Calcium-fortified foods and beverages such as soy beverages or orange juice may provide calcium, but may not provide the other nutrients found in milk and milk products.

Tips For Making Wise Choices

- Include milk as a beverage at meals. Choose fat-free or low-fat milk.

- If you usually drink whole milk, switch gradually to fat-free milk, to lower saturated fat and calories. Try reduced fat (2%), then low-fat (1%), and finally fat-free (skim).

- If you drink cappuccinos or lattes—ask for them with fat-free (skim) milk.

- Add fat-free or low-fat milk instead of water to oatmeal and hot cereals

- Use fat-free or low-fat milk when making condensed cream soups (such as cream of tomato).

- Have fat-free or low-fat yogurt as a snack.

- Make a dip for fruits or vegetables from yogurt.

- Make fruit-yogurt smoothies in the blender.

- For dessert, make chocolate or butterscotch pudding with fat-free or low-fat milk.

- Top cut-up fruit with flavored yogurt for a quick dessert.

- Top casseroles, soups, stews, or vegetables with shredded low-fat cheese.

- Top a baked potato with fat-free or low-fat yogurt.

✔ **Quick Tip**
Get Your Calcium-Rich Foods

Get 3 cups of low-fat or fat-free milk—or an equivalent amount of low-fat yogurt and/or low-fat cheese (1½ ounces of cheese equals 1 cup of milk)—every day. If you don't or can't consume milk, choose lactose-free milk products and/or calcium-fortified foods and beverages.

Source: Excerpted from "Finding Your Way to a Healthier You," U.S. Department of Agriculture, Home and Garden Bulletin No. 232-CP, 2005.

Keep It Safe To Eat

- Avoid raw (unpasteurized) milk or any products made from unpasteurized milk.

- Chill (refrigerate) perishable food promptly and defrost foods properly. Refrigerate or freeze perishables, prepared food and leftovers as soon as possible. If food has been left at temperatures between 40° and 140° F for more than two hours, discard it, even though it may look and smell good.

- Separate raw, cooked and ready-to-eat foods.

For Those Who Choose Not To Consume Milk Products

- If you avoid milk because of lactose intolerance, the most reliable way to get the health benefits of milk is to choose lactose-free alternatives within the milk group, such as cheese, yogurt, or lactose-free milk, or to consume the enzyme lactase before consuming milk products.

- Calcium choices for those who do not consume milk products include the following:

  - Calcium fortified juices, cereals, breads, soy beverages, or rice beverages

  - Canned fish (sardines, salmon with bones) soybeans and other soy products (soy-based beverages, soy yogurt, tempeh), some other dried beans, and some leafy greens (collard and turnip greens, kale, bok choy). The amount of calcium that can be absorbed from these foods varies.

♣ **It's A Fact!!**

Does pasteurization affect the nutritional value or flavor of foods?

Pasteurization can affect the nutrient composition and flavor of foods. In the case of milk, for example, the high-temperature-short-time treatments (HTST) cause less damage to the nutrient composition and sensory characteristics of foods than the low-temperature-long-time treatments (LTLT).

Source: Excerpted from *FDA/CFSAN Food Safety A to Z Reference Guide*, U.S. Food and Drug Administration (FDA), September 2001.

♣ It's A Fact!!
What counts as 1 cup in the milk group?

In general, 1 cup of milk or yogurt, 1½ ounces of natural cheese, or 2 ounces of processed cheese can be considered as 1 cup from the milk group.

Table 21.1 lists specific amounts that count as 1 cup in the milk group towards your daily recommended intake.

Table 21.1. Milk Serving Equivalents

	Amount that counts as 1 cup in the milk group	Common portions and cup equivalents
Milk (choose fat-free or low-fat milk most often)	1 cup 1 half-pint container ½ cup evaporated milk	
Yogurt (choose fat-free or low-fat yogurt most often)	1 regular container (8 fluid ounces)	1 small container (6 ounces) = ¾ cup
	1 cup (4 ounces) = ½ cup	1 snack size container
Cheese (choose low-fat cheeses most often)	1½ ounces hard cheese (cheddar, mozzarella, Swiss, parmesan)	1 slice of hard cheese is equivalent to ½ cup milk
	⅓ cup shredded cheese	
	2 ounces processed cheese (American)	1 slice of processed cheese is equivalent to ⅓ cup milk
	½ cup ricotta cheese	
	2 cups cottage cheese	½ cup cottage cheese is equivalent to ¼ cup milk
Milk-based desserts (choose fat-free or low-fat types most often)	1 cup pudding made with milk	
	1 cup frozen yogurt	
	1½ cups ice cream	1 scoop ice cream is equivalent to ⅓ cup milk

Source: U.S. Department of Agriculture (MyPyramid.gov), 2005.

Chapter 22

Hydration: Why Water Is Important

Dietary Intake Levels For Water

The vast majority of healthy people adequately meet their daily hydration needs by letting thirst be their guide, says the newest report on nutrient recommendations from the Institute of Medicine of the National Academies. The report set general recommendations for water intake based on detailed national data, which showed that women who appear to be adequately hydrated consume an average of approximately 2.7 liters (91 ounces) of total water—from all beverages and foods—each day, and men average approximately 3.7 liters (125 ounces) daily. These values represent adequate intake levels, the panel said; those who are very physically active or who live in hot climates may need to consume more water. About 80 percent of people's total water comes from drinking water and beverages—including caffeinated beverages—and the other 20 percent is derived from food.

About This Chapter: This chapter begins with "Dietary Intake Levels For Water," excerpted from "Report Sets Dietary Intake Levels for Water, Salt, and Potassium to Maintain Health and Reduce Chronic Disease Risk," February 11, 2004. © 2004 National Academy of Sciences. Reprinted with permission. The chapter continues with "Dehydration." This information was provided by TeensHealth, one of the largest resources online for medically reviewed health information written for parents, kids, and teens. For more articles like this one, visit www.TeensHealth.org, or www.KidsHealth.org. © 2004 The Nemours Center for Children's Health Media, a division of The Nemours Foundation.

We don't offer any rule of thumb based on how many glasses of water people should drink each day because our hydration needs can be met through a variety of sources in addition to drinking water," said Lawrence Appel, chair of the panel that wrote the report and professor of medicine, epidemiology, and international health, Johns Hopkins University, Baltimore. "While drinking water is a frequently choice for hydration, people also get water from juice, milk, coffee, tea, soda, fruits, vegetables, and other foods and beverages as well. Moreover, we concluded that on a daily basis, people get adequate amounts of water from normal drinking behavior—consumption at meals and in other social situations—and by letting their thirst guide them."

This report refers to total water, which includes the water contained in beverages and the moisture in foods, to avoid confusion with drinking water only.

Total water intake at the reference level of 3.7 liters for adult men and 2.7 liters for adult women per day covers the expected needs of healthy, sedentary people in temperate climates. Temporary underconsumption of water can occur due to heat exposure, high levels of physical activity, or decreased food and fluid intake. However, on a daily basis, fluid intake driven by thirst and the habitual consumption of beverages at meals is sufficient for the average person to maintain adequate hydration.

Prolonged physical activity and heat exposure will increase water losses and, therefore, may rise daily fluid needs. Very active individuals who are continually exposed to hot weather often have daily total water needs of six liters or more, according to several studies.

> **♣ It's A Fact!!**
>
> What you put into your body has a huge effect on how the outside looks and feels. Eating healthy foods is important. It is also important to drink plenty of water. Over half of your body is water, and you lose one to three quarts per day without even sweating heavily. Imagine how much more you will lose when you exercise. You need to drink enough water to keep your body hydrated so that your skin is hydrated. Drinking water keeps your internal systems clean and lets your body work right.
>
> Source: From "Sound Skin Care," *Bodywise* (www.girlpower.gov), U.S. Department of Health and Human Services, 2004.

While concerns have been raised that caffeine has a diuretic effect, available evidence indicates that this effect may be transient, and there is no convincing evidence that caffeine leads to a cumulative total body water deficits. Therefore, the panel concluded that when it comes to meeting daily hydration needs, caffeinated beverages can contribute as much as noncaffeinated options.

Some athletes who engage in strenuous activity and some individuals with certain psychiatric disorders occasionally drink water in excessive amounts that can be life-threatening. However, such occurrences are highly unusual. Therefore, the panel did not set an upper limit for water consumption.

Dehydration

Dehydration is a condition that occurs when a person loses more fluids (such as urine or sweat) than he or she takes in. Dehydration isn't as serious a problem for teens as it can be for babies or young children, but if you ignore your thirst, dehydration can slow you down.

When someone gets dehydrated, it means the amount of water in his or her body has dropped below its adequate level (our bodies are about two thirds water). Small decreases don't cause problems, and in most cases, they go completely unnoticed. But losing larger amounts of water can sometimes make a person feel quite sick.

How Do People Get Dehydrated?

One common cause of dehydration in teens is gastrointestinal illness. When you're flattened by a stomach bug, you may lose fluid through vomiting and diarrhea. You can also become dehydrated from lots of physical activity if you don't replace fluid as you go, although it's rare to reach a level of even moderate dehydration during sports or other normal outdoor activity.

Some athletes dehydrate themselves on purpose to drop weight quickly before a big game or event by sweating in saunas or using laxatives or diuretics, which make you go to the bathroom more. This practice usually hurts more than it helps, though. Athletes who do this feel weaker, which affects performance and can lead to more serious problems, like abnormalities in the salt and potassium levels in the body. Such changes can also lead to problems with the heart's rhythm.

Dieting can sap a person's water reserves as well. Beware of diets that emphasize shedding "water weight" as a quick way to lose weight.

Dealing With Dehydration

To counter dehydration, you need to restore the proper balance of water in your body. First, though, you have to recognize the problem. Thirst is the best, and earliest, indicator of potential dehydration. Although thirst is one indicator of dehydration, it is not an early warning sign. By the time you feel thirsty, you might already be dehydrated. Other symptoms of dehydration include the following:

- feeling dizzy and light-headed

♣ It's A Fact!!
Is it possible to drink too much water?

Yes, there is a condition known as "water intoxication." It is usually associated with long distance events like running and cycling. And it's not an unusual problem. For example, water intoxication was reported in 18% of marathon runners and in 29% of the finishers in a Hawaiian Ironman Triathlon in studies published recently in the *Annals of Internal Medicine* and in *Medicine & Science in Sports & Exercise* respectively.

What happens is that as the athlete consumes large amounts of water over the course of the event, blood plasma (the liquid part of blood) increases. As this takes place, the salt content of the blood is diluted. At the same time, the athlete is losing salt by sweating. Consequently, the amount of salt available to the body tissues decreases over time to a point where the loss interferes with brain, heart, and muscle function.

The official name for this condition is hyponatremia. The symptoms generally mirror those of dehydration (apathy, confusion, nausea, and fatigue), although some individuals show no symptoms at all. If untreated, hyponatremia can lead to coma and even death.

Enough, but not too much. The fluid requirement for the majority of endurance athletes, under most conditions, is about 8 to 16 ounces per hour. There is considerable variation here, of course, due to individual sweating rates, body

- having a dry or sticky mouth

- producing less urine and darker urine

As the condition progresses, a person will start to feel much sicker as more body systems (or organs) are affected by the dehydration.

The easiest way to avoid dehydration is to drink lots of fluids, especially on hot, dry, windy days. This might mean as many as six to eight cups (1.4 to 1.9 liters) a day for some people, depending on factors like how much water they're getting from foods and other liquids and how much they're sweating from physical exertion. Remember that drinking water adds no calories to your diet and can be great for your health.

size and weight, heat and humidity, and running speed, and other factors. Still, much more than this amount of fluid is, in most instances, probably physiologically excessive as well as uncomfortable, as liquid sloshes around in the gut during the activity.

One way to test if you are drinking too much water is to compare your body weight before and after a long run. Normally, people lose weight during the course of a distance event. But over-hydrated individuals typically either gain weight or maintain their starting weight. It is interesting to note, too, that this problem tends to be more of a concern with slower runners, because they are exercising at a lower intensity, and therefore have a lower fluid requirement. Also, the slower runner has more opportunity to consume fluid.

End Note: Water intoxication is a problem not only among athletes. For instance, it has become one of the most common causes of serious heat illness in the Grand Canyon. Some people hiking the canyon drink large amounts of water and do not eat enough food to provide for electrolyte (salt, potassium) replacement and energy. Fears of dehydration has led to a mistaken belief that the safe thing to do is to drink as much and as often as possible. But even with drinking water, there can be too much of a good thing.

Source: From "You Can Drink Too Much Water," by Patrick Bird, Ph.D., Dean Emeritus of the College of Human Health and Performance, University of Florida, Gainesville, © 2000. Reprinted with permission.

When you're going to be outside on a warm day, dress appropriately for your activity. Wear loose-fitting clothes and a hat if you can. That will keep you cooler and cut down on sweating. If you do find yourself feeling parched or dizzy, take a break for a few minutes. Sit in the shade or someplace cool and drink water.

If you're participating in sports or strenuous activities, you should drink some fluids before the activity begins. You should also drink at regular intervals (every 20 minutes or so) during the course of the activity and after the activity ends. The best time to train or play sports is in the early morning or late afternoon to avoid the hottest part of the day.

If you have a stomach bug and you're spending too much time getting acquainted with the toilet, you probably don't feel like eating or drinking anything. Putting anything in your mouth is probably the farthest thing from your mind, but you still need to drink. Take lots of tiny sips of fluids. For some people, ice pops may be easier to tolerate.

Staying away from caffeine in coffee, sodas, and tea can also help you avoid dehydration. Caffeine is a diuretic (it makes you urinate more frequently than you usually need to).

When To See A Doctor

Dehydration can usually be treated by drinking fluids. But if you faint or you feel faint every time you stand up (even after a couple of hours) or if you have very little urine output, you should tell an adult and visit your doctor. The doctor will probably just have you drink more fluids, but if you're more dehydrated than you realized, you may need to receive fluids through an IV to speed up the rehydration process. An IV is an intravenous tube that goes directly into a vein.

Occasionally, dehydration might be a sign of something more serious, such as diabetes, so your doctor may run tests to rule out any other potential problems.

In general, dehydration is preventable. So just keep guzzling that H_2O for healthy hydration.

Chapter 23

Why Are Oils Important?

Why is it important to consume oils?

Most of the fats you eat should be polyunsaturated (PUFA) or monounsaturated (MUFA) fats. Oils are the major source of MUFAs and PUFAs in the diet. PUFAs contain some fatty acids that are necessary for health—called "essential fatty acids."

Because oils contain these essential fatty acids, there is an allowance for oils in the food guide separate from the discretionary calorie allowance.

The MUFAs and PUFAs found in fish, nuts, and vegetable oils do not raise LDL ("bad") cholesterol levels in the blood. In addition to the essential fatty acids they contain, oils are the major source of vitamin E in typical American diets.

While consuming some oil is needed for health, oils still contain calories. In fact, oils and solid fats both contain about 120 calories per tablespoon. Therefore, the amount of oil consumed needs to be limited to balance total calorie intake. The Nutrition Facts label provides information to help you make smart choices.

About This Chapter: Excerpted from "Inside the Pyramid: Oils," U.S. Department of Agriculture (MyPyramid.gov), 2005.

What are "oils"?

Oils are fats that are liquid at room temperature, like the vegetable oils used in cooking. Oils come from many different plants and from fish. The following are some common oils:

- canola oil
- corn oil
- cottonseed oil
- olive oil
- safflower oil
- soybean oil
- sunflower oil

Some oils are used mainly as flavorings, such as walnut oil and sesame oil. A number of foods are naturally high in oils, like the following:

- nuts
- olives
- some fish
- avocados

Foods that are mainly oil include mayonnaise, certain salad dressings, and soft

> ### ♣ It's A Fact!!
> ### How are oils different from solid fats?
>
> All fats and oils are a mixture of saturated fatty acids and unsaturated fatty acids. Solid fats contain more saturated fats and/or *trans* fats than oils. Oils contain more monounsaturated (MUFA) and polyunsaturated (PUFA) fats. Saturated fats, *trans* fats, and cholesterol tend to raise "bad" (LDL) cholesterol levels in the blood, which in turn increases the risk for heart disease. To lower risk for heart disease, cut back on foods containing saturated fats, *trans* fats, and cholesterol.
>
> Source: U.S. Department of Agriculture (MyPyramid.gov), 2005.

(tub or squeeze) margarine with no *trans* fats. Check the Nutrition Facts label to find margarines with 0 grams of *trans* fat. As of 2006, amounts of *trans* fat are required on labels.

Most oils are high in monounsaturated or polyunsaturated fats, and low in saturated fats. Oils from plant sources (vegetable and nut oils) do not contain any cholesterol. In fact, no foods from plants sources contain cholesterol.

A few plant oils, however, including coconut oil and palm kernel oil, are high in saturated fats and for nutritional purposes should be considered to be solid fats.

Solid fats are fats that are solid at room temperature, like butter and shortening. Solid fats come from many animal foods and can be made from vegetable oils through a process called hydrogenation. Some common solid fats are as follows:

- butter
- beef fat (tallow, suet)
- chicken fat
- pork fat (lard)
- stick margarine
- shortening

Chapter 24

What Are Solid Fats?

Solid fats are fats that are solid at room temperature, like butter and shortening. Solid fats come from many animal foods and can be made from vegetable oils through a process called hydrogenation. Some common solid fats are as follows:

- butter
- chicken fat
- stick margarine

- beef fat (tallow, suet)
- pork fat (lard)
- shortening

Foods high in solid fats include the following:

- many cheeses
- ice creams
- regular ground beef
- sausages

- creams
- well-marbled cuts of meats
- bacon
- poultry skin

- many baked goods (such as cookies, crackers, donuts, pastries, and croissants)

About This Chapter: This chapter begins with excerpts from "Inside the Pyramid: Oils and Discretionary Calories," U.S. Department of Agriculture (MyPyramid.gov), 2005. "Revealing *Trans* Fats" is from the U.S. Food and Drug Administration's *FDA Consumer* magazine, September-October 2003 issue, with revisions made in September 2003 and May 2004. "Fat-Free Versus Regular Calorie Consumption" and "Low-Calorie, Lower-Fat Alternative Foods" are from the National Heart, Lung, and Blood Institute's Obesity Education Initiative, December 2004.

In some cases, the fat in these foods is invisible. Regular cheese and whole milk are high in solid fat, even though it is not visible.

Most solid fats are high in saturated fats and/or *trans* fats and have less monounsaturated or polyunsaturated fats. Animal products containing solid fats also contain cholesterol.

In contrast to solid fats, oils are fats that are liquid at room temperature, like the vegetable oils used in cooking. Oils come from many different plants

✎ What's It Mean?

Cholesterol: A chemical compound manufactured in the body. It is used to build cell membranes and brain and nerve tissues. Cholesterol also helps the body make steroid hormones and bile acids.

Dietary cholesterol: Cholesterol found in animal products that are part of the human diet. Egg yolks, liver, meat, some shellfish, and whole-milk dairy products are all sources of dietary cholesterol.

Fatty acid: A molecule composed mostly of carbon and hydrogen atoms. Fatty acids are the building blocks of fats.

Fat: A chemical compound containing one or more fatty acids. Fat is one of the three main constituents of food (the others are protein and carbohydrate). It is also the principal form in which energy is stored in the body.

Hydrogenated fat: A fat that has been chemically altered by the addition of hydrogen atoms (see *trans* fatty acid). Vegetable shortening and margarine are hydrogenated fats.

Lipid: A chemical compound characterized by the fact that it is insoluble in water. Both fat and cholesterol are members of the lipid family.

Lipoprotein: A chemical compound made of fat and protein. Lipoproteins that have more fat than protein are called low-density lipoproteins (LDLs). Lipoproteins that have more protein than fat are called high-density lipoproteins (HDLs). Lipoproteins are found in the blood, where their main function is to carry cholesterol.

and from fish. Some common oils include canola oil, corn oil, olive oil, peanut oil, safflower oil, soybean oil, and sunflower oil.

Some oils are used mainly as flavorings, such as walnut oil and sesame oil. A number of foods are naturally high in oils, including nuts, olives, some fish, and avocados.

A few plant oils, including coconut oil and palm kernel oil, are high in saturated fats and for nutritional purposes should be considered solid fats.

Monounsaturated fatty acid: A fatty acid that is missing one pair of hydrogen atoms in the middle of the molecule. The gap is called an "unsaturation." Monounsaturated fatty acids are found mostly in plant and sea foods. Olive oil and canola oil are high in monounsaturated fatty acids. Monounsaturated fatty acids tend to lower levels of LDL-cholesterol in the blood.

Polyunsaturated fatty acid: A fatty acid that is missing more than one pair of hydrogen atoms. Polyunsaturated fatty acids are mostly found in plant and sea foods. Safflower oil and corn oil are high in polyunsaturated fatty acids. Polyunsaturated fatty acids tend to lower levels of both HDL-cholesterol and LDL-cholesterol in the blood.

Saturated fatty acid: A fatty acid that has the maximum possible number of hydrogen atoms attached to every carbon atom. It is said to be "saturated" with hydrogen atoms. Saturated fatty acids are mostly found in animal products such as meat and whole milk. Butter and lard are high in saturated fatty acids. Saturated fatty acids tend to raise levels of LDL-cholesterol ("bad" cholesterol) in the blood. Elevated levels of LDL-cholesterol are associated with heart disease.

Trans fatty acid: A polyunsaturated fatty acid in which some of the missing hydrogen atoms have been put back in a chemical process called hydrogenation, resulting in "straighter" fatty acids that solidify at higher temperatures.

Source: Excerpted from "A Consumer's Guide to Fats," by Eleanor Mayfield, *FDA Consumer*, May 1994 revised January 1999.

Revealing *Trans* Fats

Scientific evidence shows that consumption of saturated fat, *trans* fat, and dietary cholesterol raises low-density lipoprotein (LDL), or "bad" cholesterol, levels, which increases the risk of coronary heart disease (CHD). According to the National Heart, Lung, and Blood Institute of the National Institutes of Health, more than 12.5 million Americans have CHD, and more than 500,000 die each year. That makes CHD one of the leading causes of death in the United States.

The Food and Drug Administration has required that saturated fat and dietary cholesterol be listed on food labels since 1993. Starting January 1, 2006, a new regulation required the listing of *trans* fat as well. With *trans* fat added to the Nutrition Facts panel, you will know for the first time how much of all three—saturated fat, *trans* fat, and cholesterol—are in the foods you choose. Identifying saturated fat, *trans* fat, and cholesterol on the food label gives you information you need to make food choices that help reduce the risk of CHD. This revised label will be of particular interest to people concerned about high blood cholesterol and heart disease.

However, everyone should be aware of the risk posed by consuming too much saturated fat, *trans* fat, and cholesterol. But what is *trans* fat, and how can you limit the amount of this fat in your diet?

What is *trans* fat?

Basically, *trans* fat is made when manufacturers add hydrogen to vegetable oil—a process called hydrogenation. Hydrogenation increases the shelf life and flavor stability of foods containing these fats.

Trans fat can be found in vegetable shortenings, some margarines, crackers, cookies, snack foods, and other foods made with or fried in partially hydrogenated oils. Unlike other fats, the majority of *trans* fat is formed when food manufacturers turn liquid oils into solid fats like shortening and hard margarine. A small amount of *trans* fat is found naturally, primarily in dairy products, some meat, and other animal-based foods.

Trans fat, like saturated fat and dietary cholesterol, raises the LDL cholesterol that increases your risk for CHD. Americans consume on average four to five times as much saturated fat as *trans* fat in their diets.

Although saturated fat is the main dietary culprit that raises LDL, *trans* fat and dietary cholesterol also contribute significantly.

Are all fats the same?

Simply put: No. Fat is a major source of energy for the body and aids in the absorption of vitamins A, D, E, and K and carotenoids. Both animal- and plant-derived food products contain fat, and when eaten in moderation, fat is important for proper growth, development, and maintenance of good health. As a food ingredient, fat provides taste, consistency, and stability and helps you feel full. In addition, parents should be aware that fats are an especially important source of calories and nutrients for infants and toddlers (up to two years of age), who have the highest energy needs per unit of body weight of any age group.

While unsaturated fats (monounsaturated and polyunsaturated) are beneficial when consumed in moderation, saturated and *trans* fats are not. Saturated fat and *trans* fat raise LDL cholesterol levels in the blood. Dietary cholesterol also contributes to heart disease. Therefore, it is advisable to choose foods low in saturated fat, *trans* fat, and cholesterol as part of a healthful diet.

What can you do about saturated fat, *trans* fat, and cholesterol?

When comparing foods, look at the Nutrition Facts panel, and choose the food with the lower amounts of saturated fat, *trans* fat, and cholesterol. Health experts recommend that you keep your intake of saturated fat, *trans* fat, and cholesterol as low as possible while consuming a nutritionally adequate diet. However, these experts recognize that eliminating these three components entirely from your diet is not practical because they are unavoidable in ordinary diets.

How do your choices stack up?

With the addition of *trans* fat to the Nutrition Facts panel, you can review your food choices and see how they stack up. Table 24.1 illustrates total fat, saturated fat, *trans* fat, and cholesterol content per serving for selected food products.

Table 24.1. Total Fat, Saturated Fat, *Trans* Fat, And Cholesterol Content Per Serving*

Product	Common Serving Size	Total Fat g	Sat. Fat g	%DV for Sat. Fat g	*Trans* Fat g.	Combined Sat. & *Trans* Fat g	Chol. Mg	%DV for Chol.
French Fried Potatoes‡ (Fast Food)	Medium (147 g)	27	7	35%	8	15	0	0%
Butter**	1 tbsp	11	7	35%	0	7	30	10%
Margarine, stick†	1 tbsp	11	2	10%	3	5	0	0%
Margarine, tub†	1 tbsp	7	1	5%	0.5	1.5	0	0%
Mayonnaise†† (Soybean Oil)	1 tbsp	11	1.5	8%	0	1.5	5	2%
Shortening‡	1 tbsp	13	3.5	18%	4	7.5	0	0%
Potato Chips‡	Small bag (42.5 g)	11	2	10%	3	5	0	0%
Milk, whole‡	1 cup	7	4.5	23%	0	4.5	35	12%
Milk, skim†	1 cup	0	0	0%	0	0	5	2%
Doughnut‡	1	18	4.5	23%	5	9.5	25	8%
Cookies‡ (Cream Filled)	3 (30 g)	6	1	5%	2	3	0	0%
Candy Bar‡	1 (40 g)	10	4	20%	3	7	<5	1%
Cake, pound‡	1 slice (80 g)	16	3.5	18%	4.5	8	0	0%

*Nutrient values rounded based on FDA's nutrition labeling regulations.   ‡ 1995 USDA Composition Data.

** Butter values from FDA Table of *Trans* Values, 1/30/95.

† Values derived from 2002 USDA National Nutrient Database for Standard Reference, Release 15.

†† Prerelease values derived from 2003 USDA National Nutrient Database for Standard Reference, Release 16.

Don't assume similar products are the same. Be sure to check the Nutrition Facts panel because even similar foods can vary in calories, ingredients, nutrients, and the size and number of servings in a package. Even if you continue to buy the same brand of a product, check the Nutrition Facts panel frequently because ingredients can change at any time.

How can you use the label to make heart-healthy food choices?

The Nutrition Facts panel can help you choose foods lower in saturated fat, *trans* fat, and cholesterol. Compare similar foods and choose the food with the lower combined saturated and *trans* fats and the lower amount of cholesterol.

Although the updated Nutrition Facts panel will list the amount of *trans* fat in a product, it will not show a Percent Daily Value (%DV). While scientific reports have confirmed the relationship between *trans* fat and an increased risk of CHD, none has provided a reference value for *trans* fat or any other information that the U.S. Food and Drug Administration (FDA) believes is sufficient to establish a Daily Reference Value or a %DV.

There is, however, a %DV shown for saturated fat and cholesterol. To choose foods low in saturated fat and cholesterol, use the general rule of thumb that 5 percent of the Daily Value or less is low and 20 percent or more is high.

You can also use the %DV to make dietary trade-offs with other foods throughout the day. You don't have to give up a favorite food to eat a healthy diet. When a food you like is high in saturated fat or cholesterol, balance it with foods that are low in saturated fat and cholesterol at other times of the day.

Do dietary supplements contain *trans* fat?

Would it surprise you to know that some dietary supplements contain *trans* fat from partially hydrogenated vegetable oil as well as saturated fat or cholesterol? It's true. As a result of the FDA's new label requirement, if a dietary supplement contains a reportable amount of *trans* or saturated fat, which is 0.5 gram or more, dietary supplement manufacturers must list the amounts on the Supplement Facts panel. Some dietary supplements that may contain saturated fat, *trans* fat, and cholesterol include energy and nutrition bars.

✔ Quick Tip

Fat Tips

Here are some practical tips you can use every day to keep your consumption of saturated fat, *trans* fat, and cholesterol low while consuming a nutritionally adequate diet.

- Check the Nutrition Facts panel to compare foods because the serving sizes are generally consistent in similar types of foods. Choose foods lower in saturated fat, *trans* fat, and cholesterol. For saturated fat and cholesterol, keep in mind that 5 percent of the daily value (%DV) or less is low and 20 percent or more is high. (There is no %DV for *trans* fat.)

- Choose alternative fats. Replace saturated and *trans* fats in your diet with monounsaturated and polyunsaturated fats. These fats do not raise LDL cholesterol levels and have health benefits when eaten in moderation. Sources of monounsaturated fats include olive and canola oils.

- Sources of polyunsaturated fats include soybean oil, corn oil, sunflower oil and foods like nuts and fish.

- Choose vegetable oils (except coconut and palm kernel oils) and soft margarines (liquid, tub, or spray) more often because the amounts of saturated fat, *trans* fat, and cholesterol are lower than the amounts in solid shortenings, hard margarines, and animal fats, including butter.

- Consider fish. Most fish are lower in saturated fat than meat. Some fish, such as mackerel, sardines, and salmon, contain omega-3 fatty acids, which are being studied to determine if they offer protection against heart disease.

- Choose lean meats, such as poultry without the skin and not fried and lean beef and pork, not fried, with visible fat trimmed.

- Ask before you order when eating out. A good tip to remember is to ask which fats are being used in the preparation of your food when eating or ordering out.

- Watch calories. Don't be fooled. Fats are high in calories. All sources of fat contain 9 calories per gram, making fat the most concentrated source of calories. By comparison, carbohydrates and protein have only 4 calories per gram.

Source: U.S. Food and Drug Administration, May 2004.

Table 24.2. Calorie Comparisons Of Regular, Reduced-Fat, And Fat-Free Products

Fat-Free or Reduced-Fat	Calories	Regular	Calories
Reduced-fat peanut butter, 2 T	187	Regular peanut butter, 2T	191
Reduced fat chocolate chip cookies, 3 cookies (30 g)	118	Regular chocolate chip cookies, 3 cookies (30 g)	142
Fat free fig cookies, 2 cookies (30 g)	102	Regular fig cookies, 2 cookies (30 g)	111
Nonfat vanilla frozen yogurt (<1% fat) ½ cup	100	Regular whole milk vanilla frozen yogurt (3-4% fat) ½ cup	104
Light vanilla ice cream, (7%) fat, ½ cup	111	Regular vanilla ice cream, (11%) fat, ½ cup	133
Fat free caramel topping, 2 T	103	Caramel topping, homemade with butter, 2 T	103
Lowfat granola cereal, approx. ½ cup (55 g)	213	Regular granola cereal, approx. ½ cup (55 g)	257
Lowfat blueberry muffin, 1 small (2½ inch)	131	Regular blueberry muffin, 1 small (2½ inch)	138
Baked tortilla chips, 1 oz.	113	Regular tortilla chips, 1 oz.	143
Lowfat cereal bar, 1 bar (1.3 oz.)	130	Regular cereal bar, 1 bar (1.3 oz.)	140

Nutrient data taken from Nutrient Data System for Research, Version v4.02/30, Nutrition Coordinating Center, University of Minnesota. Source of table: NHLBI, December 2004.

Table 24.3. Higher-Fat And Lower-Fat Foods

Higher-Fat Foods	Lower-Fat Foods
Dairy Products	
Evaporated whole milk	Evaporated fat-free (skim) or reduced-fat (2%) milk
Whole milk	Low-fat (1%), reduced-fat (2%), or fat-free (skim) milk
Ice cream	Sorbet, sherbet, low fat or fat-free frozen yogurt, or ice
Whipping cream	Imitation whipped cream (made with fat-free [skim] milk)
Sour cream	Plain low-fat yogurt
Cream cheese	Neufchatel or "light" cream cheese or fat-free cream cheese
Cheese (cheddar, Swiss, jack)	Reduced-calorie cheese, low-calorie processed cheeses, etc.
	Fat-free cheese
American cheese	Fat-free American cheese or other types of fat-free cheeses
Regular (4%) cottage cheese	Low-fat (1%) or reduced-fat (2%) cottage cheese
Whole milk mozzarella cheese	Part-skim milk, low-moisture mozzarella cheese
Whole milk ricotta cheese	Part-skim milk ricotta cheese
Coffee cream (½ and ½) or nondairy creamer (liquid, powder)	Low-fat (1%) or reduced-fat (2%) milk or non-fat dry milk powder
Cereals, Grains, and Pastas	
Ramen noodles	Rice or noodles (spaghetti, macaroni, etc.)
Pasta with white sauce (alfredo)	Pasta with red sauce (marinara)
Pasta with cheese sauce	Pasta with vegetables (primavera)
Granola	Bran flakes, crispy rice, etc.
	Cooked grits or oatmeal
	Reduced-fat granola

continued on next pages

Table 24.3. Higher-Fat And Lower-Fat Foods (continued from previous page)

Higher-Fat Foods	Lower-Fat Foods
Meat, Fish and Poultry	
Coldcuts or lunch meats (bologna, salami, liverwurst, etc.)	Low-fat coldcuts (95 to 97% fat-free lunch meats, low-fat pressed meats)
Hot dogs (regular)	Lower-fat hot dogs
Bacon or sausage	Canadian bacon or lean ham
Regular ground beef	Extra lean ground beef such as ground round or ground turkey (read labels)
Chicken or turkey with skin, duck, or goose	Chicken or turkey without skin (white meat)
Oil-packed tuna	Water-packed tuna (rinse to reduce sodium content)
Beef (chuck, rib, brisket)	Beef (round, loin) (trimmed of external fat) (choose select
Pork (spareribs, untrimmed loin)	Pork tenderloin or trimmed, lean smoked ham
Frozen breaded fish or fried fish (homemade or commercial)	Fish or shellfish, unbreaded (fresh, frozen, canned in water)
Whole eggs	Egg whites or egg substitutes
Frozen TV dinners (containing more than 13 grams of fat per serving)	Frozen TV dinners (containing less than 13 grams of fat per serving and lower in sodium)
Chorizo sausage	Turkey sausage, drained well (read label)
	Vegetarian sausage (made with tofu)
Baked Goods	
Croissants, brioches, etc.	Hard french rolls or soft brown 'n serve rolls
Donuts, sweet rolls, muffins, scones, or pastries	English muffins, bagels, reduced-fat or fat-free muffins or scones
Party crackers	Low-fat crackers (choose lower in sodium)
	Saltine or soda crackers (choose lower in sodium)
Cake (pound, chocolate, yellow)	Cake (angel food, white, gingerbread)

continued on next page

Table 24.3. Higher-Fat And Lower-Fat Foods (continued from previous pages)

Higher-Fat Foods	Lower-Fat Foods
Cookies	Reduced-fat or fat-free cookies (graham crackers, ginger snaps, fig bars) (compare calorie level)
Snacks and Sweets	
Nuts	Popcorn (air-popped or light microwave), fruits, vegetables
Ice cream, e.g., cones or bars	Frozen yogurt, frozen fruit or chocolate pudding bars
Custards or puddings (made with whole milk)	Puddings (made with skim milk)
Fats, Oils, and Salad Dressings	
Regular margarine or butter	Light spread margarines, diet margarine, or whipped butter, tub or squeeze bottle
Regular mayonnaise	Light or diet mayonnaise or mustard
Regular salad dressings	Reduced-calorie or fat-free salad dressings, lemon juice, or plain, herb flavored, or wine vinegar
Butter or margarine on toast or bread	Jelly, jam, or honey on bread or toast
Oils, shortening, or lard	Nonstick cooking spray for stir-frying or sautéing
	As a substitute for oil or butter, use applesauce or prune puree in baked goods
Miscellaneous	
Canned cream soups	Canned broth-based soups
Canned beans and franks	Canned baked beans in tomato sauce
Gravy (homemade with fat and/or milk)	Gravy mixes made with water or homemade with the fat skimmed off and fat-free milk
Fudge sauce	Chocolate syrup
Avocado on sandwiches	Cucumber slices or lettuce leaves
Guacamole dip or refried beans with lard	Salsa

Fat-Free Versus Regular: Calorie Comparison

A calorie is a calorie is a calorie whether it comes from fat or carbohydrate. Anything eaten in excess can lead to weight gain. You can lose weight by eating less calories and by increasing your physical activity. Reducing the amount of fat and saturated fat that you eat is one easy way to limit your overall calorie intake. However, eating fat-free or reduced-fat foods isn't always the answer to weight loss. This is especially true when you eat more of the reduced fat food than you would of the regular item. For example, if you eat twice as many fat-free cookies you have actually increased your overall calorie intake. The list of foods shown in Table 24.2 and their reduced fat varieties will show you that just because a product is fat-free, it doesn't mean that it is "calorie-free." And, calories do count.

Low-Calorie, Lower-Fat Alternative Foods

Low-calorie alternatives provide new ideas for old favorites. When making a food choice, remember to consider vitamins and minerals. Some foods provide most of their calories from sugar and fat but give you few, if any, vitamins and minerals.

Table 24.3 is a guide it is not meant to be an exhaustive list. We stress reading labels to find out just how many calories are in the specific products you decide to buy.

✔ **Quick Tip**

To keep your intake of saturated fat, *trans* fat, and cholesterol low:

- Look at the Nutrition Facts panel when comparing products. Choose foods low in the combined amount of saturated fat and *trans* fat and low in cholesterol as part of a nutritionally adequate diet.

  - Substitute alternative fats that are higher in mono- and polyunsaturated fats like olive oil, canola oil, soybean oil, corn oil, and sunflower oil.

Source: U.S. Food and Drug Administration, May 2004.

✤ It's A Fact!!
How are solid fats different from oils?

Solid fats contain more saturated fats and/or *trans* fats than oils. Oils contain more monounsaturated (MUFA) and polyunsaturated (PUFA) fats. Look for foods that are low in saturated fats, *trans* fats and cholesterol, to help reduce your risk of heart disease. *Trans* fats can be found in many cakes, cookies, crackers, icings, margarines, and microwave popcorns. Foods containing partially-hydrogenated vegetable oils usually contain *trans* fats.

Saturated fats, *trans* fats, and cholesterol tend to raise "bad" (LDL) cholesterol levels in the blood, which in turn increases the risk for heart disease. To lower risk for heart disease, cut back on foods containing saturated fats, *trans* fats and cholesterol.

Source: U.S. Department of Agriculture
(MyPyramid.gov), 2005.

Chapter 25

Caffeine: It's Really A Drug

It's 11:00 p.m. and you've already had a full day of school and after-school activities. You're tired and you know you could use some sleep, but you still haven't finished your homework or watched the movie that's due back tomorrow. So instead of catching a few ZZZs, you reach for the remote—and the caffeine.

What Is Caffeine?

Caffeine is a drug that is naturally produced in the leaves and seeds of many plants. It's also produced artificially and added to certain foods. It's part of the same group of drugs sometimes used to treat asthma.

Caffeine is defined as a drug because it stimulates the central nervous system, causing increased heart rate and alertness. Most people who are sensitive to caffeine experience a temporary increase in energy and elevation in mood.

Caffeine is in tea leaves, coffee beans, chocolate, many soft drinks, pain relievers, and other over-the-counter pills. In its natural form, caffeine tastes

About This Chapter: This information was provided by TeensHealth, one of the largest resources online for medically reviewed health information written for parents, kids, and teens. For more articles like this one, visit www.TeensHealth.org, or www.KidsHealth.org. © 2004 The Nemours Center for Children's Health Media, a division of The Nemours Foundation.

very bitter. But most caffeinated drinks have gone through enough processing to camouflage the bitter taste. Most teens get the majority of their caffeine intake through soft drinks, which can also have added sugar and artificial flavors.

Got The Jitters?

If taken in moderate amounts (like a single can of soda or cup of coffee), many people feel that caffeine increases their mental alertness. Higher doses of caffeine can cause anxiety, dizziness, headaches, and the jitters and can interfere with normal sleep, though. And very high doses of caffeine—like taking a whole box of alertness pills—would be harmful to the body.

Caffeine is addictive and may cause withdrawal symptoms for those who abruptly stop consuming it. These include severe headaches, muscle aches, temporary depression, and irritability. Although scientists once worried that caffeine could stunt growth, this concern is not supported by research.

Caffeine sensitivity refers to the amount of caffeine that will produce an effect in someone. This amount varies from person to person. On average, the smaller the person, the less caffeine necessary to produce side effects. However, caffeine sensitivity is most affected by the amount of daily caffeine use. People who regularly drink

✔ Quick Tip

Caffeine is a mildly addictive drug in colas, Mt. Dew, Sunkist Orange, Barq's Rootbeer, coffee, and tea. If you drink these items, pay attention to how much and be aware of your body's response. Have you been too hyper? Unable to sleep? Irritable? Anxious? Don't get hooked on caffeine without realizing it. Caffeinated drinks dehydrate the body; if you then drink more caffeinated drinks for your thirst, you lack the water balance your body needs for clear thinking, muscle function, and cleansing of waste products.

Source: Excerpted from "Nutrition Tips for Teens," © 2003 Munson Healthcare. All rights reserved. Reprinted with permission.

beverages containing caffeine soon develop a reduced sensitivity to caffeine. This means they require higher doses of caffeine to achieve the same effects as someone who doesn't drink caffeinated drinks every day. In short, the more caffeine you take in, the more caffeine you'll need to feel the same effects.

Caffeine moves through the body within a few hours after it's consumed and is then passed through the urine. It's not stored in the body, but you may feel its effects for up to six hours if you're sensitive to it.

Although you may think you're getting plenty of liquids when you drink caffeinated beverages, caffeine works against the body in two ways: It has a mild dehydrating effect because it increases the need to urinate. And large amounts of caffeine may cause the body to lose calcium and potassium, causing sore muscles and delayed recovery times after exercise.

Caffeine has health risks for certain users. Small children are more sensitive to caffeine because they have not been exposed to it as much as older children or adults. Pregnant women or nursing mothers should consider decreasing their caffeine intake, although in small or moderate amounts there is no evidence that it causes a problem for the baby. Caffeine can aggravate heart problems or nervous disorders, and some teens may not be aware that they're at risk.

Moderation Is The Key

Although the effects of caffeine vary from one person to the next, doctors recommend that people should consume no more than about 100 milligrams (mg) of caffeine daily. That might sound like a lot, but one espresso contains about 100 milligrams of caffeine! The chart shown in Table 25.1 includes common caffeinated products and the amounts of caffeine they contain.

Cutting Back

If you're taking in too much caffeine, you may want to cut back. Kicking the caffeine habit is never easy, and the best way is to cut back slowly. Otherwise you could get headaches and feel achy, depressed, or lousy.

Try cutting your intake by substituting noncaffeinated drinks for caffeinated sodas and coffee. Examples include water, caffeine-free sodas, and caffeine-free teas. Keep track of how many caffeinated drinks you have each day, and substitute one drink per week with a caffeine-free alternative until you've gotten below the 100-milligram mark.

As you cut back on the amount of caffeine you consume, you may find yourself feeling tired. Your best bet is to hit the sack, not the sodas: It's just your body's way of telling you it needs more rest. Your energy levels will return to normal in a few days.

Table 25.1. Caffeine Amounts

Drink/Food	Amt. of Drink/Food	Amt. of Caffeine
Jolt soft drink	12 ounces	71.2 mg
Mountain Dew	12 ounces	55.0 mg
Coca-Cola	2 ounces	34.0 mg
Diet Coke	12 ounces	45.0 mg
Pepsi	12 ounces	38.0 mg
7-Up	12 ounces	0 mg
Brewed coffee (drip method)	5 ounces	115 mg*
Iced tea	12 ounces	70 mg*
Dark chocolate	1 ounce	20 mg*
Milk chocolate	1 ounce	6 mg*
Cocoa beverage	5 ounces	4 mg*
Chocolate milk beverage	8 ounces	5 mg*
Cold relief medication	1 tablet	30 mg*
Vivarin	1 tablet	200 mg

* denotes average amount of caffeine

Source: U.S. Food and Drug Administration and National Soft Drink Association

Chapter 26

Sugar And Other Sweeteners

It's not easy to find someone who doesn't like sweet tastes. Indeed, the human preference for sweets is thought to be a basic survival adaptation. When presented with a variety of basic tastes such as sweet, salty, bitter, or sour, infants favor the sweet choice. Scientists believe this preference may be an evolutionary design that ensures infants accept life-sustaining milk, with its slightly sweet taste that comes from milk sugar (lactose).

Sugars

While many people associate sweetness with sucrose or table sugar, sucrose is just one type of sugar that provides this taste. Fruits contain simple sugars such as glucose and fructose; other foods contain sugars such as corn syrup, honey, and high fructose corn syrup, which are combinations of glucose and fructose. Another simple sugar in milk, known as lactose, is a combination of glucose and the simple sugar galactose.

All sugars are carbohydrates containing four calories per gram and all carbohydrates are made of one or more molecules of simple sugar. After digestion, sugars travel through the bloodstream to body cells, where they are used as the primary fuel for the body, to help metabolize fat, form proteins, or store for future use.

Sugars add more than just sweetness to food. Sugars also provide unique functional characteristics such as browning and texture as well as add to the enjoyment of eating a healthful diet.

Sucrose

Sucrose—commonly referred to as table sugar—is a disaccharide comprising glucose and fructose and providing four calories per gram or about 16 calories per teaspoon. Sucrose is derived from sugar cane or sugar beets. The refining process removes impurities from the sugar plant, producing the white crystals commonly found in the sugar bowl. Molasses is simply a less refined sucrose.

♣ It's A Fact!!

The Arabs' word for it was qandi, from qand, a lump of cane sugar. It came down to us, virtually intact, through successive European languages: Old Italian (zucchero candi), Old French (sucre candi), Middle English (sugre candi). In the 1800s, Americans called it "sugar candy." Now, it's just candy.

Source: Excerpted from "Candy: How Sweet It is!" by Dodi Schultz, *FDA Consumer*, U.S. Food and Drug Administration, July-August 1994.

Fructose

Like sucrose, fructose provides four calories per gram. Fructose is a constituent of sucrose and is often referred to as fruit sugar because of its presence in fruits. Fructose is also added to foods and beverages in the form of crystalline fructose (made from corn starch) or high fructose corn syrup (HFCS) (a combination of fructose and glucose).

Sugars And Low-Calorie Sweeteners In A Healthful Diet

According to the American Dietetic Association, consumers can enjoy a range of nutritive and non-nutritive sweeteners when consumed in moderation and within the context of a diet consistent with the Dietary Guidelines for Americans.

Low-Calorie Sweeteners

Low-calorie sweeteners provide a sweet taste with few or no accompanying calories. Before being approved by the FDA for use in the United States, sweeteners must undergo extensive safety testing. All FDA-approved low-calorie sweeteners meet the same standard of safety. They are safe for consumption by pregnant women and children. The six intense, low-calorie sweeteners currently approved for use in the United States are acesulfame potassium (Ace-K), aspartame, neotame, saccharin, sucralose, and tagatose. The FDA is considering petitions to approve other low-calorie sweeteners for use in the U.S. food supply: alitame and cyclamate. Both alitame and cyclamate have been approved for use in numerous other countries.

♣ It's A Fact!!

What are "added sugars"?

Added sugars are sugars and syrups that are added to foods or beverages during processing or preparation. This does not include naturally occurring sugars such as those that occur in milk and fruits.

Foods that contain most of the added sugars in American diets are as follows:

- regular soft drinks
- candy
- cakes
- cookies
- pies
- fruit drinks, such as fruitades and fruit punch
- milk-based desserts and products, such as ice cream, sweetened yogurt and sweetened milk
- grain products such as sweet rolls and cinnamon toast

Reading the ingredient label on processed foods can help to identify added sugars. Names for added sugars on food labels include the following:

- brown sugar
- corn sweetener
- corn syrup
- dextrose
- fructose
- fruit juice concentrates
- glucose
- high-fructose corn syrup
- honey
- invert sugar
- lactose
- maltose
- malt syrup
- molasses
- raw sugar
- sucrose
- sugar
- syrup

Source: U.S. Department of Agriculture (MyPyramid.gov), 2005.

Aspartame is widely used in numerous foods and beverages and as a tabletop sweetener. It contains four calories per gram but because, measure for measure, it is 200 times sweeter than sugar, very little aspartame is needed to adequately sweeten foods, and hence adds minimal calories to foods. Saccharin is the oldest of low-calorie sweeteners and contains no calories. Acesulfame potassium (or Ace-K) is also used in numerous foods and beverages and was additionally approved as a flavor enhancer in 2003. It contains no calories, is heat stable and, when blended with other low-calorie sweeteners, has a synergistic effect that helps improve the taste, sweetness, and stability of low-calorie foods and beverages. Sucralose is the only low-calorie sweetener that is made from sugar. It is approximately 600 times sweeter, does not contain calories, and is highly stable under a wide variety of processing conditions. The FDA has approved sucralose for use in foods and beverages; in cooking and baking; and as a tabletop sweetener.

> ### ♣ It's A Fact!!
>
> Also called liquid candy, sodapop packs an automatic three strikes against you:
>
> - Acid + sugar attacks enamel on teeth and causes tooth decay.
>
> - Sodapop replaces healthier drinks, such as milk, which you need for calcium.
>
> - Sodapop contains almost one teaspoon of sugar per ounce (17 teaspoons in a 20-ounce can or bottle). Sugar is a source of empty calories that can use up vitamins and minerals in your body if taken in large amounts. It also adds extra calories without making you feel full, so you eat more which may just lead to extra fat stores.
>
> Source: Excerpted from "Nutrition Tips for Teens," © 2003 Munson Healthcare. All rights reserved. Reprinted with permission.

Neotame is a non-caloric sweetener and flavor enhancer with a clean, sweet, sugar-like taste. Since it is about 8,000 times sweeter than sugar, only very small amounts are needed to sweeten foods and beverages. Neotame was granted approval by FDA in 2002 for general use in foods and beverages after an extensive review of more than 100 studies confirming its safety and functionality. Neotame is rapidly metabolized, completely eliminated, and does not accumulate in the body. It is safe for use by the general population, including pregnant and lactating women, children, and people with diabetes.

Tagatose, technically known as D-tagatose, is a low-calorie sweetener derived from lactose, which occurs naturally in some dairy products and other foods. Tagatose has been determined to be a generally recognized as safe (GRAS) substance in the United States, permitting its use in foods and beverages.

Low-Calorie Sweetener Blends

Blends of low-calorie sweeteners in foods and beverages may act synergistically to produce the desired level of sweetness at lower levels than the sweeteners used singly. The resulting taste often better meets consumer expectations of a sweetness profile close to that of sugar or other caloric sweeteners. The products may also have better sweetness stability over the life of the product. Health authorities around the world have reasonably concluded that there is no scientific basis to expect any physiological effects to emerge from blended sweeteners separate and apart from those that occur with the individual sweeteners, and none have been reported.

☞ **Remember!!**
Sweeteners And Health

Whether it is sugars, low-calorie sweeteners, sweetener blends, or sugar alcohols at work to produce the prized taste of many favorite foods, nutrition experts agree sweet foods can be part of a healthful diet. The key is moderation of calories to ensure that sweet foods, some of which may contribute few nutrients to the diet, do not crowd out more nutrient-dense foods.

Denial of sweet foods can increase their attractiveness with the potential for overeating and guilt when people "give in." Subsequent attempts at elimination can establish a cycle of denial and overindulgence, which can ultimately lead to failure in achieving dietary goals.

Source: © 2005 International Food Information Council.

Sugar Alcohols

While sweet flavors have traditionally come from sugars, today there are many other types of sweeteners that add to the enjoyment of foods. Sugar alcohols (or polyols) such as erythritol, isomalt, maltitol, mannitol, sorbitol, and xylitol provide the sweet taste found in many sugar-free candies, cookies, and chewing gums. Sugar alcohols occur naturally in a wide variety of fruits and vegetables, but are made from other carbohydrates such as sucrose, glucose, and starch when produced commercially.

Chapter 27

Salt: Flavor Enhancer Or Health Hazard?

Salt is one of the four basic taste qualities—sweet, sour, bitter, and salty. So, it is no wonder that historically salt has been the most valued flavor enhancer in our society. Despite its marked place in our kitchens, many health authorities have recommended that individuals limit their salt intake to no more than 2400 milligrams (mg) per day. The average American consumes 4000 mg per day. It is estimated that nearly one in four Americans have hypertension and middle-aged Americans have a 90% chance of developing high blood pressure at some time during their lifetime.

Sources Of Salt And Sodium In Your Diet

While some foods naturally contain sodium, most of the sodium in the typical American diet comes from salt added to foods during processing or preparation. Food processors add salt or other sodium derivatives during production as a preservative and for flavor. Popular foods with high sodium content include pickled foods, canned vegetables and soups, snack foods, cured meats, packaged mixes, and frozen dinners. To moderate your sodium intake from processed food, read the Nutrition Label on food packages. Look for no added salt or low sodium versions of your favorite foods.

About This Chapter: Text in this chapter is from "Flavor: A Matter of Taste," reprinted with permission from the American Dietetic Association, http://www.eatright.org, © 2004. All rights reserved.

Know The Label Lingo, Look For

- Sodium Free—a product that contains 5 milligrams or less of sodium per serving

- Very Low Sodium—a product that contains 35 milligrams or less of sodium per serving

- Low Sodium—a product that contains 140 milligrams or less of sodium per serving

- Reduced Sodium—a product that the usual sodium level was reduced by at least 25%

- No Added Salt, Unsalted—a product that no salt was added during processing; however this does not mean that the product does not contain sodium.

♣ **It's A Fact!!**

You weren't born with a love for salt. The good news is that you can retrain your taste buds. If you gradually decrease the sodium and salt in your diet, you will find that your taste for salt declines. The less you consume, the less you want. By using spice and herb blends instead of salt you can add satisfying flavor to just about any recipe.

Source: Reprinted with permission from the American Dietetic Association, http://www.eatright.org, © 2004. All rights reserved.

Salt, whether added during food preparation or at the table, is the most common source of sodium. One teaspoon of salt contains about 2,400 milligrams of sodium. So think before you reach for that salt shaker. Instead, jazz up food with herbs and spices. Salt-free seasoning blends provide an easy way to give great flavor without the guesswork or added salt.

Salt-Free Seasoning Guide

Vegetables

- Asparagus—lemon pepper, onion and herb salt-free seasoning

- Broccoli—Italian or multi-purpose salt-free seasoning

- Carrots—garlic and herb salt-free seasoning

- Corn—extra spicy or tomato, basil, garlic salt-free seasoning

✔ **Quick Tip**

Roasted Red Potatoes

Ingredients

1 Tablespoon (15 mL) olive oil

1 Tablespoon (15 mL) unsalted butter

12 small red potatoes, cut into wedges

1½ Tablespoons (22.5 mL) salt-free seasoning blend, split

Instructions

Preheat oven to 400°F (200°C). Add olive oil and melted butter to a large bowl, add potatoes, 1 tablespoon salt-free seasoning blend and toss. Place on a cookie sheet, and roast for 30 minutes. Increase heat to 450°F (220°C). Sprinkle with remaining salt-free seasoning blend and continue to roast for 5–10 minutes or until tender and browned.

Preparation Time: 0:10

Cooking Time: 0:40

Nutrition Information

Per Serving:

Calories: 273

Fat: 7 grams (g)

Cholesterol: 8 mg

Sodium: 17 mg

Carbohydrates: 50 g

Protein: 6 g

Fiber: 4 g

Potassium: 1500 mg

For more great tips and recipes visit http://www.mrsdash.com or call 800-622-DASH.

- Greens—onion and herb, lemon pepper salt-free seasoning

- Potatoes—garlic and herb, onion and herb, tomato, basil, garlic salt-free seasoning

- Tomatoes—Italian, extra spicy, lemon pepper salt free seasoning

Meat, Fish And Poultry

- Beef—steak grilling blend or garlic and herb salt-free seasoning

- Fish—mesquite grilling blend or lemon pepper

♣ It's A Fact!!

Why should you eat less salt and sodium?

You should cut back on salt and sodium in your diet to help prevent or lower high blood pressure. If you have high blood pressure, lowering it can reduce your chances of heart disease and stroke.

Is salt a concern for people who don't have high blood pressure?

Results from study supported by the National Heart, Lung, and Blood Institute published in *Hypertension: Journal of the American Heart Association* (2/16/01), show that sensitivity to salt increases the risk of death even for people with normal blood pressure. Although salt has been associated with hypertension for years, new research reveals that salt sensitivity (a measure of how blood pressure responds to salt intake) increases risks of developing other conditions such kidney problems.

According to Dr. Myron Weinberger, Director of the Hypertension Research Center at the Indiana University School of Medicine and the study's principal investigator, about 26 percent of Americans with normal blood pressure and about 58 percent of those with hypertension are salt sensitive. Because there is no easy way to test for salt sensitivity, Dr. Weinberger advises all Americans with normal blood pressure to follow the federal recommendation of having no more than 2,400 milligrams of sodium a day.

- Lamb—garlic and herb or Italian salt-free seasoning

- Pork—onion and herb, garlic and herb, or mesquite grilling blend

- Poultry—garlic and herb, lemon pepper, or chicken grilling blend

When experts recommend that your diet should be lower in salt and sodium, this does not mean that you have to restrict your food choices or compromise the flavor of food. Simply by altering an existing recipe using herbs, spices and salt-free seasoning blends provides satisfying, flavorful, and healthier dishes.

Because only 10 percent of dietary sodium is added by salting food at the table, Americans interested in reducing their sodium consumption should be careful about the sodium content of processed foods.

How do salt and sodium compare?

Salt is also labeled as sodium chloride. Baking soda, soda, sodium bicarbonate, and the symbol "Na" on food labels mean the product contains sodium.

- ¼ teaspoon salt = 600 milligrams (mg) sodium

- ½ teaspoon salt = 1,200 mg sodium

- ¾ teaspoon salt = 1,800 mg sodium

- 1 tsp salt = 2,400 mg sodium

- 1 tsp baking soda = 1,000 mg sodium

Source: First question from "Spice Up Your Life! Eat Less Salt and Sodium," National Heart, Lung, and Blood Institute (NHLBI), 1997; second question from "Study Reveals Link Between Salt Sensitivity and Risk of Death in People without Hypertension," *FYI from the NHLBI*, Vol. 2, Issue 1, May 2001; third question from "Body Image and Your Health," National Women's Health Information Center, August 2004.

☞ Remember!!

For food and nutrition information or for a referral to a dietetics professional in your area call: 800-366-1655 or visit: www.eatright.org

Part Three

Weight Control

Chapter 28

What Is The Right Weight?

"What's the right weight for my height?" is one of the most common questions girls and guys have. It seems like a simple question. But, for teens, it's not always an easy one to answer. Why not? People have different body types, so there's no single number that's the right weight for everyone. Even among people who are the same height and age, some are more muscular or more developed than others. That's because not all teens have the same body type or develop at the same time.

It is possible to find out if you are in a healthy weight range for your height, though—it just takes a little effort. Read on to discover how this works. You'll also be able to put your measurements into our calculator and get an idea of how you are doing.

Growth And Puberty

Not everyone grows and develops on the same schedule, but teens do go through a period of faster growth. During puberty, the body begins making hormones that spark physical changes like faster muscle growth (particularly in guys) and spurts in height and weight gain in both guys and girls. Once

About This Chapter: This information was provided by TeensHealth, one of the largest resources online for medically reviewed health information written for parents, kids, and teens. For more articles like this one, visit www.TeensHealth.org, or www.KidsHealth.org. © 2005 The Nemours Center for Children's Health Media, a division of The Nemours Foundation.

these changes start, they continue for several years. The average person can expect to grow as much as 10 inches (25 centimeters) during puberty before he or she reaches full adult height.

Most guys and girls gain weight more rapidly during this time as the amounts of muscle, fat, and bone in their bodies changes. All that new weight gain can be perfectly fine—as long as body fat, muscle, and bone are in the right proportion. Because some kids start developing as early as age eight and some not until age 14 or so, it can be normal for two people who are the same height and age to have very different weights.

♣ **It's A Fact!!**
Why You Need More Than A Scale

People overweight for their height can have major differences in body composition (the amounts of muscle, fat, and bone they have). An athlete might be considered overweight because of extra muscle, while a less fit person of the same height and weight might have less muscle but be overweight because of too much body fat.

Source: © 2005 The Nemours Center for Children's Health Media, a division of The Nemours Foundation.

It can feel quite strange adjusting to suddenly feeling heavier or taller. So it's perfectly normal to feel self-conscious about weight during adolescence— a lot of people do.

Figuring Out Fat Using BMI

Experts have developed a way to help figure out if a person is in the healthy weight range for his or her height. It's called the body mass index, or BMI. BMI is a formula that doctors use to estimate how much body fat a person has based on his or her weight and height.

The BMI formula uses height and weight measurements to calculate a BMI number. This number is then plotted on a chart, which tells a person whether he or she is underweight, average weight, at risk of becoming over-weight, or overweight.

Figuring out the body mass index is a little more complicated for teens than it is for adults (that puberty thing again). BMI charts for teens use percentile lines to help individuals compare their BMIs to those of a very large group of people the same age and gender. There are different BMI charts for guys and girls under the age of 20.

A person's BMI number is plotted on the chart for their age and gender. Each BMI chart has eight percentile lines for 5th, 10th, 25th, 50th, 75th, 85th, 90th, and 95th percentiles. A teen whose BMI is at the 50th percentile is close to the average of the age group. A teen above the 95th percentile is considered overweight because 95% of the age group has a BMI less than he or she does. A teen below the 5th percentile is considered underweight because 95% of the age group has a higher BMI.

To figure out your BMI, use the online tool available at http:// teenshealth.org/teen/food_fitness/dieting/weight_height.html. Before you start, you'll need an accurate height and weight measurement. Bathroom scales and tape measures aren't always precise. So the best way to get accurate measurements is by being weighed and measured at your doctor's office or school.

What Does BMI Tell Us?

Although you can calculate BMI on your own, it's a good idea to ask your doctor, school nurse, or fitness counselor to help you figure out what it means. That's because a doctor can do more than just use BMI to assess a person's current weight. He or she can take into account where a girl or guy is during puberty and use BMI results from past years to track whether that person

♣ It's A Fact!!

Some teens, especially those who go through puberty on a later time schedule, may feel too skinny. The good news is that their growth, development, and weight gain almost always catch up to other people their age later on.

Source: © 2005 The Nemours Center for Children's Health Media, a division of The Nemours Foundation.

may be at risk for becoming overweight. Spotting this risk early on can be helpful because the person can then make changes in diet and exercise before he or she goes on to develop a weight problem.

People don't like looking overweight, but weight problems get more serious than just how a person looks. People who are overweight as teens increase their risk of developing health problems, such as diabetes and high blood

---

♣ It's A Fact!!
BMI Is Used Differently With Children And Teens Than It Is With Adults

In children and teens, body mass index is used to assess underweight, overweight, and risk for overweight. Children's body fatness changes over the years as they grow. Also, girls and boys differ in their body fatness as they mature. This is why BMI for children, also referred to as BMI-for-age, is gender and age specific. BMI-for-age is plotted on gender specific growth charts. These charts are used for children and teens 2–20 years of age.

Each of the CDC BMI-for-age gender specific charts contains a series of curved lines indicating specific percentiles. Healthcare professionals use the following established percentile cutoff points to identify underweight and overweight in children.

Table 28.1. Body Mass Index For Children And Teens

Underweight	BMI-for-age < 5th percentile
Normal	BMI-for-age 5th percentile to < 85th percentile
At risk of overweight	BMI-for-age 85th percentile to < 95th percentile
Overweight	BMI-for-age > 95th percentile

BMI decreases during the preschool years, then increases into adulthood. The percentile curves show this pattern of growth.

Source: From "BMI—Body Mass Index: BMI for Children and Teens," Centers for Disease Control and Prevention, June 2005.

pressure. Being overweight as a teen also makes a person more likely to be overweight as an adult. And adults who are overweight may develop other serious health conditions, such as heart disease.

Although BMI can be a good indicator of a person's body fat, it doesn't always tell the full story. Someone can have a high BMI because he or she has a large frame or a lot of muscle (like a bodybuilder or athlete) instead of excess fat. Likewise, a small person with a small frame may have a normal BMI but could still have too much body fat. These are other good reasons to talk about your BMI with your doctor.

How Can I Be Sure I'm Not Overweight Or Underweight?

If you think you've gained too much weight or are too skinny, a doctor should help you decide whether it's normal for you or whether you really have a weight problem. Your doctor has measured your height and weight over time and knows whether you're growing normally.

If your doctor has a concern about your height, weight, or BMI, he or she may ask questions about your health, physical activity and eating habits. Your doctor may also ask about your family background to find out if you've inherited traits that might make you taller, shorter, or a late bloomer (a person who develops later than other people the same age). The doctor can then put all this information together to decide whether you might have a weight or growth problem.

If your doctor thinks your weight isn't in a healthy range, you will probably get specific dietary and exercise recommendations based on your individual needs. Following a doctor's or dietitian's plan that's designed especially for you will work way better than following fad diets. For teens, fad diets or starvation plans can actually slow down growth and sexual development, and the weight loss usually doesn't last.

What if you're worried about being too skinny? Most teens who weigh less than other teens their age are just fine. They may be going through puberty on a different schedule than some of their peers, and their bodies may be growing and changing at a different rate. Most underweight teens catch up in weight as they finish puberty during their later teen years and there's rarely a need to try to gain weight.

In a few cases, teens can be underweight because of a health problem that needs treatment. If you feel tired or ill a lot, or if you have symptoms like a cough, stomachache, diarrhea, or other problems that have lasted for more than a week or two, be sure to let your parents or your doctor know. Some teens are underweight because of eating disorders, like anorexia or bulimia, that require attention.

Getting Into Your Genes

Heredity plays a role in body shape and what a person weighs. People from different races, ethnic groups, and nationalities tend to have different

---

♣ It's A Fact!!

If you don't have access to the internet, you can still figure out your body mass index, but you may want to use a calculator to help you with the numbers.

Calculate your body mass index:

- Step 1: How tall are you in inches? Take this number and multiply it by itself. For example, if you are 60" tall, multiply 60 x 60. This equals 3600.

- Step 2: How much do you weight in pounds?

- Divide this number by your answer in Step 1.

- For example, if you weigh 112 pounds and are 60" tall (exactly 5'), divide 112 by 3600. This equals 0.0311

- Step 3: Multiply the answer you got in Step 1 by 703.

- For example: 0.02311 x 703 = 20.9 (rounded to one decimal point)

- To find out whether or not this represents a healthy weight for a person of your age, check the "Body mass index-for-age percentiles" (there are different charts for boys and girls). If the number is under the 5th percentile, you may be underweight; if the number is above the 95th percentile, you may be overweight.

In the example we've been using:

- If you are an 8-year old girl, are 60" tall and weigh 112 pounds, you are a little over the 95th percentile for people your age. You may be overweight.

- If you are an 8-year old boy, are 60" tall and weigh 112 pounds, you are a body fat distribution (meaning they accumulate fat in different parts of their bodies) or body composition (amounts of bone and muscle versus fat). But genes are not destiny. (That may be a relief if you're looking at Aunt Mildred and wondering if you'll end up with her physique!) No matter whose genes you inherit, you can have a healthy body and keep your weight at a level that's normal for you by eating right and being active.

Genes aren't the only things that family members may share. It's also true that unhealthy eating habits can be passed down, too. The eating and exercise habits of people in the same household probably have an even greater

---

little under the 95th percentile for people your age. You are not overweight, but you may be at risk for becoming overweight because you are over the 85th percentile.

- If you are a girl older than 11 or a boy older than 12, at this same height and weight, you are under the 85th percentile and are neither overweight nor considered at risk.

Sometimes girls in the teen years have misperceptions about the range of weights that are considered normal. Here are some examples of heights and weights that are considered underweight:

- A 14-year old girl who is 60" tall and weighs 80 pounds is underweight.
- A 15-year old girl who is 63" tall and weighs 90 pounds is underweight
- A 16-year old girl who is 65" tall and weighs 100 pounds is underweight

How much would these example girls have to weigh before they surpassed the 95th percentile to fall into the "overweight" category?

- A 14-year old girl who is 60" tall and weighs 142 has a body mass of 27.7, just over the 95th percentile
- A 15-year old girl who is 63" tall and weighs 160 has a body mass of 28.3, just over the 95th percentile
- A 16-year old girl who is 65" tall and weighs 174 has a body mass of 28.9, just over the 95th percentile

—KB

CDC Growth Charts: United States

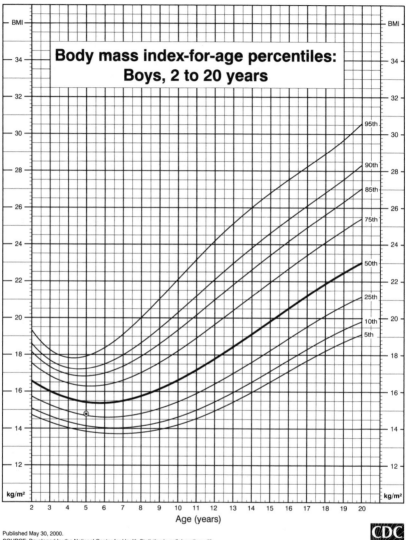

Body mass index-for-age percentiles:
Boys, 2 to 20 years

Published May 30, 2000.
SOURCE: Developed by the National Center for Health Statistics in collaboration with
the National Center for Chronic Disease Prevention and Health Promotion (2000).

Figure 28.1. BMI-for-Age, Boys.

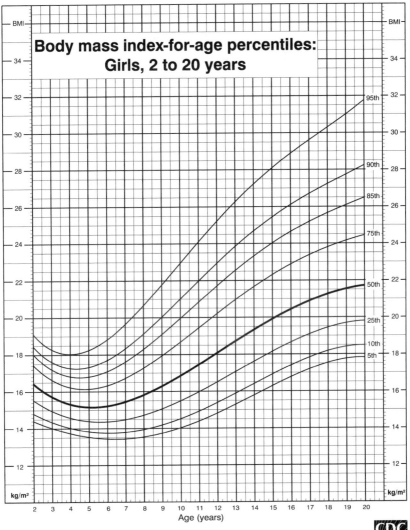

Figure 28.2. BMI-for-Age, Girls.

effect than genes on a person's risk of becoming overweight. If your family eats a lot of high-fat foods or snacks or doesn't get much exercise, you may tend to do the same. The good news is these habits can be changed for the better. Even simple forms of exercise, such as walking, have huge benefits for a person's health.

It can be tough dealing with the physical changes our bodies go through during puberty. But at this time, more than any other, it's not a specific number on the scale that's important. It's keeping your body healthy—inside and out.

♣ It's A Fact!!

Body Mass Index For Adults

BMI is just one of many factors related to developing a chronic disease (such as heart disease, cancer, or diabetes). Other factors that may be important to look at when assessing your risk for chronic disease include the following:

- Diet
- Physical activity
- Waist circumference
- Blood pressure
- Blood sugar level
- Cholesterol level
- Family history of disease

Table 28.2. Body Mass Index for Adults

BMI	Weight Status
Below 18.5	Underweight
18.5–24.9	Normal
25.0–29.9	Overweight
30.0 and Above	Obese

Common Myths

Myth: BMI Measures Body Fat

Two people can have the same BMI, but a different percent body fat. A bodybuilder with a large muscle mass and a low percent body fat may have the same BMI as a person who has more body fat because BMI is calculated using weight and height only.

Myth: BMI is a diagnostic tool

BMI alone is not diagnostic. It is one of many risk factors for disease and death.

Source: Excerpted from "Body Mass Index: BMI for Adults: What Does This All Mean?" Centers for Disease Control and Prevention, December 2004.

Chapter 29

Body Image

Concern with appearance is not new. Every period of history has had a standard of beauty, and every society has had its concept of ideal physical characteristics. For many centuries art depicted female beauty as being soft and curvaceous. The word "Rubenesque," which is used for large, beautiful women, comes from the 17th century paintings of Flemish artist Peter Paul Rubens.

Just a little over a century ago, a pale complexion was considered beautiful and women used umbrellas to protect their skin from the sun. They certainly wouldn't have gone to tanning parlors. Curves were created by corsets and bustles. Plumpness signified wealth and an abundance of food.

In the Roaring Twenties we saw the era of the flat-chested, slim-hipped flapper. By the 50s, full-figures were back in style, like Marilyn Monroe. A model of the 50s was 5'8" and weighed 132 pounds, a very healthy weight. Just one decade later, Twiggy was the beginning of the ultra thin ideal.

Ever since the 60s, ideal has been underweight. Look at how Miss America has changed. For the first 40 years Miss Americas were a healthy weight; for

About This Chapter: Excerpted from "What's Your Make and Model?" by Barbara J. Mayfield, the Maryland State Department of Education, © 2005 Maryland State Department of Education. Non-Exclusive Permission to Use Granted to Omnigraphics, Inc. Detroit, Michigan, 48226. All Other Rights Reserved by MSDE.

the past 40 years they have been underweight. In the 70s and 80s, 'ideal' became taller and more toned. The typical model was 5'8" as in the 50s, but now weighed only 117 pounds, which is classified as underweight.

The early 90s popularized the waif-like look of Kate Moss, tall and very thin, a nearly unattainable figure for most women, no matter how hard they tried. The decade of the 90s also glamorized large breasts. A tall, thin woman doesn't often have large breasts, so this is usually achieved with the help of cosmetic surgery. According to the American Society of Plastic Surgeons, nearly a quarter of a million women have breast augmentation surgery each year in the United States.

> ### ♣ It's A Fact!!
> ### What is body image?
>
> - body image is how you experience your body mentally, emotionally, and physically
> - body image is the way you think about your body
> - body image is the way you feel about your body
> - body image is how you experience living in your body
>
> Source: © 2005 Maryland State Department of Education.

The average woman in North America is 5'4" tall, weighs more than 150 pounds, and has more than 32% body fat. The average model or actress is much taller, rarely weighs over 120 pounds, and has less than 18% body fat.

Culture makes a big difference in the definition of beauty. Unlike white women, women of other cultures—African-American, Asian, Latino—have a much broader definition of beauty and are much more likely to have a positive body image. In a study at Washington University, black women rated themselves as more attractive than pictures of supposedly 'beautiful' white fashion models. Another study of overweight black women, found that 40% of these women rated their figures as attractive or very attractive.

Although African-American women in general are more comfortable with rounder body shapes than white women, many black models and actresses portray the same unrealistic thinness as white models. For example, actress Halle Berry, is 5'7" tall and weighs just 103 pounds.

In case you young men thought society only had an unrealistic definition of the 'ideal' female, here are some descriptions of the 'ideal' male: He is tall, a couple of inches taller than an average man. He has broad shoulders and a narrow waist, a good 5" smaller than an average man's waist. He is muscular and has only 15% body fat. Strength and vitality have long been the ideal for men, but Michelangelo's David, portrays muscular leanness that is more realistic than the men on the cover of muscle magazines today.

There is no question society's definition of the 'ideal' body affects our body image. Thanks to the media, we have become accustomed to a narrow definition of beauty, and we see a lot of it. We see 'beautiful' people all the time. The average American sees 3,000 ads every day. (J. Kilbourne, 2000 *Killing Us Softly 3: Advertisings Image of Women*.) It has been estimated that young women today see more images of outstandingly beautiful women in one day than their grandmothers saw throughout their entire adolescence.

These ads and media images are not pictures of people who look like us. But, because we see them so much, it makes us believe these images are real, normal, and attainable—when this ideal is actually unattainable by all but 4–5% of the population.

✔ Quick Tip

Accept your genetic body build instead of trying to make your body into a shape that's unrealistic for you. Aim for healthy living instead of only focusing on weight. Be physically active for 30–60 minutes most days of the week and use the food guide pyramid to judge your food choices. Explore your emotional, social, mental, and spiritual health as well. Seek help if needed. Don't go too long between meals to avoid becoming over-hungry. Aim for eating enough to feel just satisfied instead of full. Drink eight cups of water daily. If you eat many foods that are high in sugar and/or fat, try to decrease those amounts; substitute with more fruits, vegetables, and whole grains.

Source: Excerpted from "Nutrition Tips for Teens,"
© 2003 Munson Healthcare. All rights reserved. Reprinted with permission.

Thanks to the wonders of technology, many of the 'perfect' images we see are created by airbrushing. The models and actresses don't look like they appear. According to the magazine industry, nearly all magazine covers and advertising photos have been digitally retouched to remove imperfections and can even shave pounds and inches off thighs and arms and change body parts like noses and chins. The cost for retouching a cover photo may run as high as $20,000.

If we add ideal face, skin, and hair to ideal shape and size, this 'ideal' of beauty is achievable by probably 1% or less of the population. Is it any wonder that more than 75% of American women are dissatisfied with their appearance? Body dissatisfaction is so common in our culture that it is considered a 'normative discontent.'

Women are much more critical of their appearance than men are. Men looking in the mirror are more likely to be either pleased or indifferent to what they see. Studies show that men have a much more positive body image than women and in fact often overestimate their attractiveness, overlooking flaws in their appearance much more often than women.

> **✔ Quick Tip**
>
> If you start to have negative thoughts about your body and the way you look, think about all of the special traits that make you who you are. Look at your whole self—body and mind—in a positive way and write down what you see. Focus on the good things in your life (you may want to use the 4Girls log online at http://www.4girls.gov/mind/just4me.htm). If you are struggling with an eating disorder or just can't seem to feel better, talk to an adult you trust right away.
>
> Remember:
> - You are beautiful.
> - You are one of a kind.
> - Real beauty comes from inside.
>
> Source: From "Body Image and Eating Disorders," U.S. Department of Health and Human Services, 4GirlsHealth (www.4girls.gov), August 2005.

Studies show that female dissatisfaction with appearance begins at a very early age. Toddlers can recognize themselves in a mirror at age 2, and young girls begin to dislike their image only a few years later. Surveys of young children show girls as young as 6 years old are going on diets because they think they are fat. By the age of 9, half of all girls have already gone on a diet.

Remember!!

- Body image dissatisfaction affects our mental health. It is associated with low self-esteem, anxiety, and the development of depression.

- Body image dissatisfaction affects our eating behavior. It is associated with disordered eating, such as extreme dieting behaviors and eating disorders like anorexia and bulimia.

- Body image dissatisfaction affects our physical activity behaviors. A poor body image makes participation in activities less enjoyable and may lead many adolescents to opt out of physical activities for sport or recreation.

- Body image dissatisfaction can affect weight management. A poor body image can contribute to the development of overweight in several related ways. A high degree of body dissatisfaction is linked to dieting and binge eating, combined with reduced physical activity. Together these can lead to an unhealthy weight gain.

Source: © 2005 Maryland State Department of Education.

Boys have been shown to go through a period of body dissatisfaction prior to adolescence, but the changes that come with puberty help move boys closer to the masculine ideal because boys grow taller, get broader shoulders, and become more muscular overall.

The normal changes of puberty have the opposite effect on girls. Normal physical maturity brings an increase in weight and fat, especially on the hips and thighs, which takes girls further from society's ideal of thinness.

One of the ways you are sent the message of what is the 'ideal' body, are the toys you grew up with. How many of you played with action figures like GI Joe or fashion dolls like Barbie? According to Mattel, Inc., the average U.S. girl between 3 and 10 years old owns 8 Barbie dolls.

Barbie is the 11" plastic symbol of Americana. She was created in 1959 and since then has never had thighs that rub together. She didn't start smiling until 1971, the year Malibu Barbie came out, one of the most popular Barbies of all time.

If Barbie were a real person, she would stand 6' tall, weigh 101 pounds, wear a size 4, and her measurements would be 39-19-33, hardly realistic (source: www.anred.com). If GI Joe were real, his biceps would be 27" in circumference and his chest would measure 55".

Chapter 30

Do You Need To Gain Weight?

"I want to play hockey, like I did in middle school, but now that I'm in high school, the other guys have bulked up and I haven't. What can I do?"

"All of my friends have broad shoulders and look like they lift weights. No matter what I do, I just look scrawny. What can I do?"

"It's not like I want to gain a lot of weight, but I'd like to look like I have some curves, like the girls I see on TV. What can I do?"

A lot of teens think that they're too skinny, and wonder if they should do something about it. But before you start any kind of plan to gain weight, there's an important question to answer: Why?

Why Do People Want To Gain Weight?

Before you do anything to try to gain weight, it's a good idea to look at your reasons for wanting to do so. Some of the reasons people give for wanting to gain weight are:

I'm worried that there's something wrong with me. If you want to gain weight because you think you have a medical problem, talk to your doctor.

About This Chapter: This information, from "Should I Gain Weight?" was provided by TeensHealth, one of the largest resources online for medically reviewed health information written for parents, kids, and teens. For more articles like this one, visit www.TeensHealth.org, or www.KidsHealth.org. © 2005 The Nemours Center for Children's Health Media, a division of The Nemours Foundation.

Although certain health conditions can cause a person to be underweight, most of them have symptoms other than skinniness, like stomach pain or diarrhea. So it's likely that if some kind of medical problem is making you skinny, you probably wouldn't feel well.

I'm worried because all of my friends have filled out and I haven't. Many guys and girls are really skinny until they start to go through puberty. The changes that come with puberty include weight gain, and, in guys, broader shoulders and increased muscle mass.

Because everyone is on a different schedule, some of your friends may have started to fill out when they were as young as eight (if they are girls) or ten (if they are boys). But for some normal kids, puberty may not start until 12 for girls or 14 for guys. And even if you start puberty then, it may take three or four years for you to fully develop and gain all of the weight and muscle mass you will have as an adult.

Some people experience what's called delayed puberty. This usually can be explained simply as being a "late bloomer" (you may find that some relatives of yours developed late, too). Most teens who experience delayed puberty don't need to do anything; they'll eventually develop normally—and that includes gaining weight and muscle. If you are concerned about delayed puberty, though, talk to your doctor.

Our genes play an important role in determining our body type. Adult bodies come in all different shapes and sizes, and some people stay lean their entire lives, no matter what they do.

I've always wanted to play a certain sport—now I don't know if I can. Lots of people come to love a sport in grade school or middle school—and then find themselves on the bench when their teammates develop faster. If you've always envisioned yourself playing football, it can be tough when your body doesn't seem to want to measure up. You may need to wait until your body goes through puberty before you can play football on the varsity squad.

Another option to consider is switching your ambitions to another sport. If it seems that your body type is long and lean and you were the fastest defensive player on your middle school football team, maybe track and field is for you. Many adults find that the sports they love the most are those that fit their body types the best.

I just hate the way I look! Developing can be tough enough without the pressure to be perfect. Your body changes (or doesn't change), your friends' bodies change (or don't), and you all spend a lot of time noticing. It's easy to judge both yourself and others based on appearances. It can feel like life is some kind of beauty contest.

Your body is your own, and as frustrating as it may seem to begin with, there are certain things you can't speed up or change. But there is one thing you can do to help: Work to keep your body healthy so that you can grow and develop properly. Self-esteem can play a part here, too. People who learn to love their bodies and accept them for what they are carry themselves well and project a type of self-confidence that helps them look attractive.

If you're having trouble with your body image, talk about how you feel with someone you like and trust who's been through it—a parent, doctor, counselor, coach, or teacher.

It's The Growth, Not The Gain

No matter what your reason is for wanting to gain weight, here's a simple fact: The majority of teens have no reason—medical or otherwise—to try to gain weight. An effort like this will at best simply not work and at worst increase your body fat, putting you at risk for health problems.

So focus on growing strong, not gaining weight. Keeping your body healthy and fit so that it grows well is an important part of your job as a teen. Here are some things you can do to help this happen:

Make nutrition your mission. Your friends who want to slim down are eating more salads and fruit. Here's a surprise: So should you. You can do more for your body by eating a variety of healthier foods instead of trying to pack on body fat by forcing yourself to eat a lot of unhealthy high-fat, high-sugar foods. Chances are, high-fat foods won't help you gain weight anyway. Eating a variety of healthy foods, making time for regular meals and snacks, and eating only until you are full will give your body its best chance to stay healthy as it gets the fuel and nutrients it needs.

Good nutrition doesn't have to be complicated. Here are some simple tips:

- Eat lots of vegetables, fruits, and whole grains.

- Eat breakfast every day.

- Eat regular snacks.

- Eat a variety of foods. That can sometimes include less nutritious ones, like chips and soda. But try to limit them so you don't crowd out healthier food and drinks.

✔ **Quick Tip**   **Gaining Weight**

Being underweight can have just as many health risks as being overweight. If you are underweight, you are at risk for a nutrient deficiency, which has several implications such as anemia, osteoporosis, skin disorders, muscle wasting, mental confusion, physical fatigue, and an overall "drained" appearance.

Below are a few suggestions that may help you increase calories along with nutrients and help you gain weight:

- Spread peanut butter on anything with which it is compatible. You may swirl peanut butter into ice cream, shakes or hot cereal, or use it as a dip for fruits and vegetables.

- Add powdered milk to whole milk, shakes, gravies, pudding, mashed potatoes, scrambled eggs, casseroles, and even meat loaf.

- Drink two to three instant breakfasts or other nutritional supplements daily in addition to your normal intake.

- Drink as many calories as you can. Drinking calories is less filling and allows more room for additional high-calorie food.

- Use eggs to make French toast or add them to pancake batter, casseroles, soups, gravy, and sauces. Add chopped boiled eggs to salads. You can also use egg substitute to enhance foods with protein.

- Melt cheese on hamburgers, hot dogs, other meats, vegetables, tortillas, noodles, and scrambled eggs—anything with which it is compatible. Add

Eating well at this point in your life is important for lots of reasons. It's a key part of normal growth and development. It's also good to learn good habits now—they'll become second nature, which will help you stay healthy and fit without even thinking about it.

Keep on moving. Another way to keep your body healthy is to incorporate regular exercise. This can simply be a matter of walking to school, playing Frisbee with your friends, or helping out with some household chores. Or you might choose to work out at a gym or with a sports team. A good rule of thumb for exercise amounts during the teen years: Try to get 30 to 60 minutes

---

sliced cheese to sandwiches. Melt it in soups, casseroles, and mashed potatoes, or use it as a topping for salads and crackers.

- Use cream cheese on breads or graham crackers. Try melting it on vegetables, such as spinach, with cream cheese mixed in. Mix cream cheese with gravies or use as a dip for fruits and vegetables.

- Make trail mixes with high-calorie peanuts, almonds, cashews, granola and other cereals, and dried fruit. Place trail mix in a convenient spot and, every time you see it, you can grab a handful.

- Use oils to fry foods. Use butter on vegetables and in hot cereal. Use mayonnaise on sandwiches and in mashed potatoes. Use bacon on sandwiches and crumbled on salads and baked potatoes. Use avocados as a dip or sliced on sandwiches. Use regular salad dressings and sour cream on potatoes, in soups, or as a dip.

If you remain underweight or begin to lose more weight, please consult a physician.

Hyperthyroidism and several other disorders can cause underweight status and, if left untreated, can result in a far more serious threat to your life.

Source: Excerpted from "Gaining Weight," by 1st Lt. Cheryl Chmielewski, General Leonard Wood Army Community Hospital, Fort Leonard Wood, Mo. (Reprinted from the Fort Leonard Wood *Guidon*), Health Tips from Army Medicine, November 2003.

of activity every day (like walking to school or around the mall) and get more vigorous activity (like playing soccer or skating) for at 20 minutes or more at least three times a week.

> **Remember!!**
> Focus on feeling good. It can help to know that your body is likely to change in the months and years ahead. Few of us look at 25 like we did at 15. But, it's also important to realize that feeling good about yourself can make you more attractive to others, too.

Strength training, when done safely, is a healthy way to exercise, but it won't necessarily bulk you up. Guys especially get more muscular during puberty, but puberty is no guarantee that you'll turn into a cover model for *Muscle & Fitness* in a couple of years—some people just don't have the kind of body type for this to happen.

If you've hit puberty, the right amount of weight training will help your muscles become stronger and have more endurance. And, once a person's reached puberty, proper weight training can help him or her bulk up a bit, if that's the goal. Be sure to work with a certified trainer, who can show you how to do it without injuring yourself. It can be easy to overdo strength training, especially during the teenage years when there's more risk of injuring bones that haven't finished growing yet.

Get the skinny on supplements. Thinking about drinking something from a can or taking a pill to turn you buff overnight? Guess again. Supplements or pills that make promises like this are at best a waste of money and at worst potentially harmful to your health.

The best way to get the fuel you need to build muscle is by eating well. Before you take any kind of supplement at all—even if it's just a vitamin pill—you should talk to your doctor.

Sleep your way to stunning. Sleep is an important component of normal growth and development. If you get enough, you'll have the energy to fuel your growth. Your body is at work while it sleeps—oxygen moves to the brain, growth hormones are released, and your bones keep on developing, even while you're resting.

Chapter 31

Myths About Nutrition And Weight Loss

Diet Myths

Myth: Fad diets work for permanent weight loss.

Fact: Fad diets are not the best way to lose weight and keep it off. Fad diets often promise quick weight loss or tell you to cut certain foods out of your diet. You may lose weight at first on one of these diets. But diets that strictly limit calories or food choices are hard to follow. Most people quickly get tired of them and regain any lost weight.

Fad diets may be unhealthy because they may not provide all of the nutrients your body needs. Also, losing weight at a very rapid rate (more than three pounds a week after the first couple weeks) may increase your risk for developing gallstones (clusters of solid material in the gallbladder that can be painful). Diets that provide less than 800 calories per day also could result in heart rhythm abnormalities, which can be fatal.

Tip: Research suggests that losing ½ to 2 pounds a week by making healthy food choices, eating moderate portions, and building physical activity into your daily life is the best way to lose weight and keep it off. By adopting

About This Chapter: From "Weight-loss and Nutrition Myths: How Much Do You Really Know?" Weight-Control Information Network, an information service of the National Institute of Diabetes and Digestive and Kidney Diseases, NIH Pub. No. 04-4561, March 2004.

healthy eating and physical activity habits, you may also lower your risk for developing type 2 diabetes, heart disease, and high blood pressure.

Myth: High-protein/low-carbohydrate diets are a healthy way to lose weight.

Fact: The long-term health effects of a high-protein/low-carbohydrate diet are unknown. But getting most of your daily calories from high-protein foods like meat, eggs, and cheese is not a balanced eating plan. You may be eating too much fat and cholesterol, which may raise heart disease risk. You may be eating too few fruits, vegetables, and whole grains, which may lead to constipation due to lack of dietary fiber. Following a high-protein/low-carbohydrate diet may also make you feel nauseous, tired, and weak.

Eating fewer than 130 grams of carbohydrate a day can lead to the buildup of ketones (partially broken-down fats) in your blood. A buildup of ketones in your blood (called ketosis) can cause your body to produce high levels of uric acid, which is a risk factor for gout (a painful swelling of the joints) and kidney stones. Ketosis may be especially risky for pregnant women and people with diabetes or kidney disease.

Tip: High-protein/low-carbohydrate diets are often low in calories because food choices are strictly limited, so they may cause short-term weight loss. But a reduced-calorie eating plan that includes

---

♣ It's A Fact!!

- "Lose 30 pounds in 30 days!"

- "Eat as much as you want and still lose weight!"

- "Try the thigh buster and lose inches fast!"

An so on, and so on, and so on. With so many products and weight-loss theories out there, it's easy to get confused.

The information in this chapter will help clear up confusion about weight loss, nutrition, and physical activity. It may also help you make healthy changes in your eating and physical activity habits. If you have questions not answered here, or if you want to lose weight, talk to your health care provider. A registered dietitian or other qualified health professional can give you advice on how to follow a healthy eating plan, lose weight safely, and keep it off.

Source: NIDDK, 2004.

recommended amounts of carbohydrate, protein, and fat will also allow you to lose weight. By following a balanced eating plan, you will not have to stop eating whole classes of foods, such as whole grains, fruits, and vegetables—and miss the key nutrients they contain. You may also find it easier to stick with a diet or eating plan that includes a greater variety of foods.

Myth: Starches are fattening and should be limited when trying to lose weight.

Fact: Many foods high in starch, like bread, rice, pasta, cereals, beans, fruits, and some vegetables (like potatoes and yams) are low in fat and calories. They become high in fat and calories when eaten in large portion sizes or when covered with high-fat toppings like butter, sour cream, or mayonnaise. Foods high in starch (also called complex carbohydrates) are an important source of energy for your body.

Tip: The Dietary Guidelines for Americans recommends eating 6 to 11 servings a day, depending on your calorie needs, from the bread, cereal, rice, and pasta group—even when trying to lose weight. Pay attention to your serving sizes—one serving is equal to one slice of bread, 1 ounce of ready-to-eat cereal, or ½ cup of pasta, rice, or cooked cereal. Try to avoid high-fat toppings and choose whole grains, like whole wheat bread, brown rice, oatmeal, and bran cereal. Choose other starchy foods that are high in dietary fiber too, like beans, peas, and vegetables.

Myth: Certain foods, like grapefruit, celery, or cabbage soup, can burn fat and make you lose weight.

Fact: No foods can burn fat. Some foods with caffeine may speed up your metabolism (the way your body uses energy, or calories) for a short time, but they do not cause weight loss.

Tip: The best way to lose weight is to cut back on the number of calories you eat and be more physically active.

Myth: Natural or herbal weight-loss products are safe and effective.

Fact: A weight-loss product that claims to be "natural" or "herbal" is not necessarily safe. These products are not usually scientifically tested to prove that they are safe or that they work. For example, herbal products containing ephedra (now banned by the U.S. Government) have caused serious health problems and even death. Newer products that claim to be ephedra-free are not necessarily danger-free, because they may contain ingredients similar to ephedra.

Tip: Talk with your health care provider before using any weight-loss product. Some natural or herbal weight-loss products can be harmful.

Meal Myths

Myth: "I can lose weight while eating whatever I want."

Fact: To lose weight, you need to use more calories than you eat. It is possible to eat any kind of food you want and lose weight. You need to limit the number of calories you eat every day and/or increase your daily physical activity. Portion control is the key. Try eating smaller amounts of food and choosing foods that are low in calories.

Tip: When trying to lose weight, you can still eat your favorite foods—as long as you pay attention to the total number of calories that you eat.

Myth: Low-fat or nonfat means no calories.

Fact: A low-fat or nonfat food is often lower in calories than the same size portion of the full-fat product. But many processed low-fat or nonfat foods have just as many calories as the full-fat version of the same food or even more calories. They may contain added sugar, flour, or starch thickeners to improve flavor and texture after fat is removed. These ingredients add calories.

Tip: Read the Nutrition Facts Label on a food package to find out how many calories are in a serving. Check the serving size too it may be less than you are used to eating.

Myth: Fast foods are always an unhealthy choice and you should not eat them when dieting.

Fact: Fast foods can be part of a healthy weight-loss program with a little bit of know-how.

Tip: Avoid supersize combo meals, or split one with a friend. Sip on water or nonfat milk instead of soda. Choose salads and grilled foods, like a grilled chicken breast sandwich or small hamburger. Try a "fresco" taco (with salsa instead of cheese or sauce) at taco stands. Fried foods, like French fries and fried chicken, are high in fat and calories, so order them only once in a while, order a small portion, or split an order with a friend. Also, use only small amounts of high-fat, high-calorie toppings, like regular mayonnaise, salad dressings, bacon, and cheese.

Myth: Skipping meals is a good way to lose weight.

Fact: Studies show that people who skip breakfast and eat fewer times during the day tend to be heavier than people who eat a healthy breakfast and eat four or five times a day. This may be because people who skip meals tend to feel hungrier later on and eat more than they normally would. It may also be that eating many small meals throughout the day helps people control their appetites.

Tip: Eat small meals throughout the day that include a variety of healthy, low-fat, low-calorie foods.

✔ Quick Tip
Eat Breakfast

Tests show students perform better mentally and physically when they eat breakfast. Give it a try for one week and see if you feel a difference. Grab-n-go breakfast items include: a fruit smoothie made the night before, trail mix, yogurt, cheese stick and crackers, bread, fruit, peanut butter sandwich, and leftovers.

Source: Excerpted from "Nutrition Tips for Teens," © 2003 Munson Healthcare. All rights reserved. Reprinted with permission.

Myth: Eating after 8 p.m. causes weight gain.

Fact: It does not matter what time of day you eat. It is what and how much you eat and how much physical activity you do during the whole day that determines whether you gain, lose, or maintain your weight. No matter when you eat, your body will store extra calories as fat.

Tip: If you want to have a snack before bedtime, think first about how many calories you have eaten that day. And try to avoid snacking in front of the TV at night it may be easier to overeat when you are distracted by the television.

Physical Activity Myth

Myth: Lifting weights is not good to do if you want to lose weight, because it will make you "bulk up."

Fact: Lifting weights or doing strengthening activities like push-ups and crunches on a regular basis can actually help you maintain or lose weight. These activities can help you build muscle, and muscle burns more calories than body fat. So if you have more muscle, you burn more calories—even sitting still. Doing strengthening activities two or three days a week will not "bulk you up." Only intense strength training, combined with a certain genetic background, can build very large muscles.

Tip: In addition to doing at least 30 minutes of moderate-intensity physical activity (like walking two miles in 30 minutes) on most days of the week, try to do strengthening activities two to three days a week. You can lift weights, use large rubber bands (resistance bands), do push-ups or sit-ups, or do household or garden tasks that make you lift or dig.

Food Myths

Myth: Nuts are fattening and you should not eat them if you want to lose weight.

Fact: In small amounts, nuts can be part of a healthy weight-loss program. Nuts are high in calories and fat. However, most nuts contain healthy fats that do not clog arteries. Nuts are also good sources of protein, dietary fiber, and minerals including magnesium and copper.

Tip: Enjoy small portions of nuts. One-third cup of mixed nuts has about 270 calories.

Myth: Eating red meat is bad for your health and makes it harder to lose weight.

Fact: Eating lean meat in small amounts can be part of a healthy weight-loss plan. Red meat, pork, chicken, and fish contain some cholesterol and saturated fat (the least healthy kind of fat). They also contain healthy nutrients like protein, iron, and zinc.

Tip: Choose cuts of meat that are lower in fat and trim all visible fat. Lower fat meats include pork tenderloin and beef round steak, tenderloin, sirloin tip, flank steak, and extra lean ground beef. Also, pay attention to portion size. One serving is two to three ounces of cooked meat—about the size of a deck of cards.

Myth: Dairy products are fattening and unhealthy.

Fact: Low-fat and nonfat milk, yogurt, and cheese are just as nutritious as whole milk dairy products, but they are lower in fat and calories. Dairy products have many nutrients your body needs. They offer protein to build muscles and help organs work properly, and calcium to strengthen bones. Most milks and some yogurts are fortified with vitamin D to help your body use calcium.

Tip: The *Dietary Guidelines for Americans* recommend that people aged 9 to 18 and over age 50 have three servings of milk, yogurt, and cheese a day. Adults aged 19 to 49 need two servings a day, even when trying to lose weight. A serving is equal to 1 cup of milk or yogurt, 1½ ounces of natural cheese such as cheddar, or 2 ounces of processed cheese such as American. Choose low-fat or nonfat dairy products including milk, yogurt, cheese, and ice cream.

If you cannot digest lactose (the sugar found in dairy products), choose low-lactose or lactose-free dairy products, or other foods and beverages that offer calcium and vitamin D.

- Calcium: fortified fruit juice, soy-based beverage, or tofu made with calcium sulfate; canned salmon; dark leafy greens like collards or kale

- Vitamin D: fortified fruit juice, soy-based beverage, or cereal (getting some sunlight on your skin also gives you a small amount of vitamin D

Myth: "Going vegetarian" means you are sure to lose weight and be healthier.

Fact: Research shows that people who follow a vegetarian eating plan, on average, eat fewer calories and less fat than non-vegetarians. They also tend to have lower body weights relative to their heights than non-vegetarians. Choosing a vegetarian eating plan with a low fat content may be helpful for weight loss. But vegetarians—like non-vegetarians—can make food choices that contribute to weight gain, like eating large amounts of high-fat, high-calorie foods or foods with little or no nutritional value.

Vegetarian diets should be as carefully planned as non-vegetarian diets to make sure they are balanced. Nutrients that non-vegetarians normally get from animal products, but that are not always found in a vegetarian eating plan, are iron, calcium, vitamin D, vitamin B_{12}, zinc, and protein.

> ☞ **Remember!!**
>
> If you don't know whether or not to believe a weight-loss or nutrition claim, check it out! The Federal Trade Commission (www.ftc.gov/bcp/conline/features/wgtloss.htm) has information on deceptive weight-loss advertising claims. You can also find out more about nutrition and weight loss by talking with a registered dietitian. To find a registered dietitian in your area, visit the American Dietetic Association (www.eatright.org) online or call 1-800-877-1600.
>
> Source: NIDDK, 2004.

Tip: Choose a vegetarian eating plan that is low in fat and that provides all of the nutrients your body needs. Food and beverage sources of nutrients that may be lacking in a vegetarian diet are as follows.

- Iron: cashews, spinach, lentils, garbanzo beans, fortified bread or cereal

- Calcium: dairy products, fortified soy-based beverages or fruit juices, tofu made with calcium sulfate, collard greens, kale, broccoli

- Vitamin D: fortified foods and beverages including milk, soy-based beverages, fruit juices, or cereal

- Vitamin B_{12}: eggs, dairy products, fortified cereal or soy-based beverages, tempeh, miso (tempeh and miso are foods made from soybeans)

- Zinc: whole grains (especially the germ and bran of the grain), nuts, tofu, leafy vegetables (spinach, cabbage, lettuce)

- Protein: eggs, dairy products, beans, peas, nuts, seeds, tofu, tempeh, soy-based burgers.

Chapter 32

Weight-Loss Ads Heavy On Deception

A report from the Federal Trade Commission (FTC) finds that many weight-loss ads need some toning.

The review of 300 ads that ran during 2001 found that many made claims promising more than the product or service could likely deliver. The ads often boasted "miraculous" results—quick, easy, and effective weight loss—while ignoring and often contradicting the basic tenets of successful weight loss and weight maintenance—calorie reduction and exercise. Many ads lacked scientific evidence to support their performance claims, instead using misleading consumer testimonials and expert endorsements and other deceptive techniques to bolster the credibility of their products.

And, the report found, the use of exaggerated weight-loss claims is on the rise.

"This report confirms that consumers really need to read these ads with a big dollop of skepticism," said Richard Cleland, an Assistant Director for the FTC's Division of Advertising Practices and the report's lead author. "False and misleading claims in weight-loss ads are widespread."

About This Chapter: From "Tipping the Scales? Weight-Loss Ads Found Heavy on Deception," Federal Trade Commission, September 2002.

The report, he says, shows that the media, advertisers, and even consumers need to assess the role each plays in ensuring the accuracy of weight-loss ads. "Deceptive ads do nothing to address an individual's weight problem," he says. "If anything, they compound an already serious national health crisis by steering consumers away from weight-loss methods that have demonstrated benefits."

♣ It's A Fact!!

The FTC works for the consumer to prevent fraudulent, deceptive and unfair business practices in the marketplace and to provide information to help consumers spot, stop, and avoid them. To file a complaint or to get free information on consumer issues, visit http://www.ftc.gov or call toll-free, 1-877-FTC-HELP (1-877-382-4357); TTY: 1-866-653-4261.

Source: Federal Trade Commission, September 2002.

Quick Fixes And Other Claims

The FTC report involved a review of 300 ads from TV, radio, magazines, newspapers, direct mail solicitations, commercial e-mail, and internet websites, as well as a comparison of weight-loss ads from eight national magazines published in 1992 and 2001. FTC staff, with help from the Partnership for Healthy Weight Management—a coalition of representatives from science, academia, healthcare professions, government, commercial enterprises, and other organizations—collected and reviewed the ads.

Among the 300 ads that ran in 2001, the researchers found that 55 percent made at least one false or unsubstantiated claim. The claims generally promised:

- **Rapid weight loss:** Claims like "You can lose 18 pounds in one week!" and "You only have to stay on it 2 DAYS TO SEE RESULTS" were the most common; they appeared in 56 percent of the ads. Claims of quick weight loss also were alluded to in product names, like "Redu-Quick" and "Slim Down Fast." In reality, substantial weight loss in a short period is highly unlikely and potentially harmful. Experts generally recommend a maximum weight loss of one to two pounds a week.

- **No need for dietary restrictions or exercise:** Claims like "Lose up to 8 to 10 pounds per week ... no dieting, no strenuous exercise" and "Eat as much as you want—the more you eat, the more you'll lose" appeared in 44 percent of the ads. Though tempting, these claims contradict scientific evidence that stresses exercise and moderate calorie intake for long-term weight loss.

- **Permanent weight loss:** Claims like "Discover the secret to permanent weight loss" and "Get weight off and keep it off" appeared in 23 percent of the ads, apparently to target consumers who had lost weight but gained it back. Long-term weight loss is extremely hard to achieve, and little evidence exists to show that popular dietary supplements are more successful than lifestyle changes in achieving it. In the FTC's experience, few marketers have the scientific studies to support their long-term weight-loss claims.

- **Lose weight despite previous failures:** Apparently recognizing the low rate of weight-loss success, nearly 33 percent of the ads tried to appeal to frustrated dieters with statements like "Are you tired of fad diets that never seem to work?" and "You want to lose weight, and you've been successful before. But after a while, you're right back where you started." The advertised product or service was then touted as the one that would finally work.

- **Scientifically proven or doctor-endorsed:** Almost 40 percent of the ads claimed that their product or service was "clinically tested" or "scientifically proven." Many claimed their products were tested at "respected," "major," or "leading" medical centers or universities. However, most of the ads did not provide details—such as where the referenced study was conducted and by whom or where it was published—to help consumers assess the claims' validity. In addition, almost one-fourth of the ads stated that the product was "recommended," "approved," or "discovered" by a health professional—endorsements that can be misleading because the ads may not disclose that the medical professional has a financial interest in the product, because the health professional may not have reviewed the scientific evidence or because, if the health professional did, he or she may not have used acceptable review standards. The "professionals" also can be fictional.

- **Money-back guarantees:** About 50 percent of the ads promised money-back guarantees, apparently in an attempt to break down consumers' resistance to buying new products and services. Some ads made specific guarantees like "You will lose up to 35 pounds in three weeks. Yes. Guaranteed! You lose or it doesn't cost you a penny." While money-back guarantees—if honored—may benefit consumers, there is no reason for consumers to have any more confidence in them than in a claim that the product will actually work. And the FTC frequently has sued companies that "guaranteed" to give consumers their money back but didn't.

- **Safety:** Some 43 percent of the ads made safety-related claims, such as "proven 100% safe," "safe, immediate weight loss" and "safest weight management system in the world." The term "natural" accompanied three-fourths of these claims, perhaps relying on a perception that "natural" products are safer than prescription or over-the-counter medicines. Many ads also implied safety with claims like "not a prescription weight-loss drug" and "no dangerous pills or tablets to take." Despite the safety assurances, the FTC's Cleland says, there is little evidence on safety, particularly with long-term use of the products. "Many ads handicap consumers by not even revealing what the active ingredients are in the products being sold," he says.

Before-And-After Testimonials

Unsupported claims often appeared in consumer testimonials—that is, personal accounts of success with the product or service. One testimonial said, "7 weeks ago I weighed 268 pounds; now I'm down to just 148 pounds! ... I didn't change my eating habits ...."

Before-and-after photos appeared in 39 percent of the ads. In the before photo, the person usually appeared with poor posture, a neutral facial expression, unkempt hair, unfashionable clothes, and washed-out skin tones. The after photo, however, was better lit, almost of studio-quality. The person was smiling, wearing fashionable clothes or skimpily clad, carefully made up and stylishly coifed, and standing with shoulders held back and tummy tucked in.

At least 10 percent of the testimonials claimed an amount of weight loss that is extremely unlikely—if not impossible. The rest probably provided results that occurred in only a small percentage of users, Cleland says.

"There's nothing wrong with using testimonials, as long as they are truthful and not misleading," he says. "But in our experience, testimonials generally provide little reliable information about what consumers can expect from using the product."

Changes In Weight-Loss Ads

In comparing weight-loss ads from eight national magazines published in 1992 and 2001, the reviewers found that the use of testimonials and before-and-after photos had increased. The percentage of weight-loss ads using testimonials climbed from 12.5 percent in 1992 to 76 percent in 2001. Use of before-and-after photos increased from 12.5 percent to 48 percent.

Another difference noted was that dietary supplements comprised two-thirds of the weight-loss products advertised in 2001. In 1992, meal replacement products were the most commonly advertised product.

♣ It's A Fact!!

A claim is too good to be true if it says the product will:

- Cause weight loss of two pounds or more a week for a month or more without dieting or exercise;

- Cause substantial weight loss no matter what or how much the consumer eats;

- Cause permanent weight loss (even when the consumer stops using product);

- Block the absorption of fat or calories to enable consumers to lose substantial weight;

- Safely enable consumers to lose more than three pounds per week for more than four weeks;

- Cause substantial weight loss for all users;

- Cause substantial weight loss by wearing it on the body or rubbing it into the skin.

Source: From "Red Flag: Bogus Weight Loss Claims," Federal Trade Commission, 2003.

In addition, the number of times weight-loss ads appeared in the magazines more than doubled between 1992 and 2001, and the 2001 ads generally included more highly questionable claims.

Need For Critical Evaluation

The FTC's report notes that deception in weight-loss advertising has worsened despite an "unprecedented level of FTC enforcement." Since 1990, the FTC has brought more than 80 cases against advertisers for allegedly false and misleading weight-loss claims—more than half the total number filed since the FTC's first weight-loss case in 1927.

☞ Remember!!

If the claim looks too good to be true, it probably is.

Despite claims to the contrary, there are no magic bullets or effortless ways to burn off fat. The only way to lose weight is to lower caloric intake and/or increase physical activity. Claims for diet products or programs that promise weight loss without sacrifice or effort are bogus. And some can even be dangerous.

These facts do not keep fraudulent advertisers from preying on consumers and reaping billions of dollars each year. While the scams may vary (for example, pills, patches, clips, body wraps, insoles or "diet teas"), the claims are almost always the same—dramatic, effortless weight loss without diet or exercise.

Source: Federal Trade Commission, September 2002.

The report calls on government agencies, trade associations, self-regulatory groups, the media, and consumers to consider how they might help reduce the incidence of misleading weight-loss ads.

For consumers, the study provides important information on how to spot deceptive weight-loss products and services, says Walter Gross, an attorney in the FTC's Division of Enforcement and co-author of the study.

"Claims like 'rapid weight loss,' 'no diet or exercise required,' 'eat whatever you want,' and 'take it off and keep it off' are all 'hot' buttons advertisers use to get consumers to buy their products and services," he says. "Knowing how to recognize these will help consumers make more informed choices."

Chapter 33

Losing Weight Safely

Weight loss is a tricky topic. Lots of people are unhappy with their present weight, but most aren't sure how to change it—and many would be better off staying where they are. You may want to look like the models or actors in magazines and on TV, but those goals might not be healthy or realistic for you. Besides, no magical diet or pill will make you look like someone else.

So what should you do about weight control?

Being healthy is really about being at a weight that is right for you. The best way to find out if you are at a healthy weight or if you need to lose or gain weight is to talk to a doctor or dietitian. He or she can compare your weight with healthy norms to help you set realistic goals. If it turns out that you can benefit from weight loss then you can follow a few of the simple suggestions listed below to get started.

Weight management is about long-term success. People who lose weight quickly by crash dieting or other extreme measures usually gain back all (and often more) of the pounds they lost because they haven't permanently changed their habits. Therefore, the best weight management strategies are those that you

About This Chapter: This information, from "How Can I Lose Weight Safely?" was provided by TeensHealth, one of the largest resources online for medically reviewed health information written for parents, kids, and teens. For more articles like this one, visit www.TeensHealth.org, or www.KidsHealth.org. © 2005 The Nemours Center for Children's Health Media, a division of The Nemours Foundation.

can maintain for a lifetime. That's a long time, so we'll try to keep these suggestions as easy as possible.

Make it a family affair. Ask your mom or dad to lend help and support and to make dietary or lifestyle changes that might benefit the whole family, if possible. Teens who have the support of their families tend to have better results with their weight management programs. But remember, you should all work together in a friendly and helpful way—making weight loss into a competition is a recipe for disaster.

Watch your drinks. It's amazing how many extra calories can be lurking in the sodas, juices, and other drinks that you take in every day. Simply cutting out a couple of cans of soda or switching to diet soda can save you 360 calories or more each day. Drink lots of water or other sugar-free drinks to quench your thirst and stay away from sugary juices and sodas. Switching from whole to nonfat or low-fat milk is also a good idea.

Start small. Small changes are a lot easier to stick with than drastic ones. Try reducing the size of the portions you eat and giving up regular soda for

> **✔ Quick Tip**
> For good nutrition, follow and eating plan that:
>
> - is balanced overall, with foods from all groups, with lots of delicious fruits, vegetables, and grains is low in saturated fat and cholesterol and moderate in total fat intake (less than 10 percent of your daily calories should come from saturated fat, and less than 30 percent of your daily calories should come from total fat);
> - includes a variety of grains daily, especially whole grains, a good source of fiber;
> - includes enough fruits and vegetables (a variety of each, five to nine servings each day);
> - has a small number of calories from added sugars (like in candy, cookies, and cakes);
> - has foods prepared with less sodium or salt (aim for no more than 2,400 milligrams of sodium per day, or about one teaspoon of salt per day for a healthy heart).
>
> Source: Excerpted from "Healthy Eating," National Women's Health Information Center, August 2004.

a week. Once you have that down, start gradually introducing healthier foods and exercise into your life.

Stop eating when you're full. Lots of people eat when they're bored, lonely, or stressed, or keep eating long after they're full out of habit. Try to pay attention as you eat and stop when you're full. Slowing down can help because it takes about 20 minutes for your brain to recognize how much is in your stomach. Sometimes taking a break before going for seconds can keep you from eating another serving.

Avoid eating when you feel upset or bored—try to find something else to do instead (a walk around the block or a trip to the gym are good alternatives). Many people find it's helpful to keep a diary of what they eat and when. Reviewing the diary later can help them identify the emotions they have when they overeat or whether they have unhealthy habits. A registered dietitian can give you pointers on how to do this.

Eat less more often. Many people find that eating a couple of small snacks throughout the day helps them to make healthy choices at meals. Stick a couple of healthy snacks (carrot sticks, a low-fat granola bar, pretzels, or a piece of fruit) in your backpack so that you can have one or two snacks during the day. Adding healthy snacks to your three squares and eating smaller portions when you sit down to dinner can help you to cut calories without feeling deprived.

Five a day keep the pounds away. Ditch the junk food and dig out the fruits and veggies. Five servings of fruits and veggies aren't just a good idea to help you lose weight—they'll help keep your heart and the rest of your body healthy. Other suggestions for eating well: replace white bread with whole wheat, trade your sugary sodas for lots of water and a few cups of low-fat milk, and make sure you eat a healthy breakfast. Having low-sugar, whole grain cereal and low-fat milk and a piece of fruit is a much better idea than inhaling a donut as you run to the bus stop or eating no breakfast at all. A registered dietitian can give you lots of other snack and menu ideas.

Avoid fad diets. It's never a good idea to trade meals for shakes or to give up a food group in the hope that you'll lose weight—we all need a variety of foods to stay healthy. Stay away from fad diets because you're still growing and need to make sure you get proper nutrients. Avoid diet pills (even the over-the-counter or herbal variety). They can be dangerous to your health; besides, there's no evidence that they help keep weight off over the long term.

Don't banish certain foods. Don't tell yourself you'll never again eat your absolutely favorite peanut butter chocolate ice cream or a bag of chips from the vending machine at school. Making these foods forbidden is sure to make you want them even more. Also, don't go fat free: You need to have some fat in your diet to stay healthy, so giving up all fatty foods all the time isn't a good idea. The key to long-term success is making healthy choices most of the time. If you want a piece of cake at a party, go for it. But munch on the carrots rather than the chips to balance it out.

Get moving. You may find that you don't need to cut calories as much as you need to get off your behind. Don't get stuck in the rut of thinking you have to play a team sport or take an aerobics class to get exercise. Try a variety of activities from hiking to cycling to rowing until you find ones you like.

Not a jock? Find other ways to fit activity into your day: walk to school, jog up and down the stairs a couple of times before your morning shower, turn off the tube and help your parents in the garden, or take a stroll past your crush's house—anything that gets you moving. Your goal should be to work up to 60 minutes of exercise every day. But everyone has to begin somewhere. It's fine to start out by simply taking a few turns around the block before bed and building up your levels of fitness gradually.

Build muscle. Muscle burns more calories than fat. So adding strength training to your exercise routine can help you reach your weight loss goals as well as give you a toned bod. A good, well-balanced fitness routine includes aerobic workouts, strength training, and flexibility exercises.

Forgive yourself. So you were going to have one cracker with spray cheese on it and the next thing you know the can's pumping air and the box is empty? Drink some water, brush your teeth, and move on. Everyone who's ever tried to lose weight has found it challenging. When you slip up, the best idea is to get right back on track and don't look back. Avoid telling yourself that you'll get back on track tomorrow or next week or after New Year's. Start now.

🖙 Remember!!

Try to remember that losing weight isn't going to make you a better person—and it won't magically change your life. It's a good idea to maintain a healthy weight because it's just that: healthy.

Source: © 2005 The Nemours Center for Children's Health Media, a division of The Nemours Foundation.

Chapter 34

Diet-Plan Diagnosis: Is Yours Healthy And Safe?

Want to drop a few pounds before that big date on Friday? Feeling the need to lose weight to boost your athletic performance? Many people look for fast or easy ways to slim down at some point in their lives. And there are hundreds of diet plans out there to lure you. But before you choose between the all-juice diet and the no-carb diet, read on to find out exactly what these diets do—and don't do—for you.

What are popular weight-loss plans and how well do they work?

Commercial weight-loss plans typically fall into two categories: Those that drastically reduce a person's calorie intake or restrict the dieter to certain foods and those that require a person to take dietary supplements. Dietary supplements are usually pills, but they sometimes include special food bars or drinks.

Most of the popular diets on the market today rely on a person's natural tendency to want to lose weight quickly. They play into a desire for fast results, which is what happened to Jamie, 16, who followed a 5-day juice

About This Chapter: This information was provided by TeensHealth, one of the largest resources online for medically reviewed health information written for parents, kids, and teens. For more articles like this one, visit www.TeensHealth.org, or www.KidsHealth.org. © 2004 The Nemours Center for Children's Health Media, a division of The Nemours Foundation.

diet. Although Jamie lost the weight she wanted, a week later the scale showed she was back to her original weight.

It's quite common for people to quickly gain back all the weight they lose after a few days on a highly restrictive diet. Here's a doctor's answer on why: "The first thing to be aware of with quick weight-loss diets is that our bodies simply aren't designed to drop pounds quickly," says Steven Dowshen, MD, an expert in hormones and the endocrine system. In fact, doctors say that it's nearly impossible for a healthy, normally active teen or adult to lose more than about three pounds per week of actual fat from their bodies, even on a starvation diet.

So why does your scale tell you otherwise? "The trick these very low-calorie diets rely on is that your body's natural reaction to near-starvation is to dump water," Dr. Dowshen says. That means that most, if not all, of the weight you lose during the first few days on these diets is water, not fat. You may feel thinner, but you won't look it and

> **✔ Quick Tip**
> **Ditch These Diets**
>
> In general, you should avoid diets that require you to:
>
> • starve or drastically reduce your food intake.
>
> • eat only certain foods or eat foods in a specific order or combination.
>
> • skip meals or substitute beverages or energy/protein bars for meals.
>
> • cut fats, sugars, or carbohydrates from your diet completely.
>
> • use laxatives or water pills (also known as diuretics).
>
> • take pills, powders, or large doses of vitamins or herbal supplements.
>
> • wear a skin patch, body magnet, electrical stimulation device, or other apparatus.
>
> • reduce or eliminate physical activity.
>
> • focus on quick weight loss.
>
> Source: Nemours Foundation, 2004.

you'll probably bounce back up to your original weight once you start eating normally again. "What these diet plans don't tell you is that your body will just suck this lost water back up like a sponge once you start eating more calories again," Dr. Dowshen says.

Losing water weight is also the key to the quick weight-loss claims of some of the diet pills on the market. Many of these pills contain laxatives or diuretics—ingredients that force a person's body to eliminate more water. Other diet pills rely on ingredients that claim to speed up a person's metabolism (the process by which the body turns food into energy and stores unused calories as fat); suppress appetite; or block the absorption of fat, sugars, or carbohydrates.

Do these types of supplements actually do what they say they will? Unfortunately, there's usually no reliable scientific research to back up the claims provided by the product's manufacturer. In addition, there are many unknowns about the substances used in diet supplements, so dietitians and doctors consider them risky. What research studies do show is that most of the people who try one of these "crash" diets regain all the weight they lost within a few weeks or months.

Do these diets put your health at risk?

Luckily, very few people stick to a highly restrictive diet for long periods of time and most people give up on them after a few days. But what happens if you keep following extremely low-calorie diets or taking weight-loss supplements? That's when things can get a little scary.

Radically cutting back on calories can make you tired, jittery, and moody. These symptoms usually go away when you resume healthy eating habits, but over the long term, a highly restrictive diet may cause other health problems. You may lose some of your hair, your fingernails may become brittle, dark circles may appear under your eyes, and your muscles may shrink and weaken. Sometimes staying on a highly restrictive diet for a long period of time can cause lasting damage to your body, especially to the heart and kidneys. Following extreme diets over the long term or a pattern of extreme dieting followed by binge eating are both signs that a person may have an eating disorder.

Drastically reducing your food intake depletes the body's access to the vitamins, minerals, and fiber that it needs to stay healthy. If a diet requires you to cut out all dairy products, for example, you are also losing valuable calcium. Over a prolonged period, a lack of calcium puts a person at increased risk for osteoporosis (pronounced: ahs-tee-oh-puh-ro-sis), a condition in which bones become brittle and more susceptible to injury as a person ages. Some diets—like those that omit all red meat—may leave the dieter lacking iron, which can lead to anemia, especially in teen girls. And trying to replace the foods you're cutting out with vitamin pills is a bad idea. Foods like fruits and vegetables contain more than just vitamins and minerals—they are some of the best sources of fiber. Fiber can help to prevent disease.

Restricting food intake over a long period during a person's teenage years can stunt growth. Following restrictive diets over a long period can also delay some of the changes associated with puberty, such as breast development in females and muscle bulk in males. Another side effect of restrictive diets in teenage girls is irregular menstrual periods—or even not getting a period at all.

Another effect of very low-calorie diets is a decrease in resting energy expenditure, or the amount of calories a person burns at rest. One reason for this "slower metabolism" is that people on restrictive diets often lose muscle mass, and muscle burns more calories than fat—even while a person is resting. This makes continuing to lose weight even more difficult and regaining weight easier.

What about the long-term effects of taking diet pills? Common ingredients in diet pills include caffeine, alcohol, 5-hydroxytryptophan (5-HTP), chromium (or chromium picolinate), phentermine, and vanadium. These ingredients may carry health risks for certain people. Ephedrine (also known as ephedra or ma huang), an ingredient in many diet and sports supplements during the late 1990s and early 2000s, was linked to heart problems and may have played a role in the death of at least one professional athlete. The U.S. Food and Drug Administration decided the health risks associated with ephedra were too great, and it banned the substance in December 2003.

If you have any health conditions or are taking medication, always check with your doctor before taking weight-loss supplements because the ingredients in some supplements may interact with specific drugs. For example, 5-HTP may cause adverse reactions in people who take certain medications for depression.

Even ingredients that seem like a normal part of your diet can carry risks when used in weight-loss pills or other stimulants: For example, the average caffeine-based weight-loss pill contains as much caffeine as 6 cups of coffee. Imagine how wired you'd be if you took two or three of these pills each day. The side effects associated with these products include rapid heart rate, increased blood pressure, dizziness, sleeplessness, seizures, and even addiction.

Furthermore, it's important to know that most diet supplements have not been tested on teen users. Not only does this mean that the dosages prescribed may not be accurate, it could mean that taking certain supplements might carry unknown risks for teens.

How can you lose weight for the long term?

Regardless of concerns about the effectiveness and safety of restrictive diets, keeping the pounds off long term should be the major goal for anyone who wants to lose weight—and that can be more challenging than losing them in the first place. Weight loss is most likely to be successful and lasting when a person changes his or her habits to reduce the overall number of calories he or she eats while at the same time increasing the number of calories burned through exercise. Exercise not only burns calories, it also builds muscle. The more muscle you have, the more efficient your body becomes at burning calories, even when you aren't exercising. You don't have to become a gym rat, though: Walking the family dog, cycling to school, and doing other things that increase your daily level of activity can all make a difference.

Research confirms that one reason people get less exercise these days is because of an increase in "screen time"—in other words, the amount of time spent watching TV, looking at the computer, or playing video games. The American Academy of Pediatrics recommends limiting all screen time to one hour per day. If you're hanging with your friends at the mall instead of chatting to them on the computer, for example, you're getting more exercise.

A survey on health and nutrition conducted by the Centers for Disease Control and Prevention shows that serving sizes for both kids and adults have increased over the past ten years, and that this is a contributor to obesity. If you super-size your fries or always go for extra hot fudge on your sundae, you are probably taking in more calories than your body can use. Another key dietary factor in weight gain today is the increased consumption of flavored beverages, such as sodas, sweetened juice drinks, and sports drinks. Some people keep a food diary to track what they eat and drink. Writing everything you eat in a daily diary might help you identify those hidden foods that contribute to unwanted weight gain—like the candy bar you usually munch between third and fourth period.

The best way to build a weight-loss program that's right for you is to talk to your doctor or a registered dietitian. During your appointment, your doctor or dietitian may ask you what types of foods you eat, how much weight you want to lose, and the reasons why you want to lose weight. He or she will also help you figure out approximately where your weight should be based on your height and other factors and suggest a sound weight-loss plan that meets your individual needs. (Dietitians report that most guys and girls find

---

♣ **It's A Fact!!**

Fad Diet Dangers

Like many dieters anxious to shed unwanted pounds, you may have been tempted to experiment with popular or "fad" diets. Sometimes it may be hard to resist the amazing "before and after" stories and the "hype" that surrounds these diets. You may have tried several times before to lose weight, but without much long-term success. There's no point in feeling bad about yourself, because the truth is, losing weight is not easy. No magic formula will trim away extra pounds and keep them off. So, before you allow yourself to fall into the fad diet trap, consider these critical facts:

- Fad diets usually over-emphasize one food or type of food. They violate the first principle of good nutrition, which is to eat a balanced diet that includes a variety of foods.

- Those able to stay on a fad diet for more than a few weeks may develop nutritional deficiencies because no one type of food has all the nutrients necessary for good health.

weight-loss plans that take their daily schedule and food preferences into account are easier to follow.) The eating plan must include enough calories per day to keep your body working and developing properly. And if you're cutting calories to lose weight, your body will still need to get the same amount of nutrients to stay healthy.

Staying active is an important part of keeping off the weight you've lost. If you achieved your weight-loss goal by eating a variety of foods in smaller portions and exercising regularly, chances are better that you will stick with a healthier lifestyle and keep the pounds off in the long run.

There's a lot of hype out there when it comes to dieting. "Trendy new diets sell books and magazines, so of course you're going to see a lot about the 'hot' new diet of the moment," says Neil Izenberg, MD, an expert in adolescent medicine and the media. However, "the tried and true approach—cutting back on calories and increasing your level of exercise—is still the best way to lose weight and keep it off," Dr. Izenberg says.

As you have explored the options for a weight-reducing diet, you may have already noticed that many fad diets restrict you to eating primarily one type of food and that they promise unbelievable weight-loss results almost overnight. Realistically, though, gimmicks and get-thin-quick schemes don't work. That's why, over the long haul, the fads—the grapefruit diet, the very low fat diet, the low-carb diet—are not the answer. Here are several of the unavoidable facts about fad diets:

- No "superfoods" exist. That's why people should eat a balanced diet, which includes moderate amounts from all food groups, not just large amounts of a few special foods.

- Fad diets can never be a permanent solution. They are so monotonous that it's almost impossible to stay on them for long periods of time.

- Fad diets also violate the second important principle of good nutrition: eating should be enjoyable.

Source: "Fad Diet Dangers," reproduced with permission. American Heart Association. © 2005, American Heart Association.

Chapter 35

Popular Diets Reviewed

Don't Go On Fad Diets

Wipe out the word "dieting" from your vocabulary. Eating a healthy diet is not the same as dieting. Eating a healthy diet means eating nutritious foods that your body needs for good health, while eating less nutritious foods less often. Skipping meals or following weird, unhealthy eating patterns actually can keep you from getting the nutrients you need to grow as healthy as you could be. Trying to lose weight when your body is growing and changing isn't smart, unless your doctor thinks it's a good idea and helps you with it.

You've probably heard about a lot of fad diets, which allow you to only eat a few specific foods or only drink certain liquids. Fad diets are usually popular for a little while and then go out of style. They may be advertised as a quick way to lose weight, but most are not balanced or healthy in the long run. Many are not effective, and some are not even safe, especially for growing bodies. Fad diets may make you lose weight while you are on the diet, but as soon as you stop the diet and start eating normally again, you usually gain all the weight back. Also, the weight lost on a fad diet is mostly loss of normal body water that comes right back when you stop the fad diet. Some fad diets can even cause you to lose some of your precious muscle, which doesn't come back when you regain weight.

About This Chapter: "Don't Go on Fad Diets!" is from BodyWise, U.S. Department of Health and Human Services, 2004. "Popular Diets Reviewed" is reprinted with permission from the American Dietetic Association, http://www.eatright.org, © 2004. All rights reserved.

Eating a healthy diet is a way of living, one that keeps your body healthy and working, and not just a way to look thinner or something you ever finish or go off of.

So what do you do if you think you are looking chunky? If you feel that your weight is not right for you, talk to your parents, your doctor, or an adult you trust. They can help you figure out if you weigh too much and suggest changes you may need to make in your life. Remember to balance a healthy diet with physical activity. To maintain a healthy weight, you need to balance energy coming into your body (food) with energy going out of your body (physical activity.) For you to lose weight, your doctor may recommend making your energy unbalanced so that you take in less food and exercise more.

♣ **It's A Fact!!**

Reasons Not To Go On A Restrictive Diet Without A Doctor's Approval

• Diets don't make you physically fit.

• Diets slow down your metabolism (the way your body converts food and oxygen into energy).

• Diets make you sluggish.

• Diets make you crave food.

• Diets confuse your body systems.

• Diets can be dangerous.

Source: U.S. Department of Health and Human Services, 2004.

Your doctor may suggest you make changes to your diet so that you will be healthier. Listen to what your doctor has to say and follow his or her instructions. This kind of a diet is different than you deciding on your own to limit your food intake in unhealthy ways. Never go on a diet without talking to your doctor first.

Popular Diets Reviewed

By the time you read this, there may already be a new best-selling diet book heading the list, but with some help from current or former ADA media spokespeople we have put together this information to give you the scoop on current popular diets.

Dr. Phil's Ultimate Weight Solution

The Ultimate Weight Solution: The 7 Keys to Weight Loss Freedom by Phillip McGraw, PhD, Free Press, 2003.

Diet Summary: The theme of this program is that behavior modification and cognitive restructuring, along with a healthy diet and exercise, can lead to permanent weight management. Claiming an 80 percent success rate, the program's key points offer behavioral and nutritional advice ranging from portion control to supplement recommendations. Foods are divided into two categories: high response foods (good) and low response foods (bad). While some of the book's advice is good (recycling behavior modification strategies that have been used in weight control programs for decades), several of the book's points contain erroneous or outdated nutrition and dietary recommendations. Additionally, the *Ultimate Weight Solution* includes seemingly simple advice for dealing with complicated emotional, eating and family issues. Without proper supervision, managing these issues alone can lead to ultimate dietary disaster. Dr. Phil suggests enlisting a 'circle of support,' including a nutritionist with 'technical expertise;' however, this advice comes late in the book.

And For Adolescents

The Ultimate Weight Loss Solution for Teens: The 7 Keys to Weight Freedom by Jay McGraw, Free Press, 2003.

Written by Dr. Phil's son, this book is essentially a gentler version of the original *Ultimate Weight Solution*. While I do like the way it adapts the 7 Keys for kids with softer, hopeful language, this diet is still comprised of recycled behavior modification tips and unrealistically simple solutions to treating obesity and eating disorders.

—Lisa Dorfman, MS, RD, LMHC, Licensed Psychotherapist

The "New" Atkins Diet

Dr. Atkins' New Diet Revolution: Revised and Improved by Robert C. Atkins, MD, Avon, 2001.

Diet Summary: Arguably one of the most famous fad diets, the Atkins Diet program restricts carbohydrates and focuses on eating mostly protein

✎ What's It Mean?

Complex Carbohydrates: Large chains of sugar units arranged to form starches and fiber. Complex carbohydrates include vegetables, whole fruits, rice, pasta, potatoes, grains (brown rice, oats, wheat, barley, corn), and legumes (chick peas, black-eyed peas, lentils, as well as beans such as lima, kidney, pinto, soy, and black beans).

Glycemic Index: A classification proposed to quantify the relative blood glucose response to carbohydrate-containing foods.

Glycemic Load: An indicator of glucose response or insulin demand that is induced by total carbohydrate intake.

Glycemic Response: The effects that carbohydrate-containing foods have on blood glucose concentration during the digestion process.

Simple Carbohydrates: Sugars composed of a single sugar molecule (monosaccharide) or two joined sugar molecules (a disaccharide), such as glucose, fructose, lactose, and sucrose. Simple carbohydrates include white and brown sugar, fruit sugar, corn syrup, molasses, honey, and candy.

Source: Excerpted from "Appendix G-1: Glossary of Terms," *Dietary Guidelines for Americans 2005*, U.S. Department of Agriculture, 2005.

with the use of vitamin and mineral supplements. According to the program, this will alter a body's metabolism so it will burn stored fat while building muscle mass. The "new" Atkins Diet is the same diet with a more liberal maintenance plan. With the "new" Atkins diet, some of the sensationalism is gone and there is heavy promoting of low-carb bars and food products from Atkins Nutritionals, Inc. But the bottom line is still the same. Carbs are demonized and there are major restrictions on fruits and vegetables, whole grains, legumes and low-fat dairy foods, which contradicts everything we know about health promotion and disease prevention.

—Keith Ayoob, EdD, RD, FADA

✔ Quick Tip
Refuse To Use Diet Aids

Using over-the-counter diet pills, diuretics (medicine that makes you lose fluid), or laxatives to lose weight is dangerous. Just because you see ads or commercials for them doesn't mean they're safe.

Most diet pills contain stimulants like caffeine to make you less hungry. But your appetite is natural—it's the way your body lets you know it's hungry and needs nourishment. Taking diet pills deprives your body of the food it needs for growth.

Some weight-loss aids may contain a diuretic, which increases the loss of body water by going to the bathroom. This can result in a quick loss of pounds that consist of water and important minerals that aren't absorbed by your cells before the fluid leaves your body. It can make you dehydrated, and you will almost surely gain the weight back as soon as you drink liquids.

Another risk of diet pills is that the stimulant action can raise your blood pressure and heart rate to dangerous levels. Stimulants make people hyper, restless, and cranky. Diet pills also can be addictive.

Resist any temptation you have to lose weight quickly and easily through diet aids. There's always a catch.

Eating nutritious foods can be fun and easy. The benefits will last a lifetime and your body will thank you for it.

Source: BodyWise, GirlPower (www.girlpower.gov), U.S. Department of Health and Human Services.

The Zone Diet

The Zone: Revolutionary Life Plan to Put Your Body in Total Balance for Permanent Weight Loss by Barry Sears, MD, Regan Books, 1995.

Diet Summary: Promoting a "balanced nutritional approach," the Zone Diet is a complex eating plan that divides each meal into proportions of 40 percent carbohydrates, 30 percent proteins and 30 percent fats. The "Zone" refers to the state in which the body is at its physical peak, presumably from following this diet.

While the Zone Diet is closer to what most dietetics professionals would recommend compared to other fad diets, there are still better nutrition and exercise programs that are less complicated and frustrating than constantly measuring proportions and counting calories.

—Althea Zanecosky, MS, RD

South Beach Diet

The South Beach Diet: The Delicious, Doctor-Designed, Foolproof Plan for Fast and Healthy Weight Loss by Arthur Agaston, MD, Rodale Press, 2003.

Diet Summary: Comprised of three phases, the South Beach Diet begins by banning carbohydrates such as fruit, bread, rice, potatoes, pasta and baked goods and allowing normal-size portions of meat, poultry, shellfish, vegetables, eggs, and nuts. Dieters are told they will lose between eight and 13 pounds in the first two weeks during the "detoxification" phase. The second phase reintroduces "good carbs" (as defined using an online glycemic index) and dieters expect to lose one to two pounds per week until the weight goal is reached. The third phase is the least restrictive, allowing the dieters to eat pretty much anything in moderation.

The theory behind the South Beach Diet is that the faster sugars and starches are digested, the more weight is gained. Instead, the diet will cause weight loss because it is a low-calorie plan with an average intake of about 1,400 to 1,500 calories per day. The diet's first phase promotes potentially dangerous accelerated weight loss; however, the second and third phases emphasize whole grains, lean proteins and dairy, unsaturated fats and fruits and vegetables, in addition to consistent meal times, snacks, a healthy dessert and plenty of water.

—Dawn Jackson, RD, LD

Raw Food Diets

The Raw Life: Becoming Natural in an Unnatural World by Paul Nison, 343 Publishing Company, 2000, and *Raw, the Uncooked Book* by Juliano Brotman and Erika Lenkert, Regan Books, 1999.

Diet Summary: Various versions of raw food diets exist, but they share the same basic principle: Cooked foods lose the natural vitamins, nutrients, and enzymes necessary to build a strong immune system. They recommend eating only fruits and vegetables picked ripe from the tree, garden, or vine (organic preferred), nuts, or seeds. Some raw food diets claim that it is "not natural" to eat sea vegetables, and others say that they are very important to include in the diet.

Raw food diets may be high in fiber and low in total fat, saturated fat, cholesterol and calories, but they restrict so many important foods that it becomes a challenge to get all the nutrients the body needs. For example, avoiding all animal foods presents a challenge in getting enough vitamins B_{12} and D.

—Claudia M. González, MS, RD, LD/N

♣ It's A Fact!!

What is a very low-calorie diet (VLCD)?

VLCDs are commercially prepared formulas of about 800 calories that replace all usual food intake for several weeks or months. VLCDs are not the same as over-the-counter meal replacements, which are meant to substitute for one or two meals a day. VLCDs, when used under proper medical supervision, effectively produce significant short-term weight loss in patients who are moderately to extremely obese.

Studies have shown that meal replacements at higher calorie levels (800–1000 calories) produce weight loss similar to that seen with much lower calorie levels, probably due to better compliance with the diet. In addition, VLCDs are usually part of weight-loss treatment programs that include other techniques such as behavioral therapy, nutrition counseling, physical activity, and/or drug treatment.

Who should use a VLCD?

VLCDs are intended to produce rapid weight loss at the start of a weight-loss program in adults with a body mass index (BMI) greater than 30. BMI correlates significantly with total body fat content. It is calculated by dividing weight in kilograms by height in meters squared, or by dividing weight in pounds by height in inches squared and multiplying by 703.

Use of VLCDs in patients with a BMI of 27 to 30 should be reserved for those who have medical complications resulting from their overweight. VLCDs are not recommended for pregnant or breastfeeding women. **VLCDs are not appropriate for children or adolescents,** except in specialized treatment programs.

Source: Excerpted from "Very-Low-Calorie Diets," National Institute of Diabetes and Digestive and Kidney Diseases, NIH Pub. No. 03-3894, January 2003.

Sugar Busters

The New Sugar Busters! Cut Sugar to Trim Fat by H. Leighton Steward; Morrison C. Bethea, MD; Sam S. Andrews, MD; Luis A. Balart, MD, Ballatine Books, 1998.

Diet Summary: The basic tenet of Sugar Busters is that all sugars, including the sugar derived from complex carbohydrates and starches, are "toxic" because they produce excess insulin, which causes our bodies to store sugar as fat and make cholesterol. According to the book, foods with a high glycemic index produce a greater insulin response and fat storage. The book concludes with a list of acceptable foods and foods to avoid, a 14-day sample meal plan, and Sugar Busters! recipes. The diet is recommended as appropriate for children, pregnant women, people with diabetes, hypoglycemia sufferers, and persons with a history of cardiovascular disease.

The carbohydrate/insulin response theory as a cause of weight gain has become popular in fad diets, but there is no evidence that excess insulin release causes obesity in people with normal pancreatic function. Obesity is more likely a result of a decline in physical activity and increase in calorie intake than increased sugar or carbohydrate consumption. While the authors mention that protein foods and fats should also be limited, some of the recipes suggest the contrary, such as the filet mignon recipe for four that includes four 10-ounce filets, a cup of blue cheese, and a half-pound of bacon.

—Kathleen Zelman, MPH, RD, LD

> ✔ **Quick Tip**
> ## Recommended Reading
>
> *American Dietetic Association Complete Food and Nutrition Guide* by Roberta Larson Duyff, MS, RD, FADA, CFCS, John Wiley & Sons, 2002.
>
> *Dieting for Dummies,* second edition by Jane Kirby, RD, Wiley Publishing, 2004.
>
> *The Way to Eat* by David L. Katz, MD, MPH, FACPM and Maura H. Gonzalez, MS, RD, Sourcebooks, 2002.
>
> *365 Days of Healthy Eating* from the American Dietetic Association by Roberta Larson Duyff, MS, RD, FADA, CFCS, John Wiley, 2004.
>
> *ADA Guide to Healthy Eating for Kids: How Your Children Can Eat Smart from 5 to 12* by Jodie Shield, MEd, RD and Mary Catherine Mullen, MS, RD, John Wiley, 2002.
>
> *ADA Guide to Eating Right When You Have Diabetes* by Maggie Powers, MS, RD, CDE, John Wiley, 2003.
>
> *ADA Guide to Better Digestion* by Leslie Bonci, MPH, RD, John Wiley, 2003.
>
> Source: © 2004 American Dietetic Association.

Chapter 36

"Screen Time" And Weight Control

Numerous studies comparing the amount of time people of all ages spend watching TV or in other forms of "screen time" have shown that increasing media time results in increasing body weight.

- A study published in 2001 (Crespo, C. et al. *Archives of Pediatric and Adolescent Medicine*) found that the incidence of obesity was highest among children who watched four or more hours of television a day and lowest among children who watched an hour or less a day.

- Another group of researchers analyzed national survey data collected between 1988 and 1994 and found that 26% of children who watched four or more hours of television a day had much more body fat than children who watched less television. (Anderson, R.E., et al. *JAMA*, 1998)

- Another study estimated that 60% of the overweight in children aged 10 to 15 might be due to excessive TV viewing. (Gortmacher S.L. et al. *Archives of Pediatric and Adolescent Medicine*, 1996)

- Several studies have looked at how much the risk of obesity increases with the amount of television viewing. A study back in 1985, found that for every hour of television, the incidence of obesity increased by 2%. (Dietz, W.H. *Pediatrics*, 1985) A more recent study of preschoolers ages one to four, found that the risk of overweight increased by 6% for every hour of television watched per day. If the preschooler had a television set in their bedroom, their risk of overweight jumped by 31% for every hour they watched because they spent much more time watching TV every week. (Dennison M.D., et al. *Pediatrics*, 2002)

Why are we more likely to be overweight if we spend a lot of time watching TV and using computers and playing video games? We're going to look at four reasons.

1. TV viewing and other forms of screen time displaces (or takes the place of) time spent in physical activity.

If you are watching TV or sitting in front of a computer screen, you are most likely sitting still instead of standing, walking, or being more active. Let's compare how the calories expended doing a sedentary activity for six and a half hours compares with doing light or moderate activities for that same period of time:

Sedentary activity burns 0.01 kcal/min/kg, light activity burns 0.02 kcal/min/kg, and moderate activity burns 0.03 kcal/min/kg. Light activities would include sitting or standing with arm movement, bathing, or slow walking. Moderate activities include housework, moderate-paced walking, light exercising, or recreational activities like bowling or golfing.

Figure out how many calories you would burn for physical activity (this is over and above the calories burned for staying alive during that period of time) in six and a half hours (390 minutes), based on your body weight (weight in pounds ÷ 2.2 = weight in kilograms). Calculate it three times, once for calories burned being sedentary, once for calories burned if engaged in light activity, and once for calories burned if engaged in moderate activity.

Here is an example for a student weighing 125 pounds:

125 ÷ 2.2 = 56.8 kg

6½ hours = 390 minutes

Sedentary = 0.01 x 390 x 56.8 = 221.5 calories burned in 6½ hours

Light = 0.02 x 390 x 56.8 = 443 calories burned in 6½ hours

Moderate = 0.03 x 390 x 56.8 = 664.6 calories burned in 6½ hours

What is the difference in calories every day between sedentary and light? Answer: 221.5 calories

How many days would it take for this difference to equal one pound of excess body fat (3,500 calories), if you did not eat fewer calories? Answer: 16 days

2. TV viewing and other forms of screen time also displaces meaningful social interaction, which is good for our mental well-being and in turn helpful in maintaining a healthy weight.

Social research has shown that the loneliness and social isolation that the presence of electronic media creates in our lives is strongly associated with mental health problems. We spend many more hours looking at screens than at other human faces. TV and computer use disconnects us from others. Studies have shown that Americans today are more familiar with the lives of television characters than the lives of their neighbors.

3. TV viewing can also lead to "disengaged" or "mindless" eating.

Snacking while watching television or using another electronic media is very common. Whenever eating is occurring while engaged in another activity, the focus is not on eating, or on the body's hunger and satiety signals. Often, food is eaten from a package rather than from a portioned amount. It is not unusual for someone watching TV to consume an entire bag of potato chips or other snack food without being aware of it.

4. Advertising exposure on television is primarily for high-calorie, low-nutrient foods.

- How many television commercials do you think an average American child sees every year? Between 20,000 and 40,000 (Strasburger, VC, *Journal of Developmental and Behavioral Pediatrics*, 2001), which is 55–110 every day.

- What percentage of advertising aimed at children is for food? Nearly half of all advertising to children is for food. (Nestle, M. and M. Wootan, *The Food Institute Report*, 2002)

- How much is spent on food advertisements aimed at children and youth every year by food and beverage companies? $13 billion a year is spent every year just to market foods and beverages to American children. More than $230 billion is spent in the U.S. on advertising of all kinds. Advertisers spend more than $2,000 per household every year to promote their products.

♣ It's A Fact!!

Advertisers market to children and youth because they spend a lot of their own money. Youth, age 12–19, spent $155–$172 billion of their own money in 2001, according to several surveys: the National Institute on Media and the Family (www.mediaandthefamily.org) and Teen Research Unlimited, 2002.

Young children under age 12 influence $500 billion in family purchases each year, according to marketing expert James McNeal (MarketResearch.com). So, products of all kinds are marketed to children.

Advertisers want to promote "brand loyalty" from an early age. "Branding" is building a positive impression of a product, linking the product's name and/or logo to a positive image or feeling in the buyer's mind.

Studies indicate that brand loyalty may begin as early as age two (Children's Business, 2000). By age three, one in five American children request products by brand-name (www.newdream.org). A lifetime customer may be worth $100,000 to a retail company, so creating brand loyalty from "cradle to grave" is very valuable to marketers. Studies show that children who watch more television want more of what they see advertised than children who watch less television, including brand-name toys and advertised food. (Strasburger, VC and Wilson BJ. *Children, adolescents and the media*, 2002)

Chapter 37

The Importance Of Being Physically Active

Why is physical activity important?

Being physically active is a key element in living a longer, healthier, happier life. It can help relieve stress and can provide an overall feeling of well-being. Physical activity can also help you achieve and maintain a healthy weight and lower risk for chronic disease. The benefits of physical activity may include the following:

- Improves self-esteem and feelings of well-being

- Increases fitness level

- Helps build and maintain bones, muscles, and joints

- Builds endurance and muscle strength

- Enhances flexibility and posture

- Helps manage weight

- Lowers risk of heart disease, colon cancer, and type 2 diabetes

- Helps control blood pressure

- Reduces feelings of depression and anxiety

Physical activity and nutrition work together for better health. Being active increases the amount of calories burned.

About This Chapter: This chapter includes excerpts from "Inside The Pyramid," U.S. Department of Agriculture (www.mypyramid.gov), 2005.

✎ What's It Mean?

Leisure-Time Physical Activity: Physical activity that is performed during exercise, recreation, or any additional time other than that associated with one's regular job duties, occupation, or transportation.

Metabolic Equivalent (MET): A way of measuring physical activity intensity. This unit is used to estimate the amount of oxygen used by the body during physical activity. 1 MET = the energy (oxygen) used by the body as you sit quietly, perhaps while talking on the phone or reading a book. The harder your body works during the activity, the higher the MET.

Moderate Physical Activity: Any activity that burns 3.5 to 7 kcal/min or the equivalent of 3 to 6 metabolic equivalents (METs) and results in achieving 60 to 73 percent of peak heart rate. An estimate of a person's peak heart rate can be obtained by subtracting the person's age from 220. Examples of moderate physical activity include walking briskly, mowing the lawn, dancing, swimming, or bicycling on level terrain. A person should feel some exertion but should be able to carry on a conversation comfortably during the activity.

Resistance Exercise: Anaerobic training, including weight training, weight machine use, and resistance band workouts. Resistance training will increase strength, muscular endurance, and muscle size, while running and jogging will not.

Sedentary Behaviors: In scientific literature, sedentary is often defined in terms of little or no physical activity during leisure time. A sedentary lifestyle is a lifestyle characterized by little or no physical activity.

Vigorous Physical Activity: Any activity that burns more than 7 kcal/min or the equivalent of 6 or more metabolic equivalents (METs) and results in achieving 74 to 88 percent of peak heart rate. Examples of vigorous physical activity include jogging, mowing the lawn with a nonmotorized push mower, chopping wood, participating in high-impact aerobic dancing, swimming continuous laps, or bicycling uphill. Vigorous-intensity physical activity may be intense enough to represent a substantial challenge to an individual and results in a significant increase in heart and breathing rate.

Weight-Bearing Exercise: Any activity one performs that works bones and muscles against gravity, including walking, running, hiking, dancing, gymnastics, and soccer.

Source: Excerpted from "Appendix G-1: Glossary of Terms," *Dietary Guidelines for Americans 2005*, U.S. Department of Agriculture, 2005.

Some types of physical activity are especially beneficial:

- **Aerobic activities:** speeds heart rate and breathing and improves heart and lung fitness. Examples are brisk walking, jogging, and swimming.

- **Resistance, strength building, and weight-bearing activities:** helps build and maintain bones and muscles by working them against gravity. Examples are carrying a child, lifting weights, and walking. They help to build and maintain muscles and bones.

- **Balance and stretching activities:** enhances physical stability and flexibility, which reduces risk of injuries. Examples are gentle stretching, dancing, yoga, martial arts, and t'ai chi.

What is physical activity?

Physical activity simply means movement of the body that uses energy. Walking, gardening, briskly pushing a baby stroller, climbing the stairs, playing soccer, or dancing the night away are all good examples of being active. For health benefits, physical activity should be moderate or vigorous and add up to at least 30 minutes a day.

Moderate physical activities include:

- Walking briskly (about 3½ miles per hour)

- Hiking

- Gardening/yard work

- Dancing

- Golf (walking and carrying clubs)

- Bicycling (less than 10 miles per hour)

- Weight training (general light workout)

♣ **It's A Fact!!**

If you eat 100 more food calories a day than you burn, you'll gain about 1 pound in a month. That's about 10 pounds in a year. The bottom line is that to lose weight, it's important to reduce calories and increase physical activity.

Source: Excerpted from "Finding Your Way to a Healthier You," U.S. Department of Agriculture, Home and Garden Bulletin No. 232-CP, 2005.

Vigorous physical activities include:

- Running/jogging (5 miles per hour)

- Bicycling (more than 10 miles per hour)

- Swimming (freestyle laps)

- Aerobics

- Walking very fast (4½ miles per hour)

- Heavy yard work, such as chopping wood

- Weight lifting (vigorous effort)

- Basketball (competitive)

Some physical activities are not intense enough to help you meet the recommendations. Although you are moving, these activities do not increase your heart rate, so you should not count these towards the 30 or more minutes a day that you should strive for. These include walking at a casual pace, such as while grocery shopping, and doing light household chores.

> ### ✔ Quick Tip
>
> If you avoid physical activity because you do not want to ruin your hairstyle, try:
>
> - a natural hairstyle;
> - a style that can be wrapped or pulled back;
> - a short haircut;
> - braids, twists, or locs.
>
> Day-to-day activities can cause salt buildup in your hair. To remove salt, shampoo with a mild, pH-balanced product at least once a week.
>
> Source: Excerpted from "Celebrate the Beauty of Youth," National Institute of Diabetes and Digestive and Kidney Diseases, NIH Pub. No. 04-4903, June 2004.

How much physical activity is needed?

Children and teenagers should be physically active for at least 60 minutes every day, or most days. For those who have lost weight, at least 60 to 90 minutes a day may be needed to maintain the weight loss. At the same time, calorie needs should not be exceeded.

No matter what activity you choose, it can be done all at once, or divided into two or three parts during the day. Even 10-minutes bouts of activity count toward your total.

Individuals with one of the conditions below should also consult a health care provider for help in designing a safe program of physical activity.

- A chronic health problem such as heart disease, high blood pressure, diabetes, osteoporosis, asthma, or obesity.

- High risk for heart disease, such as a family history of heart disease or stroke, eating a diet high in saturated fat, trans fat and cholesterol, smoking, or having a sedentary lifestyle.

How many calories does physical activity use?

Table 37.1 shows about how many calories a 154-pound man (5'10") will use up doing each of the activities listed. Those who weigh more will use more calories, and those who weigh less will use fewer. The calorie values listed include both calories used by the activity and the calories used for normal body functioning.

Table 37.1. Approximate Calories Used By A 154 Pound Man

Moderate Physical Activities:	In 1 hour	In 30 minutes
Hiking	370	185
Light gardening/yard work	330	165
Dancing	330	165
Golf (walking and carrying clubs)	330	165
Bicycling (less than 10 miles per hour)	290	145
Walking (3½ miles per hour)	280	140
Weight training (general light workout)	220	110
Stretching	180	90

Vigorous physical activities:	In 1 hour	In 30 minutes
Running/jogging (5 miles per hour)	590	295
Bicycling (more than 10 miles per hour)	590	295
Swimming (slow freestyle laps)	510	255
Aerobics	480	240
Walking (4½ miles per hour)	460	230
Heavy yard work (chopping wood)	440	220
Weight lifting (vigorous effort)	440	220
Basketball (vigorous)	440	220

Tips For Increasing Physical Activity

Make Physical Activity A Regular Part Of The Day

Choose activities that you enjoy and can do regularly. Fitting activity into a daily routine can be easy—such as taking a brisk 10-minute walk to and from the parking lot, bus stop, or subway station. Or, join an exercise class. Keep it interesting by trying something different on alternate days. What's important is to be active most days of the week and make it part of daily routine. For example, to reach a 30-minute goal for the day, walk the dog for 10 minutes before and after school, and add a 10-minute walk at lunchtime. Or, swim three times a week and take a yoga class on the other days. Make sure to do at least 10 minutes of the activity at a time, shorter bursts of activity will not have the same health benefits. To be ready anytime, keep some comfortable clothes and a pair of walking or running shoes in the car and at the office.

✔ **Quick Tip**

Physical activity can be fun! Do things you enjoy like:

- dancing;
- rollerblading;
- fast walking;
- playing sports;
- bicycling;
- swimming.

If you can, be physically active with a friend or a group. That way, you can cheer each other on, have company, and feel safer when you are outdoors. Find a local school track where you can walk or run, go for a stroll in a local park, or join a recreation center near your home or work.

Think you do not have time for physical activity? It is easy to move more by making these small changes to your daily routine:

- Get off the bus or subway one stop early and walk the rest of the way (be sure the area is safe).
- Park your car farther away and walk to your destination.
- Walk to each end of the mall when you go shopping.

Source: Excerpted from "Celebrate the Beauty of Youth," National Institute of Diabetes and Digestive and Kidney Diseases, NIH Pub. No. 04-4903, June 2004.

✔ Quick Tip

Exercise And Bones: Weight-Bearing Exercises For Kids And Teens

Exercise helps build bone and weight-bearing exercise is particularly helpful in this task. Weight-bearing exercise includes any activity in which your feet and legs carry your own weight. Here are just some examples of weight-bearing exercise that can help you build strong bones:

- Walking

- Running

- Jumping rope

- Dancing

- Climbing stairs

- Jogging

- Aerobic dancing

- Hiking   .

- Inline skating/ice skating

- Racquet sports, such as tennis or racquetball

- Team sports such as soccer, basketball, field hockey, volleyball, and softball or baseball

Source: From "Why Calcium?" National Institute of Child Health and Human Development (NICHD), 2005.

More Ways To Increase Physical Activity

At Home

- Join a walking group in the neighborhood or at the local shopping mall. Recruit a partner for support and encouragement.

- Push a baby in a stroller.

- Get the whole family involved— enjoy an afternoon bike ride.

- Walk up and down the soccer or softball field sidelines while watching your friends play.

- Walk the dog—don't just watch the dog walk.

- Clean the house or wash the car.

- Walk, skate, or cycle more, and drive less.

- Do stretches, exercises, or pedal a stationary bike while watching television.

- Mow the lawn with a push mower.

- Plant and care for a vegetable or flower garden.

- Play with your younger siblings— tumble in the leaves, build a snowman, splash in a puddle, or dance to favorite music.

At Play

- Walk, jog, skate, or cycle.

- Swim or do water aerobics.

- Take a class in martial arts, dance, or yoga.

- Golf (pull cart or carry clubs).

- Canoe, row, or kayak.

- Play racket ball, tennis, or squash.

- Ski cross-country or downhill.

- Play basketball, softball, or soccer.

- Hand cycle or play wheelchair sports.

- Take a nature walk.

- Most important—have fun while being active!

♣ It's A Fact!!

Girls who were inactive during adolescence gained an average of 10 to 15 pounds more than active girls, according to results of a 10-year observational study of obesity. Total calorie intake increased only slightly and was not associated with the weight gains. These new results show that a previously reported steep decline in physical activity among adolescent girls is directly associated with increased fatness and an increase of body mass index (BMI), a measure of body weight adjusted for height.

Source: Excerpted from "Decline in Physical Activity Plays Key Role in Weight Gain Among Adolescent Girls," *NIH News*, National Institutes of Health, July 13, 2005.

Part Four

Medical Conditions And Special Circumstances Related To Diet

Chapter 38

Preventing Obesity And Chronic Diseases Through Good Nutrition And Physical Activity

The Reality

- Obesity in the United States is truly epidemic. In the last ten years, obesity rates have increased by more than 60% among adults. Approximately 59 million adults are obese.

- Since 1980, obesity rates have doubled among children and tripled among adolescents. Of children and adolescents aged 6–19 years, 15%—about 9 million young people—are considered overweight.

- Only about one-fourth of U.S. adults eat the recommended five or more servings of fruits and vegetables each day.

- More than 60% of young people eat too much fat, and less than 20% eat the recommended five or more servings of fruits and vegetables each day.

About This Chapter: From "Preventing Obesity and Chronic Diseases Through Good Nutrition and Physical Activity," National Center for Chronic Disease Prevention and Health Promotion, Centers for Disease Control and Prevention (CDC), reviewed August 2005.

- Despite the proven benefits of physical activity, more than 60% of American adults do not get enough physical activity to provide health benefits.

- More than a third of young people in grades 9–12 do not regularly engage in vigorous physical activity.

- Unhealthy diet and physical inactivity play an important role in many chronic diseases and conditions, including type 2 diabetes, hypertension, heart disease, stroke, breast cancer, colon cancer, gallbladder disease, and arthritis.

The Cost Of Obesity And Chronic Diseases

- Among children and adolescents, annual hospital costs related to obesity were $127 million during 1997–1999 (in 2001 constant U.S. dollars), up from $35 million during 1979–1981.

- In 2000, the total cost of obesity in the United States was estimated to be $117 billion, of which $61 billion was for direct medical costs and $56 billion was for indirect costs.

- Among U.S. adults in 1996, $31 billion of treatment costs (in year 2000 dollars)—17% of direct medical costs—for cardiovascular disease was related to overweight and obesity.

✎ What's It Mean?

Chronic Diseases: Diseases such as heart disease, cancer, and diabetes—these are the leading causes of death and disability in the United States. These diseases account for 7 of every 10 deaths and affect the quality of life of 90 million Americans. Although chronic diseases are among the most common and costly health problems, they are also among the most preventable. Adopting healthy behaviors such as eating nutritious foods, being physically active, and avoiding tobacco use can prevent or control the devastating effects of these diseases.

Source: Excerpted from "Appendix C: Glossary of Terms," *Dietary Guidelines for Americans 2005*, U.S. Department of Agriculture, 2005.

How Good Nutrition, Physical Activity, And Weight Loss Save Money

Nutrition

- Each year, over $33 billion in medical costs and $9 billion in lost productivity due to heart disease, cancer, stroke, and diabetes are attributed to diet.

Physical Activity

- In 2000, health care costs associated with physical inactivity were more than $76 billion.

- If 10% of adults began a regular walking program, $5.6 billion in heart disease costs could be saved.

- Every dollar spent on physical activity programs for older adults with hip fractures results in a $4.50 return.

Weight Loss

- A 10% weight loss will reduce an overweight person's lifetime medical costs by $2,200–$5,300.

- The lifetime medical costs of five diseases and conditions (hypertension, diabetes, heart disease, stroke, and high cholesterol) among moderately obese people are $10,000 higher than among people at a healthy weight.

Promising Approaches For Preventing Obesity

- Children who are ever breast-fed are 15%–25% less likely to become overweight, and those who are breast-fed for six months or more are 20%–40% less likely.

- Regular physical activity is a key part of any weight loss effort. Developing multiuse trails can directly affect the obesity epidemic by giving more people access to places for physical activity.

- Reducing the time spent watching television appears to be effective for treating and preventing obesity.

- Increased physical activity for overweight patients reduces many of the illnesses associated with obesity, helps maintain weight loss, and helps prevent weight gain.

🖒 Remember!!

By improving eating habits and increasing physical activity, we can reduce obesity and other chronic diseases. Increasing opportunities for healthy eating, such as making fruits and vegetables more available, will enable people to eat better. Increasing opportunities for physical activity, including multiuse trails, will help more people be active.

Source: CDC, 2004.

Chapter 39

Health Risks Of Being Overweight

Weighing too much may increase your risk for developing many health problems. If you are overweight or obese on a body mass index (BMI) chart, you may be at risk for the following:

- type 2 diabetes
- cancer
- osteoarthritis
- fatty liver disease

- heart disease and stroke
- sleep apnea
- gallbladder disease

You can lower your health risks by losing as little as 10 to 20 pounds.

Type 2 Diabetes

What is it?

Type 2 diabetes used to be called adult-onset diabetes or noninsulin-dependent diabetes. It is the most common type of diabetes in the U.S. Type 2 diabetes is a disease in which blood sugar levels are above normal. High blood sugar is a major cause of early death, heart disease, kidney disease, stroke, and blindness.

About This Chapter: From "Do You Know the Health Risks of Being Overweight?" National Institute of Diabetes and Digestive and Kidney Diseases, NIH Pub. No. 04-4098, November 2004.

How is it linked to overweight?

More than 80 percent of people with type 2 diabetes are overweight. It is not known exactly why people who are overweight are more likely to suffer from this disease. It may be that being overweight causes cells to change, making them less effective at using sugar from the blood. This then puts stress on the cells that produce insulin (a hormone that carries sugar from the blood to cells) and makes them gradually fail.

♣ It's A Fact!!
If you are overweight, you are more likely to develop certain health problems. You can improve your health by losing as little as 10 to 20 pounds.

What can weight loss do?

You can lower your risk for developing type 2 diabetes by losing weight and increasing the amount of physical activity you do. If you have type 2 diabetes, losing weight and becoming more physically active can help you control your blood sugar levels. Losing weight and exercising more may also allow you to reduce the amount of diabetes medication you take.

Heart Disease And Stroke

What is it?

Heart disease means that the heart and circulation (blood flow) are not functioning normally. If you have heart disease, you may suffer from a heart attack, congestive heart failure, sudden cardiac death, angina (chest pain), or abnormal heart rhythm. During a stroke, blood and oxygen do not flow normally to the brain, possibly causing paralysis or death. Heart disease is the leading cause of death in the U.S., and stroke is the third leading cause.

How is it linked to overweight?

People who are overweight are more likely to suffer from high blood pressure, high levels of triglycerides (blood fats) and LDL cholesterol (a fat-like substance often called the "bad cholesterol"), and low levels of HDL cholesterol (the "good cholesterol"). These are all risk factors for heart disease and stroke. In addition, people with more body fat have higher blood levels of substances that cause inflammation. Inflammation in blood vessels and throughout the body may raise heart disease risk.

What can weight loss do?

Losing 5 to 15 percent of your weight can lower your chances for developing heart disease or having a stroke. If you weigh 200 pounds, this means losing as little as 10 pounds. Weight loss may improve your blood pressure, triglyceride, and cholesterol levels; improve how your heart works and your blood flows; and decrease inflammation throughout your body.

Cancer

What is it?

Cancer occurs when cells in one part of the body, such as the colon, grow abnormally or out of control and possibly spread to other parts of the body, such as the liver. Cancer is the second leading cause of death in the U.S.

How is it linked to overweight?

Being overweight may increase the risk of developing several types of cancer, including cancers of the colon, esophagus, and kidney. Overweight is also linked with uterine and postmenopausal breast cancer in women. Gaining weight during adult life increases the risk for several of these cancers. Being overweight also may increase the risk of dying from some cancers. It is not known exactly how being overweight increases cancer risk. It may be that fat cells make hormones that affect cell growth and lead to cancer. Also, eating or physical activity habits that may lead to being overweight may also contribute to cancer risk.

What can weight loss do?

Avoiding weight gain may prevent a rise in cancer risk. Weight loss, and healthy eating and physical activity habits, may lower cancer risk.

Sleep Apnea

What is it?

Sleep apnea is a condition in which a person stops breathing for short periods during the night. A person who has sleep apnea may suffer from daytime sleepiness, difficulty concentrating, and even heart failure.

How is it linked to overweight?

The risk for sleep apnea is higher for people who are overweight. A person who is overweight may have more fat stored around his or her neck. This may make the airway smaller. A smaller airway can make breathing difficult, loud (snoring), or stop altogether. In addition, fat stored in the neck and throughout the body can produce substances that cause inflammation. Inflammation in the neck may be a risk factor for sleep apnea.

What can weight loss do?

Weight loss usually improves sleep apnea. Weight loss may help to decrease neck size and lessen inflammation.

Osteoarthritis

What is it?

Osteoarthritis is a common joint disorder. With osteoarthritis, the joint bone and cartilage (tissue that protects joints) wear away. Osteoarthritis most often affects the joints of the knees, hips, and lower back.

How is it linked to overweight?

Extra weight may place extra pressure on joints and cartilage, causing them to wear away. In addition, people with more body fat may have higher blood levels of substances that cause inflammation. Inflammation at the joints may raise the risk for osteoarthritis.

What can weight loss do?

Weight loss can decrease stress on your knees, hips, and lower back, and lessen inflammation in your body. If you have osteoarthritis, losing weight may help improve your symptoms.

> ✔ **Quick Tip**
> ## How can I lower my health risks?
>
> If you are overweight, losing as little as 5 percent of your body weight may lower your risk for several diseases, including heart disease and diabetes. If you weigh 200 pounds, this means losing 10 pounds. Slow and steady weight loss of ½ to 2 pounds per week, and not more than 3 pounds per week, is the safest way to lose weight.

Gallbladder Disease

What is it?

Gallstones are clusters of solid material that form in the gallbladder. They are made mostly of cholesterol and can sometimes cause abdominal or back pain.

How is it linked to overweight?

People who are overweight have a higher risk for developing gallbladder disease and gallstones. They may produce more cholesterol, a risk factor for gallstones. Also, people who are overweight may have an enlarged gallbladder, which may not work properly.

What can weight loss do?

Weight loss—especially fast weight loss (more than three pounds per week) or loss of a large amount of weight—can actually increase your chance of developing gallstones. Modest, slow weight loss of about ½ to 2 pounds a week is less likely to cause gallstones.

Fatty Liver Disease

What is it?

Fatty liver disease occurs when fat builds up in the liver cells and causes injury and inflammation in the liver. It can sometimes lead to severe liver damage, cirrhosis (build-up of scar tissue that blocks proper blood flow in the liver), or even liver failure. Fatty liver disease is like alcoholic liver damage, but it is not caused by alcohol and can occur in people who drink little or no alcohol. The National Digestive Diseases Information Clearinghouse (NDDIC) has more information on fatty liver disease or nonalcoholic steatohepatitis (NASH).

How is it linked to overweight?

People who have diabetes or "pre-diabetes" (when blood sugar levels are higher than normal but not yet in the diabetic range) are more likely to have fatty liver disease than people without these conditions. And people who are overweight are more likely to have diabetes (see type 2 diabetes). It is not known why some people who are overweight or diabetic get fatty liver and others do not.

What can weight loss do?

Losing weight can help you control your blood sugar levels. It can also reduce the build-up of fat in your liver and prevent further injury. People with fatty liver disease should avoid drinking alcohol.

♣ It's A Fact!!

To lose weight and keep it off over time, try to make long-term changes in your eating and physical activity habits. Choose healthy foods, such as vegetables, fruits, whole grains, and low-fat meat and dairy products, more often and eat just enough food to satisfy you. Try to do at least 30 minutes of moderate-intensity physical activity—like walking—on most days of the week, preferably every day. To lose weight, or to maintain weight loss, you may need to do more than 30 minutes of moderate physical activity daily.

The Weight-control Information Network (WIN) http://win.niddk.gov/publications/index offers many fact sheets to help you eat better and increase your physical activity. WIN fact sheets are listed as follows.

"Active at Any Size" describes the benefits of being physically active no matter what a person's size, and presents a variety of activities that very large people can enjoy safely.

"Just Enough for You: About Food Portions" describes the difference between a portion—the amount of food a person chooses to eat—and a measured serving. It offers tips for judging portion sizes and for controlling portions at home and when eating out.

"Walking...A Step in the Right Direction" offers tips for getting started on a walking program and illustrates warm-up stretching exercises. It also includes a sample walking program.

"Weight and Waist Measurement Tools for Adults" offers guidance on determining whether your weight is healthy.

"Weight Loss for Life" contains information about safe and effective weight loss programs and offers tips to help you create your own weight loss plan.

Chapter 40

What Is Obesity?

The most important part of being a normal weight isn't looking a certain way—it's feeling good and staying healthy. Having too much body fat can be harmful to the body in many ways.

The good news is that it's never too late to make changes in eating and exercise habits to control your weight, and those changes don't have to be as big as you might think. So if you or someone you know is obese or overweight, this chapter can give you information and tips for dealing with the problem by adopting a healthier lifestyle.

What is obesity?

Being obese and being overweight are not exactly the same thing. An obese person has a large amount of extra body fat, not just a few extra pounds. People who are obese are very overweight and at risk for serious health problems.

To determine if someone is obese, doctors and other health care professionals often use a measurement called body mass index (BMI). First, a doctor measures a person's height and weight. Then the doctor uses these numbers to calculate another number, the BMI.

About This Chapter: This information was provided by TeensHealth, one of the largest resources online for medically reviewed health information written for parents, kids, and teens. For more articles like this one, visit www.TeensHealth.org, or www.KidsHealth.org. © 2005 The Nemours Center for Children's Health Media, a division of The Nemours Foundation.

Once the doctor has calculated a child's or teen's BMI, he or she will plot this number on a specific chart to see how it compares to other people of the same age and gender. A person with a BMI above the 95th percentile (meaning the BMI is greater than that of 95% of people of the same age and gender) is generally considered overweight. A person with a BMI between the 85th and 95th percentiles typically is considered at risk for overweight. Obesity is the term used for extreme overweight. There are some exceptions to this formula, though. For instance, someone who is very muscular (like a bodybuilder) may have a high BMI without being obese because the excess weight is from extra muscle, not fat.

What causes obesity?

People gain weight when the body takes in more calories than it burns off. Those extra calories are stored as fat. The amount of weight gain that leads to obesity doesn't happen in a few weeks or months. Because being obese is more than just being a few pounds overweight, people who are obese have usually been getting more calories than they need for years.

Genes—small parts of the DNA that people inherit from their parents and that determine traits like hair or eye color—can play an important role in this weight gain. Some of your genes tell your body how to metabolize food and how to use extra calories or stored fat. Some people burn calories faster or slower than others do because of their genes.

Obesity can run in families, but just how much is due to genes is hard to determine. Many families eat the same foods, have the same habits (like snacking in front of the TV), and tend to think alike when it comes to weight issues (like urging children to eat a lot at dinner so they can grow "big and strong"). All of these situations can contribute to weight gain, so it can be difficult to figure out if a person is born with a tendency to be obese or overweight or learns eating and exercise habits that lead to weight gain. In most cases, weight problems arise from a combination of habits and genetic factors. Certain illnesses, like thyroid gland problems or unusual genetic disorders, are uncommon causes for people gaining weight.

Sometimes emotions can fuel obesity as well. People tend to eat more when they are upset, anxious, sad, stressed out, or even bored. Then after they eat too much, they may feel bad about it and eat more to deal with those bad feelings, creating a tough cycle to break.

One of the most important factors in weight gain is a sedentary lifestyle. People are much less active today than they used to be, with televisions, computers, and video games filling their spare time. Cars dominate our lives, and fewer people walk or ride bikes to get somewhere. As lives become busier, there is less time to cook healthy meals, so more and more people eat at restaurants, grab takeout food, or buy quick foods at the grocery store or food market to heat up at home. All of these can contain lots more fat and calories than meals prepared from fresh foods at home.

Who is at risk for becoming obese?

The number of people who are obese is rising. About 1.2 billion people in the world are overweight and at least 300 million of them are obese, even though obesity is one of the ten most preventable health risks, according to the World Health Organization. In the United States, more than 97 million adults—that's more than half—are overweight and almost one in five adults is obese. Among teenagers and kids six years and older, more than 15% are overweight—that's more than three times the number of young people who were overweight in the 1970s. At least 300,000 deaths every year in the United States can be linked to obesity.

✤ **It's A Fact!!**

As a culture, we have an excess energy crisis. Often we eat more food and get less exercise than we need. Inactive people (all ages) with lots of extra fat stores more often end up with diabetes, high blood pressure, cancer, heart disease, and stroke. Today, 50% of adults and 25% of youth are overweight, and these numbers have skyrocketed. Super-sizing, food advertising, screen time (TV, movies, computers, electronic games), and car travel all contribute. It takes a committed effort to maintain a healthy lifestyle, but people feel much better when they do.

Source: Excerpted from "Nutrition Tips for Teens," © 2003 Munson Healthcare. All rights reserved. Reprinted with permission.

In the United States, women are slightly more at risk for becoming obese than men. Race and ethnicity also can be factors—in adolescents, obesity is more common among Mexican Americans and African Americans.

How can obesity affect your health?

Obesity is bad news for both body and mind. Not only does it make a person feel tired and uncomfortable, it can wear down joints and put extra stress on other parts of the body. When a person is carrying extra weight, it's harder to keep up with friends, play sports, or just walk between classes at school. It is also associated with breathing problems such as asthma and sleep apnea and problems with hips and knee joints that may require surgery.

There can be more serious consequences as well. Obesity in young people can cause illnesses that once were thought to be problems only for adults, such as hypertension (high blood pressure), high cholesterol levels, liver disease, and type 2 diabetes, a disease in which the body has trouble converting food to energy, resulting in high blood sugar levels. As they get older, people who are obese are more likely to develop heart disease, congestive heart failure, bladder problems, and, in women, problems with the reproductive system. Obesity also can lead to stroke, greater risk for certain cancers such as breast or colon cancer, and even death.

In addition to other potential problems, people who are obese are more likely to be depressed. That can start a vicious cycle: When people are overweight, they may feel sad or even angry and eat to make themselves feel better. Then they feel worse for eating again. And when someone's feeling depressed, that person is less likely to go out and exercise.

How can you avoid becoming overweight or obese?

The best way to avoid these health problems is to maintain a healthy weight. And the keys to healthy weight are regular exercise and good eating habits.

To stay active, try to exercise 30 to 60 minutes every day. Your exercise doesn't have to be hard core, either. Walking, swimming, and stretching are all good ways to burn calories and help you stay fit. Try these activities to get moving:

- Go outside for a walk.

- Take the stairs instead of the elevator.

- Walk or bike to places (such as school or a friend's house) instead of driving.

- If you have to drive somewhere, park farther away than you need to and walk the extra distance.

- Tackle those household chores, such as vacuuming, washing the car, or cleaning the bathroom—they all burn calories.

- Alternate activities so you don't get bored: Try running, biking, skating—the possibilities are endless.

- Limit your time watching TV or playing video games; even reading a book burns more energy.

- Go dancing—it can burn more than 300 calories an hour!

Eating well doesn't mean dieting over and over again to lose a few pounds. Instead, try to make healthy choices every day:

- Soft drinks, fruit juices, and sports drinks are loaded with sugar; drink fat-free or low-fat milk or water instead.

- Eat at least five servings of fruit and vegetables a day.

- Avoid fast-food restaurants. If you can't, try to pick healthier choices like grilled chicken or salads, and stick to regular servings—don't super-size!

- If you want a snack, try carrot sticks, a piece of fruit, or a piece of whole-grain toast instead of processed foods like chips and crackers, which can be loaded with fat and calories.

- Eat when you're hungry, not when you're bored or because you can't think of anything else to do.

- Eat a healthy breakfast every day.

- Don't eat meals or snacks while watching TV because you'll probably end up eating more than you intend to.

- Pay attention to the portion sizes of what you eat.

What can you do if you are overweight or obese?

Before you start trying to lose weight, talk to a doctor, a parent, or a registered dietitian. With their help, you can come up with a safe plan, based on eating well and exercising. Remember that teenagers need to keep eating regularly. Don't starve yourself because you won't get the nutrients you need to grow and develop normally.

♣ It's A Fact!!
How Big Is A Serving?

- 1 cup (225 grams) of fruit is the size of a baseball.

- 1 ounce (28 grams) of snack foods (such as pretzels) equals a large handful.

- 3 ounces (85 grams) of meat is the size of a deck of cards.

Source: © 2005 The Nemours Center for Children's Health Media, a division of The Nemours Foundation.

You may also want to keep a food and activity journal. Keep track of what you eat, when you exercise, and how you feel. Changes can take time, but seeing your progress in writing will help you stick to your plan. You might also want to consider attending a support group; check your local hospital or the health section of a newspaper for groups that meet near you. Above all, surround yourself with friends and family who will be there for you and help you tackle these important changes in your life.

Chapter 41

What Are Eating Disorders?

Eating disorders are extreme expressions of food and weight issues experienced by many individuals, particularly girls and women. They include anorexia nervosa, bulimia nervosa, and binge eating. Eating disorders are dangerous behaviors that result in big health problems.

Teens with eating disorders can do major damage to their bodies. Restricting what you eat can make you sick—like feeling nauseous, tired, dizzy, or irritable. If this behavior goes on too long, it can mess up your menstrual cycle, dry out your hair and skin, and might even cause early osteoporosis—a disease of the bones. The physical consequences can become life threatening.

But the physical problems are only half the story. The emotional problems can be serious too. An unhealthy attitude about food and body image is the main problem. Some girls use food to make themselves feel better; others stop eating to feel like they are "in control" of their life. Both behaviors leave people feeling bad about what they are eating. And worst of all, the more people begin to obsess over what they are eating (or not eating), the less they care about other things—like school, friends, or other activities.

About This Chapter: This chapter begins with text from "What Are Eating Disorders," BodyWise, U.S. Department of Health and Human Services, 2004. Additional text is excerpted from the following publications of the National Women's Health Information Center: "Anorexia—Easy to Read," August 2004; "Bulimia—Easy to Read," August 2004; "Binge Eating Disorder," January 2005; "Boys and Eating Disorders," 2004; and "At Risk: All Ethnic And Cultural Groups," 2004.

✎ What's It Mean?

Anorexia nervosa is self-starvation. People with this disorder eat very little even though they are thin. They have an intense and overpowering fear of body fat and weight gain.

Bulimia nervosa is characterized by cycles of binge eating and purging, either by vomiting or taking laxatives or diuretics (water pills). People with bulimia have a fear of body fat even though their size and weight may be normal.

Overexercising is exercising compulsively for long periods of time as a way to burn calories from food that has just been eaten. People with anorexia or bulimia may overexercise.

Binge eating disorder means eating large amounts of food in a short period of time, usually alone, without being able to stop when full. The overeating or bingeing is often accompanied by feeling out of control and then depressed, guilty, or disgusted.

Disordered eating refers to troublesome eating behaviors, such as restrictive dieting, bingeing, or purging, which occur less frequently or are less severe than those required to meet the full criteria for the diagnosis of an eating disorder.

Source: "At Risk," National Women's Health Information Center, 2004.

How do people get eating disorders?

Experts don't know exactly how people develop eating disorders, but it is likely the result of many factors. Many people who suffer from eating disorders have low self-esteem. Most people with eating disorders share certain traits such as a fear of becoming fat, feelings of not measuring up to other people's expectations, or feeling helpless. Some people with eating disorders feel they have to be perfect in every way—having a perfect body, getting perfect grades, and being an excellent athlete. People who suffer from eating disorders may be depressed or feel they lack control over their lives. Sometimes, they also feel like they don't fit in or don't belong. Often, the problems begin when a person is dealing with a difficult transition, shock, or loss.

Frequently Asked Questions About Anorexia

What is anorexia?

Anorexia nervosa, typically called anorexia, is a type of eating disorder that mainly affects girls and young women. A person with this disorder has an intense fear of gaining weight and limits the food she eats. She:

- has a low body weight;
- refuses to keep a normal body weight;
- is extremely afraid of becoming fat;
- believes she is fat even when she's very thin;
- misses three (menstrual) periods in a row—for girls/women who have started having their periods.

What causes it?

Anorexia is more than just a problem with food. It's a way of using food or starving oneself to feel more in control of her life and to ease tension, anger, and anxiety. While there is no single known cause of anorexia, several things may contribute to the development of the disorder:

- **Biology:** Several biological factors, including genetics and other related hormones, may contribute in the onset the disorder.

- **Culture:** Some cultures in the U.S. have an ideal of extreme thinness. Women may define themselves on how beautiful they are.

- **Personal feelings:** Someone with anorexia may feel badly about herself, feel helpless, and hate the way she looks. She has unrealistic expectations of herself and strives for perfection. She feels worthless, despite achievements and perceives a social pressure to be thin.

- **Stressful events or life changes:** Things like starting a new school or job or being teased or traumatic events, like rape, can lead to the onset of anorexia.

- **Families:** People with a mother or sister with anorexia are more likely to develop the disorder. Parents who think appearance is very important, diet themselves, and criticize their children's bodies are more likely to have a child with anorexia.

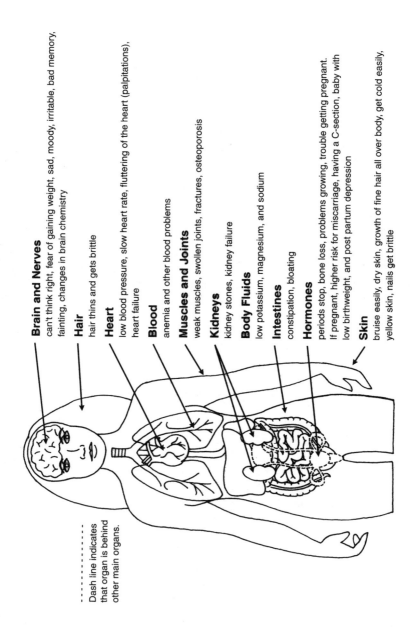

Brain and Nerves
can't think right, fear of gaining weight, sad, moody, irritable, bad memory, fainting, changes in brain chemistry

Hair
hair thins and gets brittle

Heart
low blood pressure, slow heart rate, fluttering of the heart (palpitations), heart failure

Blood
anemia and other blood problems

Muscles and Joints
weak muscles, swollen joints, fractures, osteoporosis

Kidneys
kidney stones, kidney failure

Body Fluids
low potassium, magnesium, and sodium

Intestines
constipation, bloating

Hormones
periods stop, bone loss, problems growing, trouble getting pregnant. If pregnant, higher risk for miscarriage, having a C-section, baby with low birthweight, and post partum depression

Skin
bruise easily, dry skin, growth of fine hair all over body, get cold easily, yellow skin, nails get brittle

- - - - - - - - - - - -
Dash line indicates that organ is behind other main organs.

Figure 41.1. Anorexia affects your whole body (Source: National Women's Health Information Center, August 2004).

What are signs of anorexia?

A person with anorexia will have many of the following signs:

- Looks a lot thinner
- Uses extreme measures to lose weight
    - makes herself throw up
    - takes pills to urinate or have a bowel movement (BM)
    - takes diet pills
    - doesn't eat or follows a strict diet
    - exercises a lot
    - weighs food and counts calories
    - moves food around the plate; doesn't eat it
- Has a distorted body image
    - thinks she's fat when she's too thin
    - wears baggy clothes to hide appearance
    - fears gaining weight
    - weighs herself many times a day
- Acts differently
    - talks about weight and food all the time
    - won't eat in front of others
    - acts moody or depressed
    - doesn't socialize

What happens to your body with anorexia?

The body doesn't get the energy from foods that it needs, so it slows down. Look at the picture in Figure 41.1 to find out how anorexia affects your health.

Can someone with anorexia get better?

Yes. People with this disorder can get better. The treatment depends on what the person needs. The person must get back to a healthy weight. Many times, eating disorders happen with other problems, like depression and anxiety problems. These problems are treated along with the anorexia and may involve medicines that help reduce feelings of depression and anxiety.

With outpatient care, the patient goes to the hospital during the day for treatment, but lives at home. Sometimes, the patient goes to a hospital and stays there for treatment. Different types of health care providers, like doctors, nutritionists, and therapists, will help the patient get better. These providers will help the patient regain the weight, improve physical health and nutrition, learn healthy eating patterns, and cope with thoughts and feelings related to the disorder. After leaving the hospital, the patient continues to get help from her providers. Individual counseling can also help someone with anorexia. Counseling may involve the whole family too, especially if the patient is young. Support groups may also be a part of treatment. Support groups help patients and families talk about their experiences and help each other get better.

Can women who had anorexia in the past still get pregnant?

It depends. Women who have fully recovered from anorexia have a better chance of getting pregnant. While a woman has active anorexia, she does not get her usual period and doesn't normally ovulate, so it would be harder to get pregnant. However, she may get pregnant as she regains weight because her reproductive system is getting back to normal. After they gain back some weight, some women may skip or miss their periods, which can cause problems getting pregnant. If this happens, a woman should see her doctor.

Can anorexia hurt a baby when the mother is pregnant?

If a woman with active anorexia gets pregnant, the baby and mother can be affected. The baby is more likely to be born at a low weight and born early. The mother is more likely to have a miscarriage, deliver by C-section, and have depression after the baby is born.

♣ It's A Fact!!

Girls often experiment with different ways to lose as much weight as possible or to keep their weight down. Here are some examples of unsafe methods girls use to control their weight:

- Diuretics (or water pills) make your body lose water but also important nutrients. In extreme cases, this can cause heart problems.

- Laxatives can cause stomachaches and cramps as well as other serious problems to your digestive system. Laxatives can become habit-forming.

- Self-induced vomiting, even once in a while, can pop blood vessels in your face and swell up your neck glands. Because your food isn't being digested right, you may suffer stomachaches, constipation, heartburn, or diarrhea. Also, repeated vomiting can ruin your teeth and give you cavities.

- Diet pills can cause your heart to beat faster and make you jittery. They also are habit-forming. Once they wear off, you become hungry and want to eat, so you reach for another pill to control your appetite.

- Serious over exercising is another unhealthy way some people control their weight. Exercising for long periods of time when it is not part of a program (like with your school coach) is not smart. Over exercising will make you feel tired and increase your chance of injuries.

Source: U.S. Department of Health and Human Services, 2004.

Frequently Asked Questions About Bulimia

What is bulimia?

Bulimia nervosa, typically called bulimia, is a type of eating disorder. Someone with bulimia eats a lot of food in a short amount of time (called bingeing) and then tries to prevent weight gain by purging. Purging might be done in these ways:

- making oneself throw up

- taking laxatives, pills, or liquids that increase how fast food moves through your body and leads to a bowel movement (BM)

A person with bulimia may also use these ways to prevent weight gain:

- exercising a lot

- eating very little or not at all

- taking pills to pass urine

What causes it?

Bulimia is more than just a problem with food. Purging and other behaviors to prevent weight gain are ways for people with bulimia to feel more in control of their lives and ease stress and anxiety. While there is no single known cause of bulimia, many things may have a role in its development:

- **Biology:** There are studies being done to look at many genes, hormones, and chemicals in the brain that may have an effect on the development of, and recovery from, bulimia.

- **Culture:** Some cultures in the U.S. have an ideal of extreme thinness. Women may define themselves on how beautiful they are.

- **Personal feelings:** Someone with bulimia may feel badly about herself, feel helpless, and hate the way she looks.

- **Stressful events or life changes:** Things like starting a new school or job, being teased, or traumatic events like rape can lead to the onset of bulimia.

- **Families:** The attitude of parents about appearance and diet affects their kids. Also, a person is more likely to develop bulimia if a mother or sister has it.

What are signs of bulimia?

People with bulimia may be underweight, overweight, or have a normal weight. This makes it harder to know if someone has this disorder. However, someone with bulimia may have the following signs:

- Uses extreme measures to lose weight

  - uses diet pills, or takes pills to urinate or have a bowel movement (BM)

  - goes to the bathroom all the time after she eats (to throw up)

  - exercises a lot, even during bad weather, tiredness, sickness, or injury

- Shows signs of throwing up

  - swelling of the cheeks or jaw area

  - cuts and calluses on the back of the hands and knuckles

  - teeth that look clear

- Acts differently

  - is depressed

  - doesn't see friends or participate in activities as much

What happens to someone who has bulimia?

Bulimia can be very harmful to the body. Look at the picture in Figure 41.2 to find out how bulimia affects your health.

Can someone with bulimia get better?

Yes, a person with bulimia can get better. Different types of therapy have worked to help people with bulimia. This may include individual, group, and family therapy. A class of medicines, also used for depression, like Zoloft, has been effective when used with therapy. These medicines change the way certain chemicals work in the brain.

Can women who had bulimia in the past still get pregnant?

Bulimia can cause problems with a woman's period. She may not get it every four weeks or it may stop. But researchers don't think this affects a woman's chances of getting pregnant after she recovers.

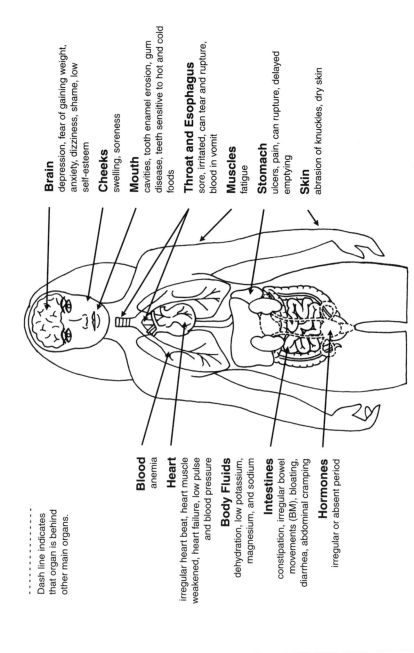

Brain
depression, fear of gaining weight, anxiety, dizziness, shame, low self-esteem

Cheeks
swelling, soreness

Mouth
cavities, tooth enamel erosion, gum disease, teeth sensitive to hot and cold foods

Throat and Esophagus
sore, irritated, can tear and rupture, blood in vomit

Muscles
fatigue

Stomach
ulcers, pain, can rupture, delayed emptying

Skin
abrasion of knuckles, dry skin

- - - - - - - - - - -
Dash line indicates that organ is behind other main organs.

Blood
anemia

Heart
irregular heart beat, heart muscle weakened, heart failure, low pulse and blood pressure

Body Fluids
dehydration, low potassium, magnesium, and sodium

Intestines
constipation, irregular bowel movements (BM), bloating, diarrhea, abdominal cramping

Hormones
irregular or absent period

Figure 41.2. Bulimia affects your whole body (Source: National Women's Health Information Center, August 2004).

Does bulimia hurt a baby when the mother is pregnant?

If a woman with active bulimia gets pregnant, the following problems may result:

- miscarriage

- high blood pressure in the mother

- baby isn't born alive

- low birth weight

- low Apgar score, which are tests done after birth to make sure the baby is healthy during the delivery, they baby tries to come out with feet or buttocks first

- birth by C-section

- baby is born early

- depression after the baby is born

Frequently Asked Questions About Binge Eating Disorder

What is binge eating disorder?

People with binge eating disorder often eat an unusually large amount of food and feel out of control during the binges. People with binge eating disorder also may:

- eat more quickly than usual during binge episodes;
- eat until they are uncomfortably full;
- eat when they are not hungry;
- eat alone because of embarrassment;
- feel disgusted, depressed, or guilty after overeating.

What causes binge eating disorder?

No one knows for sure what causes binge eating disorder. Researchers are looking at the following factors that may affect binge eating:

- **Depression:** As many as half of all people with binge eating disorder are depressed or have been depressed in the past.

- **Dieting:** Some people binge after skipping meals, not eating enough food each day, or avoiding certain kinds of food.

- **Coping skills:** Studies suggest that people with binge eating may have trouble handling some of their emotions. Many people who are binge eaters say that being angry, sad, bored, worried, or stressed can cause them to binge eat.

- **Biology:** Researchers are looking into how brain chemicals and metabolism (the way the body uses calories) affect binge eating disorder. Research also suggests that genes may be involved in binge eating, since the disorder often occurs in several members of the same family.

Certain behaviors and emotional problems are more common in people with binge eating disorder. These include abusing alcohol, acting quickly without thinking (impulsive behavior), and not feeling in charge of themselves.

What are the health consequences of binge eating disorder?

People with binge eating disorder are usually very upset by their binge eating and may become depressed. Research has shown that people with binge eating disorder report more health problems, stress, trouble sleeping, and suicidal thoughts than people without an eating disorder. People with binge eating disorder often feel badly about themselves and may miss work, school, or social activities to binge eat.

People with binge eating disorder may gain weight. Weight gain can lead to obesity, and obesity raises the risk for the following health problems:

• type 2 diabetes

• high blood pressure

• high cholesterol

• gallbladder disease

• heart disease

• certain types of cancer

What is the treatment for binge eating disorder?

People with binge eating disorder should get help from a health care provider, such as a psychiatrist, psychologist, or clinical social worker. There are several different ways to treat binge eating disorder:

• Cognitive-behavioral therapy teaches people how to keep track of their eating and change their unhealthy eating habits. It teaches them how to cope with stressful situations. It also helps them feel better about their body shape and weight.

• Interpersonal psychotherapy helps people look at their relationships with friends and family and make changes in problem areas.

• Drug therapy, such as antidepressants, may be helpful for some people.

Other treatments include dialectical behavior therapy, which helps people regulate their emotions; drug therapy with the anti-seizure medication topiramate; exercise in combination with cognitive-behavioral therapy; and support groups.

Many people with binge eating disorder also have a problem with obesity. There are treatments for obesity, like weight loss surgery (gastrointestinal surgery), but these treatments will not treat the underlying problem of binge eating disorder.

Boys And Eating Disorders

Eating disorders often are seen as problems affecting only girls. However, studies suggest that hundreds of thousands of boys are experiencing these disorders. Although bulimia is not common among males, one in four pre-adolescent cases of anorexia have been found to occur in boys. Studies also suggest that boys may be as likely as girls to develop binge eating disorder.

Males make up the majority of people identified as having muscle dysmorphia, a type of body image disorder characterized by extreme concern with becoming more muscular. People with this disorder, which has been found to occur among bodybuilders, see themselves as puny despite being very muscular, and are likely to use steroids and other drugs to gain muscle mass.

Factors Associated With Eating Disorders Are Similar For Males And Females

The characteristics of males with eating disorders are similar to those seen in females with eating disorders. These factors include low self-esteem, the need to be accepted, an inability to cope with emotional pressures, and family and relationship problems. Homosexuality also appears to be a risk factor for males because it may include them in a subculture that places a premium on appearance.

Both males and females with eating disorders are likely to experience depression, substance abuse, anxiety disorders, and personality disorders. However, substance abuse is more common among males than females with eating disorders. Male patients with eating disorders have been found to be more severely affected by osteoporosis than female patients.

The signs and symptoms of eating disorders are similar for boys and girls. They are described elsewhere in this chapter under the headings for the different types of eating disorders.

Students of all ethnic and cultural groups are vulnerable to developing eating disorders. For example, Black and Hispanic boys have been found to be more likely to binge eat than Caucasian boys.

Boys May Try To Lose Fat And Gain Muscle To Improve Body Image And/Or Athletic Performance

While the female body ideal is thin, the male ideal is lean, V-shaped, and muscular. Unlike girls, who generally want to lose weight, boys are equally divided between those who want to lose weight and those who want to gain weight. Boys who consider themselves overweight want to lose weight, while those who think they are too thin want to gain weight. All want to be more muscular.

Boys may try to lose fat and/or gain muscle for many reasons. Some of these are: to avoid being teased about being fat; to improve body image; to increase strength and/or to improve athletic performance in wrestling, track, swimming, or other sports.

✔ **Quick Tip**
Where To Go For Help

If you think that you or somebody you know may have an eating disorder, get help! Don't wait and don't try to deal with the problem by yourself. Talk to a parent or other trusted adult like a counselor, coach, relative, or teacher.

Confronting someone who has an eating disorder is very hard. Your friend may not want to admit she has a problem and may get angry with you for trying to help. If you think a friend has an eating disorder, let her know that you care about her, you're worried, and you want to help. Urge her to tell a trusted adult about her eating disorder. If she won't do it, you need to talk to an adult yourself. She needs as much support and understanding from the people in her life as possible. Reaching out to get help could save your friend's life.

Source: From BodyWise, GirlPower (http://www.girl power.gov), U.S. Department of Health and Human Services, 2004.

Overweight boys are at a higher risk for dieting than those who are not overweight. Boys who think they are too small, on the other hand, may be at a greater risk than other boys for using steroids or taking untested nutritional supplements such as protein and creatine to increase muscle mass.

Boys Are Less Likely To Be Diagnosed Early With An Eating Disorder

Doctors reportedly are less likely to make a diagnosis of eating disorders in males than females. Other adults who work with young people and parents also may be less likely to suspect an eating disorder in boys, thereby delaying detection and treatment. A study of 135 males hospitalized with an eating disorder noted that the males with bulimia felt ashamed of having a stereotypically "female" disorder, which might explain their delay in seeking treatment. Binge eating disorder may go unrecognized in males because a male who overeats is less likely to provoke attention than a female who overeats.

Here Are Some Ideas About What To Do

• Communicate openly about body image issues using messages that support acceptance of body diversity, discourage disordered eating, and promote self-esteem.

• Do not tolerate teasing and bullying in school, particularly when focused on a boy's body size or masculinity.

♣ **It's A Fact!!**
Action Figures Are Bulking Up

A recent study noted that some of the most popular male action figures have grown extremely muscular over time. Researchers compared action toys today—including GI Joe and Star Wars' Luke Skywalker and Hans Solo—with their original counterparts. They found that many action figures have acquired the physiques of bodybuilders, with particularly impressive gains in the shoulder and chest areas. Some of the action toys have not only grown more muscular but have also developed increasingly sharp muscle definition, such as rippled abdominals. As noted in the study, if the GI Joe Extreme were 70 inches in size, he would sport larger biceps than any bodybuilder in history.

Source: "Boys," National Women's Health Information Center, 2004.

- Conduct media literacy activities that explore the extremely lean and muscular body shape as the cultural ideal and that build skills to resist such messages.

- Develop policies that prohibit student athletes from engaging in harmful weight control or bodybuilding measures.

- Connect young men with positive role models who will encourage personal growth and development.

At Risk: All Ethnic And Cultural Groups

Boys And Girls Of All Ethnic Groups Are Susceptible To Eating Disorders

Many people believe that eating disorders commonly occur among affluent white females. Although the prevalence of these disorders elsewhere in the population is much lower, an increasing number of males and minorities are also suffering from eating disorders.

Girls and boys from all ethnic and racial groups may suffer from eating disorders and disordered eating. The specific nature of the most common eating problems, as well as risk and protective factors, may vary from group to group but no population is exempt. Research findings regarding prevalence rates and specific types of problems among particular groups are limited, but it is evident that disturbed eating behaviors and attitudes occur across all cultures.

Large percentages of African American, American Indian, and Hispanic females are overweight. Being overweight is a risk factor for engaging in disordered eating behaviors. Risk factors and incidence rates for eating disorders can vary dramatically among subgroups of a specific population.

Cultural Norms Regarding Body Size Can Play A Role In The Development Of Eating Disorders

In Western cultures, the ideal female body is thin. Membership in ethnic groups and cultures that do not value a thin body may protect girls from body dissatisfaction and weight concerns. However, young people who identify with cultures that prefer larger body sizes may be at risk for becoming overweight or obese. Research also suggests that women who think they are smaller than the body size favored by their cultural group may be at risk for binge eating.

Eating Disorders Among Ethnically And Culturally Diverse Girls May Be Underreported And Undetected

Eating disorders among ethnically and culturally diverse girls may be underreported due to the lack of population-based studies that include representatives from these groups. The perception that non-white females are at decreased risk may also contribute to the lack of detection. Stereotyped body images of ethnically diverse women (for example, petite Asian American, heavier African American) can also deter detection. In addition, for some ethnic and cultural groups, seeking professional help for emotional problems is not a common practice.

✔ Quick Tip

Here are some things schools can do to help fight eating disorders:

- Provide students with diverse role models of all shapes and sizes who are praised for their accomplishments, not their appearance.

- Invite community representatives to speak about specific cultural attitudes toward food preferences, dietary practices, and body image.

- Provide students with information on the relationship between nutrition and overall health.

- Gather and disseminate culturally sensitive materials on eating disorders, puberty, and other adolescent health issues.

- Conduct media literacy activities that allow students to examine critically how magazines, television, and other media—including those targeting specific cultural groups—present the concept of beauty.

- Encourage children and adolescents of all ethnic and cultural groups to exercise and participate in sports and other athletic activities.

- Advocate for a safe and respectful school environment that prohibits gender, cultural, and racial stereotyping as well as sexual harassment, teasing, and bullying.

Source: "At Risk," National Women's Health Information Center, 2004.

☞ Remember!!

Eating disorders are treatable and people do recover from them. They are most successfully treated when treated early. While most patients can be treated as outpatients, some need hospitalized care. Because eating disorders are both an emotional and physical problem, a range of professionals are important for recovery. A therapist helps with the underlying emotional issues and a nutritionist or doctor helps with choosing nutritious foods to maintain a normal weight. A doctor also treats any medical complications of an eating disorder.

Source: From "Treatment," BodyWise, GirlPower (http://www.girlpower.gov), U.S. Department of Health and Human Services, 2004.

Girls of different ethnic and cultural groups often receive treatment for the accompanying symptoms of an eating disorder, such as depression or malnutrition, rather than for the eating disorder itself. When these girls are finally diagnosed as having an eating disorder, the disorder (especially anorexia), tends to be more severe. This problem is exacerbated by the difficulty they may have in locating culturally sensitive treatment centers.

Chapter 42

Eating For A Healthy Heart

The Food and Drug Administration (FDA) is a U. S. government agency that makes sure foods are safe, wholesome, and honestly labeled.

Eat Healthy To Help Prevent Heart Disease

What kills Americans most?

Heart disease. It's the No. 1 cause of death in this country.

You can lower your chances of getting heart disease. One way is to choose foods carefully. For a healthy heart, follow these dietary tips:

- eat less fat
- eat less sodium
- eat fewer calories
- eat more fiber

Eat Less Fat

Some fats are more likely to cause heart disease. These fats are usually found in foods from animals, such as meat, milk, cheese, and butter. They also are found in foods with palm and coconut oils.

About This Chapter: From "Eating for a Healthy Heart," U.S. Food and Drug Administration (FDA), February 2000.

Eat Less Sodium

Eating less sodium can help lower some people's blood pressure. This can help reduce the risk of heart disease.

Sodium is something we need in our diets, but most of us eat too much of it. Much of the sodium we eat comes from salt we add to our food at the table or that food companies add to their foods. So, avoid adding salt to foods at the table.

Eat Fewer Calories

When we eat more calories than we need, we gain weight. Being overweight can cause heart disease.

When we eat fewer calories than we need, we lose weight.

Eat More Fiber

Eating fiber from fruits, vegetables and grains may help lower your chances of getting heart disease.

✎ What's It Mean?

Cardiovascular Disease: Refers to diseases of the heart and diseases of the blood vessel system (arteries, capillaries, veins) within a person's entire body, such as the brain, legs, and lungs.

Coronary Heart Disease: A narrowing of the small blood vessels that supply blood and oxygen to the heart (coronary arteries).

Source: Excerpted from "Appendix C: Glossary of Terms," *Dietary Guidelines for Americans 2005*, U.S. Department of Agriculture, 2005.

Diet Tips For A Healthy Heart

- Eat a diet low in saturated fat, especially animal fats and palm and coconut oils.

- Add foods to your diet that are high in monounsaturated fats, such olive oil, canola oil, and seafood.

- Eat foods containing polyunsaturated fats found in plants and seafood. Safflower oil and corn oil are high in polyunsaturated fats.

- Choose a diet moderate in salt and sodium.

- Maintain or improve your weight.

- Eat plenty of grain products, fruits and vegetables.

Eating this way does not mean you have to spend more money on food. You can still eat many foods that cost the same or less than what you're eating now.

Tips For Losing Weight

- Eat smaller portions

- Avoid second helpings

- Eat less fat by staying away from fried foods, rich desserts, and chocolate candy. Foods with a lot of fat have a lot of calories

- Eat more fruits and vegetables

- Eat "low-calorie" foods, such as low-calorie salad dressings

Read The Food Label

The food label can help you eat less fat and sodium, fewer calories, and more fiber.

Look for certain words on food labels: The words can help you spot foods that may help reduce your chances of getting heart disease. FDA has set rules on how these words can be used. So, if the label says "low-fat," the food must be low in fat.

Look at the side or back of the package: Here, you will find "Nutrition Facts." Look for the following words:

- Total fat

- Saturated fat

- Cholesterol

- Sodium

Look at the %Daily Value listed next to each term. If it is 5% or less for fat, saturated fat, cholesterol, and sodium, the food is low in these nutrients. That's good. It means the food fits in with a diet that may help reduce your chances of getting heart disease.

Table 42.1. Here's How To Eat Healthier Foods

Instead of	Do this
Whole or 2 percent milk, and cream	Use 1 percent or skim milk
Fried foods	Eat baked, steamed, boiled, broiled, or microwaved foods
Cooking with lard, butter, palm and coconut oils, and shortenings made with these oils	Cook with these oils only: corn, safflower, sunflower, soybean, cottonseed, olive, canola, peanut, sesame, or shortenings made from these oils
Smoked, cured, salted and canned meat, poultry and fish	Eat unsalted fresh or frozen meat, poultry and fish
Fatty cuts of meat, such as prime rib	Eat lean cuts of meat or cut off the fatty parts of meat
One whole egg in recipes	Use two egg whites
Sour cream and mayonnaise	Use plain low-fat yogurt, low-fat cottage cheese, or low-fat or "light" sour cream and mayonnaise
Sauces, butter and salt	Season vegetables, including potatoes, with herbs and spices
Regular hard and processed cheeses	Eat low-fat, low-sodium cheeses
Crackers with salted tops	Eat unsalted or low-sodium whole-wheat crackers
Regular canned soups, broths and bouillons and dry soup mixes	Eat sodium-reduced canned broths, bouillons and soups, especially those with vegetables
White bread, white rice, and cereals made with white flour	Eat whole-wheat bread, brown rice, and whole-grain cereals
Salted potato chips and other snacks	Choose low-fat, unsalted tortilla and potato chips and unsalted pretzels and popcorn

♣ It's A Fact!!
FDA Allows Qualified Health Claim To Decrease Risk Of Coronary Heart Disease

The Food and Drug Administration (FDA) announced, on November 1, 2004, the availability of a qualified health claim for monounsaturated fat from olive oil and reduced risk of coronary heart disease (CHD).

There is limited but not conclusive evidence that suggests that consumers may reduce their risk of CHD if they consume monounsaturated fat from olive oil and olive oil-containing foods in place of foods high in saturated fat, while at the same time not increasing the total number of calories consumed daily.

"With this claim, consumers can make more informed decisions about maintaining healthy dietary practices," said Dr. Lester M. Crawford, Acting FDA Commissioner. "Since CHD is the number one killer of both men and women in the U.S., it is a public health priority to make sure that consumers have accurate and useful information on reducing their risk."

A qualified health claim on a conventional food must be supported by credible scientific evidence. Based on a systematic evaluation of the available scientific data, as outlined in FDA's "Interim Procedures for Qualified Health Claims in the Labeling of Conventional Human Food and Human Dietary Supplements", FDA is announcing the availability of this claim on food labels and the labeling of olive oil and certain foods that contain olive oil.

Although this research is not conclusive, the FDA intends to exercise its enforcement discretion with respect to the following qualified health claim:

Limited and not conclusive scientific evidence suggests that eating about 2 tablespoons (23 grams) of olive oil daily may reduce the risk of coronary heart disease due to the monounsaturated fat in olive oil. To achieve this possible benefit, olive oil is to replace a similar amount of saturated fat and not increase the total number of calories you eat in a day. One serving of this product [Name of food] contains [x] grams of olive oil."

This claim is the third qualified health claim FDA has announced for conventional food since the process for establishing such claims took effect last year. Additional information about qualified health claims is available online at www.cfsan.fda.gov/~dms/qhcolive.html.

Source: U.S. Food and Drug Administration (FDA), *FDA News*, press release dated 11/1/2004.

Here Are Some Other Things You Can Do To Keep Your Heart Healthy

Ask your doctor to check your cholesterol level. This is done with a blood test. The test will show the amount of cholesterol in your blood with a number. Below 200 is good. The test will also show the amount of "good" and "bad" cholesterol. Your doctor can tell you more about what these numbers mean.

If your cholesterol is high, your doctor may suggest diet changes, exercise, or drugs to bring it down.

Regular exercise—like walking, swimming, or gardening—can help you keep your weight and cholesterol down.

☞ **Remember!!**
You can lower your chances of getting heart disease. One way is through your diet.

- Eat less fat.

- Eat less sodium.

- Reduce your calories if you're overweight.

- Eat more fiber.

- Eat a variety of foods.

- Eat plenty of bread, rice, and cereal. Also eat lots of vegetables and fruit.

- Teens should not drink alcohol.

Chapter 43

Healthy Eating Habits To Help Manage And Prevent Type 2 Diabetes

What Is Type 2 Diabetes?

Food is fuel for daily life—your body uses food to produce energy. With diabetes, the body has difficulty using food properly because it either fails to make enough insulin or doesn't use insulin correctly. Insulin is a hormone that helps convert food into energy. Diabetes makes it hard for the body to control blood sugar levels.

Type 2 diabetes is the most common form of the disease. Type 2 usually appears after age 40, but younger and younger people, even children, are being diagnosed with the condition.

This form of diabetes is linked closely to obesity and physical inactivity—two factors you can do something about.

Nutrition Is Key

In many cases, you can control type 2 diabetes through better nutrition, weight loss, increased physical activity, and regular checkups with your health care team.

About This Chapter: "Healthy Habits to Help Manage and Prevent Type 2 Diabetes," reprinted with permission from the American Dietetic Association, http://www.eatright.org, © 2002. All rights reserved.

What, when and how much you eat are all important factors in managing type 2 diabetes.

With the help of your registered dietitian or health care professional, you should develop and follow a meal plan based on your individual needs.

Nutrition Tips For People With Type 2 Diabetes

While no single plan will work for everyone, the following general tips can help:

- Follow a consistent meal plan and schedule.

- Eat a balanced diet with a variety of foods, including fruits, vegetables, whole grain foods, low-fat dairy products, and lean meat, poultry, fish, or meat alternatives. This will help keep your blood sugar levels steady.

- Choose lower fat options and limit saturated fats.

- Use sugar in moderation. Consider lower sugar options if available.

- Check nutrition labels.

- Get your fiber. The American Dietetic Association recommends that all people eat 20–35 grams of fiber per day. Fruits, vegetables, beans, and whole grain foods are good sources of fiber.

- Drink plenty of water.

- Use less salt.

Get Active

Everyone knows that physical activity is good for your health. But it's especially important for people with type 2 diabetes or those trying to prevent the disease.

> ### ♣ It's A Fact!!
>
> - Seventeen million Americans have diabetes, and nearly six million more do not know they have the disease. The number of Americans with diabetes is growing every year.
>
> - 90%–95% of people with diabetes have type 2 diabetes. This condition has been closely linked to obesity and physical inactivity.
>
> - But there's good news: Better nutrition and physical activity can help you deal with type 2 diabetes and may prevent the disease.

♣ It's A Fact!!
Children And Type 2 Diabetes: Facts For Parents

Did you know that 12.5% of American children between six and 17 years old are overweight? Children who are overweight often have pre-diabetes and insulin resistance, conditions that may lead to type 2 diabetes. In fact, there has recently been a sharp increase in reported cases of diabetes in children and adolescents.

If you are concerned that your child may be at risk, consider the following:

1. Find out if your family has a history of type 2 diabetes.

2. Encourage your kids to be physically active.

3. Present food as fuel for your child's body, not a reward for good behavior.

4. Trade regular sodas and other sweet drinks for water or low-fat milk.

5. Keep serving sizes reasonable.

6. Make healthy eating habits and increased physical activity a family goal—lead by example.

7. Talk to a health care professional about a blood glucose test and nutrition recommendations for your child.

To find a registered dietitian in your area to help you develop a balanced eating plan for your child, contact the American Dietetic Association at 800-366-1655 or go to http://www.eatright.org.

Type 2 diabetes is closely linked to being overweight. Research demonstrates that along with healthy eating habits, regular physical activity helps the body to use insulin better, which helps to improve the symptoms—or even reduce the risk—of type 2 diabetes.

Physical activity has an insulin-like effect—it can help lower blood sugar levels.

Everyone benefits from physical activity—those who have type 2 diabetes and those trying to prevent the disease.

In addition to improving blood sugar control, decreasing the risk of diabetes, and maintaining overall good health, being active boosts brain activity, helps you deal with stress and improves your mood.

A Sweet Discovery

Numerous studies have shown that old beliefs about sugar and diabetes may have been incorrect.

For a long time, experts thought people with diabetes couldn't have foods containing sugar, like candy and desserts. Researchers thought that these foods in particular made blood sugar levels rise too quickly, faster than starches.

Research now shows that candy and sweets don't raise blood sugar levels any higher or any more quickly than certain starches, such as white bread, white rice, and white potatoes.

So, you can have starches, sugars, and sweets—just be sure that you eat them in moderation. Most importantly, make sure that you eat a balanced diet so your body gets the nutrients it needs.

Talk to your registered dietitian or health care professional about how much and when to include all of these foods in your meal plan.

Chapter 44

Dieting And Gallstones

If you are overweight or obese, you can lower your risk for type 2 diabetes, heart disease, stroke, and some forms of cancer by losing weight. People who are overweight are at greater risk for developing gallstones than people who are at a healthy weight. When choosing a weight-loss program, be aware that the risk for developing gallstones increases with quick weight loss or a large weight loss. Gradual weight loss can lower the risk for obesity-related gallstones.

What are gallstones?

Gallstones are clusters of solid material that form in the gallbladder. They are made mostly of cholesterol. Gallstones may occur as one large stone or as many small ones. They vary in size and may be as large as a golf ball or as small as a grain of sand.

Experts estimate that 16 to 22 million people in the United States have gallstones—as many as one in every 12 Americans. Most people with gallstones do not know that they have them and experience no symptoms. Painless gallstones are called silent gallstones. Sometimes gallstones can cause abdominal or back pain. These are called symptomatic gallstones. In rare

About This Chapter: From "Dieting and Gallstones," National Institutes of Diabetes and Digestive and Kidney Diseases, NIH Pub. No. 02-3677, February 2002.

cases, gallstones can cause serious health problems. Symptomatic gallstones result in about 800,000 hospitalizations and more than 500,000 operations each year in the U.S.

What causes gallstones?

Gallstones develop in the gallbladder, a small pear-shaped organ beneath the liver on the right side of the abdomen. The gallbladder is about 3 inches long and an inch wide at its thickest part. It stores and releases bile into the intestine to help digestion. Bile is a liquid made by the liver. It contains water, cholesterol, bile salts, fats, proteins, and bilirubin, a bile pigment. During digestion, the gallbladder contracts to release bile into the intestine where the bile salts help to break down fat. Bile also dissolves excess cholesterol.

According to researchers, gallstones may form in one of three ways: when bile contains more cholesterol than it can dissolve, when there is too much of certain proteins or other substance in the bile that causes cholesterol to form hard crystals, or when the gallbladder does not contract and empty its bile regularly.

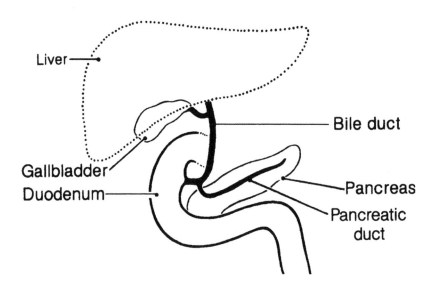

Figure 44.1. The gallbladder is about three inches long and is located beneath the liver on the right side of the abdomen.

Is obesity a risk factor for gallstones?

Obesity is a strong risk factor for gallstones, especially among women. People who are obese are more likely to have gallstones than people who are at a healthy weight.

Researchers have found that people who are obese may produce high levels of cholesterol. This leads to the production of bile containing more cholesterol than it can dissolve. When this happens, gallstones can form. People who are obese may also have large gallbladders that do not empty normally or completely. Some studies have shown that men and women who carry fat around their midsections may be at a greater risk for developing gallstones than those who carry fat around their hips and thighs.

♣ **It's A Fact!!**

Some common symptoms of gallstones or gallstone attack include the following:

- Severe pain in the upper abdomen that starts suddenly and lasts from 30 minutes to many hours
- Pain under the right shoulder or in the right shoulder blade
- Nausea or vomiting
- Indigestion after eating high-fat foods, such as fried foods or desserts

Is weight-loss dieting a risk factor for gallstones?

Weight-loss dieting increases the risk of developing gallstones. People who lose a large amount of weight quickly are at greater risk than those who lose weight more slowly. Rapid weight loss may also cause silent gallstones to become symptomatic. Studies have shown that people who lose more than 3 pounds per week may have a greater risk of developing gallstones than those who lose weight at slower rates.

A very low-calorie diet (VLCD) allows a person who is obese to quickly lose a large amount of weight. VLCDs usually provide about 800 calories or less per day in food or liquid form, and are followed for 12 to 16 weeks under the supervision of a health care provider. Studies have shown that 10 to 25 percent of people on a VLCD developed gallstones. These gallstones were usually silent—they did not produce any symptoms. About one-third of the dieters who developed gallstones, however, did have symptoms and some of these required gallbladder surgery. [VLCDs are not appropriate for children or adolescents, except in specialized treatment programs.]

Experts believe dieting may cause a shift in the balance of bile salts and cholesterol in the gallbladder. The cholesterol level is increased and the amount of bile salts is decreased. Following a diet too low in fat or going for long periods without eating (skipping breakfast, for example), a common practice among dieters, may also decrease gallbladder contractions. If the gallbladder does not contract often enough to empty out the bile, gallstones may form.

Is weight cycling a risk factor for gallstones?

Weight cycling, or losing and regaining weight repeatedly, may increase the risk of developing gallstones. People who weight cycle—especially with losses and gains of more than 10 pounds—have a higher risk for gallstones than people who lose weight and maintain their weight loss. In addition, the more weight a person loses and regains during a cycle, the greater the risk of developing gallstones.

Why weight cycling is a risk factor for gallstones is unclear. The rise in cholesterol levels during the weight loss phase of a weight cycle may be responsible.

Is surgery to treat obesity a risk factor for gallstones?

Gallstones are common among people who undergo gastrointestinal surgery to lose weight, also called bariatric surgery. Experts estimate that one-third of patients who have bariatric surgery develop gallstones. The gallstones usually develop in the first few months after surgery and are symptomatic.

How can I safely lose weight and decrease the risk of gallstones?

You can take several measures to decrease the risk of developing gallstones during weight loss. Losing weight gradually, instead of losing a large amount of weight quickly, lowers your risk. Experts recommend losing 1 to 2 pounds per week. You can also decrease the risk of gallstones associated with weight cycling by aiming for a modest weight loss that you can maintain. Even a loss of 10 percent of body weight over a period of six months or more can improve the health of an adult who is overweight or obese.

Your food choices can also affect your gallstone risk. Experts recommend including some fat in your diet to stimulate gallbladder contracting and emptying. However, no more than 30 percent of your total calories should come from fat. Studies have also shown that diets high in fiber and calcium may reduce the risk of gallstone development. Finally, regular physical activity is related to a lower risk for gallstones.

What is the treatment for gallstones?

Silent gallstones are usually left alone and sometimes disappear on their own. Symptomatic gallstones are usually treated. The most common treatment is surgery to remove the gallbladder. This operation is called a cholecystectomy. In other cases, drugs are used to dissolve the gallstones. Your health care provider can help determine which option is best for you.

☞ Remember!!

If you are thinking about starting an eating and physical activity plan to lose weight, talk with your health care provider first. Together, you can discuss various eating and exercise programs, your medical history, and the benefits and risks of losing weight including the risk of developing gallstones.

Are the benefits of weight loss greater than the risk of getting gallstones?

Although weight loss increases the risk of developing gallstones, obesity poses an even greater risk. In addition to gallstones, obesity is linked to many serious health problems including the following:

- type 2 diabetes

- high blood pressure

- heart disease

- stroke

- certain types of cancer

- sleep apnea (when breathing stops for short periods during sleep)

- osteoarthritis (wearing away of the joints)

- gastroesophageal reflux disease (GERD)

For people who are obese, weight loss can lower the risk of developing these illnesses. Even a small weight loss of 10 to 20 pounds can improve health and lower disease risk. In addition, weight loss can bring other benefits such as better mood and positive self-image.

Chapter 45

Food Allergies

Introduction

If you have an unpleasant reaction to something you have eaten, you might wonder if you have a food allergy. This chapter describes allergic reactions to foods and their possible causes as well as the best ways to diagnose and treat allergic reactions to food. It also describes other reactions to foods, known as food intolerances, which can be confused with food allergy, and it describes some unproven and controversial food allergy theories.

How Do Allergic Reactions Work?

An immediate allergic reaction involves two actions of your immune system.

- Your immune system produces immunoglobulin E (IgE), a type of protein that works against a specific food. This protein is called a food-specific antibody, and it circulates through the blood.

- The food-specific IgE then attaches to mast cells, cells found in all body tissues. They are more often found in areas of your body that are typical sites of allergic reactions. Those sites include your nose, throat, lungs, skin, and gastrointestinal (GI) tract.

About This Chapter: Text in this chapter is excerpted from "Food Allergy: An Overview," National Institute of Allergy and Infectious Diseases, NIH Publication No. 04-5518, July 2004.

Generally, your immune system will form IgE against a food if you come from a family in which allergies are common—not necessarily food allergies but perhaps other allergic diseases such as hay fever or asthma. If you have two allergic parents, you are more likely to develop food allergy than someone with one allergic parent.

If your immune system is inclined to form IgE to certain foods, you must be exposed to the food before you can have an allergic reaction.

- As this food is digested, it triggers certain cells in your body to produce a food-specific IgE in large amounts. The food-specific IgE is then released and attaches to the surfaces of mast cells.

✦ It's A Fact!!
What Is Food Allergy?

Food allergy is an abnormal response to a food triggered by the body's immune system.

Allergic reactions to food can cause serious illness and, in some cases, death. Therefore, if you have a food allergy, it is extremely important for you to work with your health care provider to find out what food(s) causes your allergic reaction.

Sometimes, a reaction to food is not an allergy at all but another type of reaction called "food intolerance." Food intolerance is more common than food allergy. The immune system does not cause the symptoms of a food intolerance, though these symptoms can look and feel like those of a food allergy.

Source: National Institute of Allergy and Infectious Diseases, 2004.

- The next time you eat that food, it interacts with food-specific IgE on the surface of the mast cells and triggers the cells to release chemicals such as histamine.

- Depending upon the tissue in which they are released, these chemicals will cause you to have various symptoms of food allergy.

Food allergens are proteins within the food that enter your bloodstream after the food is digested. From there, they go to target organs, such as your skin or nose, and cause allergic reactions.

An allergic reaction to food can take place within a few minutes to an hour. The process of eating and digesting food affects the timing and the location of a reaction.

- If you are allergic to a particular food, you may first feel itching in your mouth as you start to eat the food.

- After the food is digested in your stomach, you may have GI symptoms such as vomiting, diarrhea, or pain.

- When the food allergens enter and travel through your bloodstream, they may cause your blood pressure to drop.

- As the allergens reach your skin, they can cause hives or eczema.

- When the allergens reach your lungs, they may cause asthma.

Food Allergy Or Intolerance?

If you go to your health care provider and say, "I think I have a food allergy," your provider has to consider other possibilities that may cause symptoms and could be confused with food allergy, such as food intolerance. To find out the difference between food allergy and food intolerance, your provider will go through a list of possible causes for your symptoms. This is called a "differential diagnosis." This type of diagnosis helps confirm that you do indeed have a food allergy rather than a food intolerance or other illness.

✎ What's It Mean?

Cross-Reactivity: If you have a life-threatening reaction to a certain food, similar foods may also trigger a reaction. For example, if you have a history of allergy to shrimp, testing will usually show that you are not only allergic to shrimp but also to crab, lobster, and crayfish. This is called "cross-reactivity." Another interesting example of cross-reactivity occurs in people who are highly sensitive to ragweed. During ragweed pollen season, they sometimes find that when they try to eat melons, particularly cantaloupe, they experience itching in their mouths and simply cannot eat the melon. Similarly, people who have severe birch pollen allergy also may react to apple peels. This is called the "oral allergy syndrome."

Source: National Institute of Allergy and Infectious Diseases, 2004.

Types Of Food Intolerance

Food Poisoning: One possible cause of symptoms like those of food allergy is foods contaminated with microbes, such as bacteria, and bacterial products, such as toxins. Contaminated meat and dairy products sometimes cause symptoms, including GI discomfort, that resemble a food allergy when it is really a type of food poisoning.

Histamine Toxicity: There are substances, such as histamine present in certain foods, that cause a reaction like an allergic reaction. For example, histamine can reach high levels in cheese, some wines, and certain kinds of fish such as tuna and mackerel.

In fish, histamine is believed to come from contamination by bacteria, particularly in fish that are not refrigerated properly. If you eat one of these foods with a high level of histamine, you could have a reaction that strongly resembles an allergic reaction to food. This reaction is called "histamine toxicity."

Lactose Intolerance: Another cause of food intolerance confused with a food allergy is lactose intolerance or lactase deficiency. This common food intolerance affects at least one out of ten people.

♣ It's A Fact!!
Common Food Allergies

In adults, the foods that most often cause allergic reactions include:

- Shellfish such as shrimp, crayfish, lobster, and crab;
- Peanuts;
- Tree nuts such as walnuts;
- Fish;
- Eggs.

The most common foods that cause problems in children are:

- Eggs;
- Milk;
- Peanuts.

Tree nuts and peanuts are the leading causes of deadly food allergy reactions called anaphylaxis.

Adults usually keep their allergies for life, but children sometimes outgrow them. Children are more likely to outgrow allergies to milk or soy, however, than allergies to peanuts or shrimp. The foods to which adults or children usually react are those foods they eat often. In Japan, for example, rice allergy is more frequent. In Scandinavia, codfish allergy is more common.

Source: National Institute of Allergy and Infectious Diseases, 2004.

- Lactase is an enzyme that is in the lining of the gut.

- Lactase breaks down lactose, a sugar found in milk and most milk products.

- There is not enough lactase in the gut to digest lactose.

- Lactose, instead, is used by bacteria to form gas which causes bloating, abdominal pain, and sometimes diarrhea.

There are tests your health care provider can use to find out whether your body can digest lactose.

Food Additives: Another type of food intolerance is a reaction to certain products that are added to food to enhance taste, provide color, or protect against the growth of microbes. Several compounds, such as MSG (monosodium glutamate) and sulfites, are tied to reactions that can be confused with food allergy.

- MSG is a flavor enhancer, and, when taken in large amounts, can cause some of the following signs: flushing; sensations of warmth; headache; chest discomfort; or feelings of detachment. These passing reactions occur rapidly after eating large amounts of food to which MSG has been added.

- Sulfites occur naturally in foods or may be added to increase crispness or prevent mold growth. Sulfites in high concentrations sometimes pose problems for people with severe asthma. Sulfites can give off a gas called sulfur dioxide that the asthmatic inhales while eating the sulfited food. This irritates the lungs and can send an asthmatic into severe bronchospasm, a tightening of the lungs. The Food and Drug Administration (FDA) has banned sulfites as spray-on preservatives in fresh fruits and vegetables. Sulfites are still used in some foods, however, and occur naturally during the fermentation of wine.

Gluten Intolerance: Gluten intolerance is associated with the disease called gluten-sensitive enteropathy" or "celiac disease." It happens if your immune system responds abnormally to gluten, which is a part of wheat and some other grains.

Psychological Causes: Some people may have a food intolerance that has a psychological trigger. If your food intolerance is caused by this type of trigger, a careful psychiatric evaluation may identify an unpleasant event in your life, often during childhood, tied to eating a particular food. Eating that food years later, even as an adult, is associated with a rush of unpleasant sensations.

Other Causes: There are several other conditions, including ulcers and cancers of the GI tract, that cause some of the same symptoms as food allergy. These problems include vomiting, diarrhea, and cramping abdominal pain made worse by eating.

Diagnosis

After ruling out food intolerances and other health problems, your health care provider will use several steps to find out if you have an allergy to specific foods.

Detailed History

This technique is the most valuable. Your provider will ask you several questions and listen to your history of food reactions to decide if the facts go with a food allergy.

- What was the timing of your reaction?

- Did your reaction come on quickly, usually within an hour after eating the food?

- Did allergy medicines help? Antihistamines should relieve hives, for example.

- Is your reaction always associated with a certain food?

- Did anyone else who ate the same food get sick? For example, if you ate fish contaminated with histamine, everyone who ate the fish should be sick.

- How much did you eat before you had a reaction? The severity of a reaction is sometimes related to the amount of food eaten.

- How was the food prepared? Some people will have a violent allergic reaction only to raw or undercooked fish. Complete cooking of the fish may destroy the allergen, and they can then eat it with no allergic reaction.

- Did you eat other foods at the same time you had the reaction? Some foods may delay digestion and thus delay the start of the allergic reaction.

Elimination Diet

The next step some health care providers use is an elimination diet. Under your provider's direction:

- You don't eat a food suspected of causing the allergy, such as eggs;

- You then substitute another food—in the case of eggs, another source of protein;

- Your provider can almost always make a diagnosis if the symptoms go away after you remove the food from your diet.

The diagnosis is confirmed if you then eat the food and the symptoms come back. You should do this only when the reactions are not significant and under health care provider direction.

Your provider can't use this technique, however, if your reactions are severe or don't happen often. If you have a severe reaction, you should not eat the food again.

Skin Test

If your history, diet diary, or elimination diet suggests a specific food allergy is likely, your health care provider will then use tests to confirm the diagnosis.

One of these is a scratch skin test, during which an extract of the food is placed on the skin of your lower arm. Your provider will then scratch this portion of your skin with a needle and look for swelling or redness which would be a sign of a local allergic reaction. If the scratch test is positive, it means that there is IgE on the skin's mast cells that is specific to the food being tested. Skin tests are rapid, simple, and relatively safe.

You can have a positive skin test to a food allergen, however, without having an allergic reaction to that food. A health care provider diagnoses a food allergy only when someone has a positive skin test to a specific allergen and the history of reactions suggests an allergy to the same food.

Blood Test

If you are extremely allergic and have severe anaphylactic reactions, your health care provider cannot use skin testing because causing an allergic reaction could be dangerous. Skin testing also cannot be done if you have eczema over a large portion of your body.

♣ **It's A Fact!!**
Diet Diary

Sometimes your health care provider can't make a diagnosis solely on the basis of your history. In that case, you may be asked to keep a record of the contents of each meal you eat and whether you have a reaction. This gives more detail from which you and your provider can see if there is a consistent pattern in your reactions.

Source: National Institute of Allergy and Infectious Diseases, 2004.

In those cases, a health care provider may use blood tests such as the RAST (radioallergosorbent test) or the ELISA (enzyme-linked immunosorbent assay). These tests measure the presence of food-specific IgE in your blood. As with skin testing, positive tests do not necessarily mean you have a food allergy.

Double-Blind Food Challenge

The final method health care providers use to diagnose food allergy is double-blind food challenge. This testing has come to be the "gold standard" of allergy testing.

- Your health care provider will give you individual opaque capsules containing various foods, some of which are suspected of starting an allergic reaction.

- You swallow a capsule and are watched to see if a reaction occurs. This process is repeated until you have swallowed all the capsules.

In a true double-blind test, your health care provider is also "blinded" (the capsules having been made up by another medical person). In that case your provider does not know which capsule contains the allergen. The advantage of such a challenge is that if you react only to suspected foods and not to other foods tested, it confirms the diagnosis. You cannot be tested this way if you have a history of severe allergic reactions.

In addition, this testing is difficult because it takes a lot of time to perform and many food allergies are difficult to evaluate with this procedure. Consequently, health care providers seldom do double-blind food challenges.

This type of testing is most commonly used if your health care provider thinks the reaction you describe is not due to a specific food and wishes to obtain evidence to support this. If your provider finds that your reaction is not due to a specific food, then additional efforts may be used to find the real cause of the reaction.

Treatment

Food allergy is treated by avoiding the foods that trigger the reaction. Once you and your health care provider have identified the food(s) to which you are sensitive, you must remove them from your diet. To do this, you must read the detailed ingredient lists on each food you are considering eating.

Many allergy-producing foods such as peanuts, eggs, and milk, appear in foods one normally would not associate them with. Peanuts, for example, are often used as a protein source, and eggs are used in some salad dressings.

FDA requires ingredients in a packaged food to appear on its label. You can avoid most of the things to which you are sensitive if you read food labels carefully and avoid restaurant-prepared foods that might have ingredients to which you are allergic.

If you are highly allergic, even the tiniest amounts of a food allergen (for example, a small portion of a peanut kernel) can prompt an allergic reaction.

If you have severe food allergies, you must be prepared to treat unintentional exposure. Even people who know a lot about what they are sensitive to occasionally make a mistake. To protect yourself if you have had allergic reactions to a food, you should:

- Wear a medical alert bracelet or necklace stating that you have a food allergy and are subject to severe reactions;

- Carry a syringe of adrenaline (epinephrine), obtained by prescription from your health care provider, and be prepared to give it to yourself if you think you are getting a food allergic reaction;

- Seek medical help immediately by either calling the rescue squad or by getting transported to an emergency room.

♣ It's A Fact!!

Can foods trigger asthma?

Only a few. For years it has been suspected that foods or food ingredients may cause or exacerbate symptoms in those with asthma. After many years of scientific and clinical investigation, there are very few confirmed food triggers of asthma. Sulfites and sulfiting agents in foods (found in dried fruits, prepared potatoes, wine, bottled lemon or lime juice, and shrimp), and diagnosed food allergens (such as milk, eggs, peanuts, tree nuts, soy, wheat, fish, and shellfish) have been found to trigger asthma. Many food ingredients such as food dyes and colors, food preservatives like BHA and BHT, monosodium glutamate, aspartame, and nitrite, have not been conclusively linked to asthma.

What can individuals with asthma do to prevent a food-triggered asthma attack?

The best way to avoid food-induced asthma is to eliminate or avoid the offending food or food ingredient from the diet or from the environment. Reading ingredient information on food labels and knowing where food triggers of asthma are found are the best defenses against a food-induced asthma attack. The main objectives of an asthmatic's care and treatment are to stay healthy, to remain symptom free, to enjoy food, to exercise, to use medications properly, and to follow the care plan developed between the physician and patient.

Source: Excerpted from "Background on Food Allergies and Asthma," © 2005 International Food Information Council. All rights reserved. Reprinted with permission.

✤ **It's A Fact!!**
Exercise-Induced Food Allergy

At least one situation may require more than simply eating food with allergens to start a reaction: exercise-induced food allergy. People who have this reaction only experience it after eating a specific food before exercising. As exercise increases and body temperature rises, itching and lightheadedness start and allergic reactions such as hives may appear and even anaphylaxis may develop.

The cure for exercised-induced food allergy is simple—avoid eating for a couple of hours before exercising.

Source: National Institute of Allergy and Infectious Diseases, 2004.

There are several medicines that you can take to relieve food allergy symptoms that are not part of an anaphylactic reaction. These include:

• Antihistamines to relieve GI symptoms, hives, or sneezing and a runny nose;

• Bronchodilators to relieve asthma symptoms.

You should take these medicines if you have accidentally eaten a food to which you are allergic. They do not prevent an allergic reaction when taken before eating the food. No medicine in any form will reliably prevent an allergic reaction to that food before eating it.

Some Controversial And Unproven Theories

There are several disorders that are popularly thought by some to be caused by food allergies. There is not enough scientific evidence, or evidence that does exist goes against such claims.

Migraine Headaches: There is controversy about whether migraine headaches can be caused by food allergy. Studies show people who are prone to migraines can have their headaches brought on by histamines and other substances in foods. The more difficult issue is whether food allergies actually cause migraines in such people.

Arthritis: There is virtually no evidence that most rheumatoid arthritis or osteoarthritis can be made worse by foods, despite claims to the contrary.

Allergic Tension Fatigue Syndrome: There is no evidence that food allergies can cause a disorder called the allergic tension fatigue syndrome, in which people are tired, nervous, and may have problems concentrating, or have headaches.

Cerebral Allergy: Cerebral allergy is a term that has been given to people who have trouble concentrating and have headaches as well as other complaints. These symptoms are sometimes blamed on mast cells activated in the brain but no other place in the body. Researchers have found no evidence that such a scenario can happen. Most health experts do not recognize cerebral allergy as a disorder.

Environmental Illness: In a seemingly pristine environment, some people have many non-specific complaints such as problems concentrating or depression. Sometimes this is blamed on small amounts of allergens or toxins in the environment. There is no evidence that such problems are due to food allergies.

Childhood Hyperactivity: Some people believe hyperactivity in children is caused by food allergies. But researchers have found that this behavioral disorder in children is only occasionally associated with food additives, and then only when such additives are consumed in large amounts. There is no evidence that a true food allergy can affect a child's activity except for the possibility that if a child itches and sneezes and wheezes a lot, the child may be uncomfortable and therefore more difficult to guide. Also, children who are on antiallergy medicines that cause drowsiness may get sleepy in school or at home.

Controversial And Unproven Diagnostic Methods

Cytotoxicity Testing: One controversial diagnostic technique is cytotoxicity testing, in which a food allergen is added to your blood sample. A technician then examines the sample under the microscope to see if white cells in the blood "die." Scientists have evaluated this technique in several studies and have found it does not effectively diagnose food allergy.

Provocative Challenge: Another controversial approach is called sublingual (placed under the tongue) or subcutaneous (injected under the skin) provocative challenge. In this procedure, diluted food allergen is put under your tongue if you feel that your arthritis, for instance, is due to foods. The technician then asks you if the food allergen has made your arthritis symptoms worse. In clinical studies, researchers have not shown that this procedure can effectively diagnose food allergy.

✔ Quick Tip
How Can I Help My Friend Who Has A Food Allergy?

Here are a few guidelines to help your friend stay safe.

Do

- Learn what food or foods your friend must avoid.

- Ask about symptoms of a food allergy reaction.

- Find out what medications your friend uses to treat a reaction and how you can help in the event of an allergic emergency.

- Remind your friend to read labels.

- Wash your hands after eating.

Don't

- Pressure your friend to try a food.

- Ignore the symptoms of a reaction.

- Exclude your friend because of food allergy.

- Allow others to make fun of your friend.

Source: © 2004 The Food Allergy and Anaphylaxis Network. Reprinted with permission from the Food Allergy and Anaphylaxis Network. For additional information, visit http://www.foodallergy.org or http://www.fankids.org.

Immune Complex Assay: An immune complex assay is sometimes done on people suspected of having food allergies to see if groups, or complexes, of certain antibodies connect to the food allergen in the bloodstream. Some think that these immune groups link with food allergies. But the formation of such immune complexes is a normal offshoot of food digestion, and everyone, if tested with a sensitive enough measurement, has them. To date, no one has conclusively shown that this test links with allergies to foods.

IgG Subclass Assay: Another test is the IgG subclass assay, which looks specifically for certain kinds of IgG antibody. Again, there is no evidence that this diagnoses food allergy.

Controversial And Unproven Treatments

Controversial treatments include putting a diluted solution of a particular food under your tongue about a half hour before you eat the food suspected of causing an allergic reaction. This is an attempt to "neutralize" the subsequent exposure to the food that you believe is harmful. The results of a carefully conducted clinical study show this procedure does not prevent an allergic reaction.

Allergy Shots: Another unproven treatment involves getting shots (immunotherapy) containing small quantities of the food extracts to which you are allergic. These shots are given regularly for a long period of time with the aim of "desensitizing" you to the food allergen. Researchers have not yet proven that allergy shots reliably relieve food allergies.

Chapter 46

Lactose Intolerance

What is lactose intolerance?

Lactose intolerance is the inability to digest significant amounts of lactose, the predominant sugar of milk. This inability results from a shortage of the enzyme lactase, which is normally produced by the cells that line the small intestine. Lactase breaks down milk sugar into simpler forms that can then be absorbed into the bloodstream. When there is not enough lactase to digest the amount of lactose consumed, the results, although not usually dangerous, may be very distressing. While not all persons deficient in lactase have symptoms, those who do are considered to be lactose intolerant.

Common symptoms include nausea, cramps, bloating, gas, and diarrhea, which begin about 30 minutes to two hours after eating or drinking foods containing lactose. The severity of symptoms varies depending on the amount of lactose each individual can tolerate.

Some causes of lactose intolerance are well known. For instance, certain digestive diseases and injuries to the small intestine can reduce the amount of enzymes produced. In rare cases, children are born without the ability to

About This Chapter: "Lactose Intolerance," National Institute of Diabetes and Digestive and Kidney Diseases, NIH Publication No. 03-2715, March 2003.

produce lactase. For most people, though, lactase deficiency is a condition that develops naturally over time. After about the age of two years, the body begins to produce less lactase. However, many people may not experience symptoms until they are much older.

Between 30 and 50 million Americans are lactose intolerant. Certain ethnic and racial populations are more widely affected than others. As many as 75 percent of all African Americans and American Indians and 90 percent of Asian Americans are lactose intolerant. The condition is least common among persons of northern European descent.

Researchers have identified a genetic variation associated with lactose intolerance; this discovery may be useful in developing a diagnostic test to identify people with this condition.

How is lactose intolerance diagnosed?

The most common tests used to measure the absorption of lactose in the digestive system are the lactose tolerance test, the hydrogen breath test, and the stool acidity test. These tests are performed on an outpatient basis at a hospital, clinic, or doctor's office.

The lactose tolerance test begins with the individual fasting (not eating) before the test and then drinking a liquid that contains lactose. Several blood samples are taken over a two-hour period to measure the person's blood glucose (blood sugar) level, which indicates how well the body is able to digest lactose.

Normally, when lactose reaches the digestive system, the lactase enzyme breaks it down into glucose and galactose. The liver then changes the galactose into glucose, which enters the bloodstream and raises the person's blood glucose level. If lactose is incompletely broken down, the blood glucose level does not rise and a diagnosis of lactose intolerance is confirmed.

The hydrogen breath test measures the amount of hydrogen in a person's breath. Normally, very little hydrogen is detectable. However, undigested lactose in the colon is fermented by bacteria, and various gases, including hydrogen, are produced. The hydrogen is absorbed from the intestines, carried through the bloodstream to the lungs, and exhaled. In the test, the patient drinks a lactose-loaded beverage, and the breath is analyzed at regular intervals. Raised levels of hydrogen in the breath indicate improper digestion of lactose. Certain foods, medications, and cigarettes can affect the accuracy of the test and should be avoided before taking it. This test is available for children and adults.

The lactose tolerance and hydrogen breath tests are not given to infants and very young children who are suspected of having lactose intolerance. A large lactose load may be dangerous for the very young because they are more prone to the dehydration that can result from diarrhea caused by the lactose. If a baby or young child is experiencing symptoms of lactose intolerance, many pediatricians simply recommend changing from cow's milk to soy formula and waiting for symptoms to abate.

If necessary, a stool acidity test, which measures the amount of acid in the stool, may be given to infants and young children. Undigested lactose fermented by bacteria in the colon creates lactic acid and other short-chain fatty acids that can be detected in a stool sample. In addition, glucose may be present in the sample as a result of unabsorbed lactose in the colon.

♣ **It's A Fact!!**

Recent research shows that yogurt with active cultures may be a good source of calcium for many people with lactose intolerance, even though it is fairly high in lactose. Evidence shows that the bacterial cultures used to make yogurt produce some of the lactase enzyme required for proper digestion.

How is lactose intolerance treated?

Fortunately, lactose intolerance is relatively easy to treat. No treatment can improve the body's ability to produce lactase, but symptoms can be controlled through diet.

Young children with lactase deficiency should not eat any foods containing lactose. Most older children and adults need not avoid lactose completely, but people differ in the amounts and types of foods they can handle. For example, one person may have symptoms after drinking a small glass of milk, while another can drink one glass but not two. Others may be able to manage ice cream and aged cheeses, such as cheddar and Swiss, but not other dairy products. Dietary control of lactose intolerance depends on people learning through trial and error how much lactose they can handle.

For those who react to very small amounts of lactose or have trouble limiting their intake of foods that contain it, lactase enzymes are available without a prescription to help people digest foods that contain lactose. The tablets are taken with the first bite of dairy food. Lactase enzyme is also available as a liquid. Adding a few drops of the enzyme will convert the lactose in milk or cream, making it more digestible for people with lactose intolerance.

Lactose-reduced milk and other products are available at most supermarkets. The milk contains all of the nutrients found in regular milk and remains fresh for about the same length of time, or longer if it is super-pasteurized.

How is nutrition balanced?

Milk and other dairy products are a major source of nutrients in the American diet. The most important of these nutrients is calcium. Calcium is essential for the growth and repair of bones throughout life. In the middle and later years, a shortage of calcium may lead to thin, fragile bones that break easily, a condition called osteoporosis. A concern, then, for both children and adults with lactose intolerance, is getting enough calcium in a diet that includes little or no milk.

In 1997, the Institute of Medicine released a report recommending

Table 46.1. Calcium Requirements

Age group	Amount of calcium to consume daily, in milligrams (mg)
0–6 months	210 mg
7–12 months	270 mg
1–3 years	500 mg
4–8 years	800 mg
9–18 years	1,300 mg
19–50 years	1,000 mg
51–70+ years	1,200 mg

Pregnant and nursing women under 19 need 1,300 mg daily, while pregnant and nursing women over 19 need 1,000 mg.

✔ **Quick Tip**

Some people with lactose intolerance may think they are not getting enough calcium and vitamin D in their diet. Consultation with a doctor or dietitian may be helpful in deciding whether any dietary supplements are needed. Taking vitamins or minerals of the wrong kind or in the wrong amounts can be harmful. A dietitian can help in planning meals that will provide the most nutrients with the least chance of causing discomfort.

new requirements for daily calcium intake. How much calcium a person needs to maintain good health varies by age group. Recommendations from the report are shown in Table 46.1.

In planning meals, making sure that each day's diet includes enough calcium is important, even if the diet does not contain dairy products. Many nondairy foods are high in calcium. Green vegetables, such as broccoli and kale, and fish with soft, edible bones, such as salmon and sardines, are excellent sources of calcium. To help in planning a high-calcium and low-lactose diet, the table that follows lists some common foods that are good sources of dietary calcium and shows how much lactose they contain.

Clearly, many foods can provide the calcium and other nutrients the body needs, even when intake of milk and dairy products is limited. However, factors other than calcium and lactose content should be kept in mind when planning a diet. Some vegetables that are high in calcium (Swiss chard, spinach, and rhubarb, for instance) are not listed in the chart because the body cannot use the calcium they contain. They also contain substances called oxalates, which stop calcium absorption. Calcium is absorbed and used only when there is enough vitamin D in the body. A balanced diet should provide an adequate supply of vitamin D. Sources of vitamin D include eggs and liver. However, sunlight helps the body naturally absorb or synthesize vitamin D, and with enough exposure to the sun, food sources may not be necessary.

What is hidden lactose?

Although milk and foods made from milk are the only natural sources, lactose is often added to prepared foods. People with very low tolerance for lactose should know about the many food products that may contain even small amounts of lactose, such as the following:

• bread and other baked goods

• processed breakfast cereals

Table 46.2. Calcium and Lactose in Common Foods

	Calcium Content	Lactose Content
Vegetables		
Calcium-fortified orange juice, 1 cup	308–344 mg	0
Sardines, with edible bones, 3 oz.	270 mg	0
Salmon, canned, with edible bones, 3 oz.	205 mg	0
Soymilk, fortified, 1 cup	200 mg	0
Broccoli (raw), 1 cup	90 mg	0
Orange, 1 medium	50 mg	0
Pinto beans, 1/2 cup	40 mg	0
Tuna, canned, 3 oz.	10 mg	0
Lettuce greens, 1/2 cup	10 mg	0
Dairy Products		
Yogurt, plain, low-fat, 1 cup	415 mg	5 g
Milk, reduced fat, 1 cup	295 mg	11 g
Swiss cheese, 1 oz.	270 mg	1 g
Ice cream, 1/2 cup	85 mg	6 g
Cottage cheese, 1/2 cup	75 mg	2–3 g

Adapted from *Manual of Clinical Dietetics. 6th ed.* American Dietetic Association, 2000; and Soy Dairy Alternatives. Available at: http://www.soyfoods.org. Accessed March 5, 2002.

☞ Remember!!

Even though lactose intolerance is widespread, it need not pose a serious threat to good health. People who have trouble digesting lactose can learn which dairy products and other foods they can eat without discomfort and which ones they should avoid. Many will be able to enjoy milk, ice cream, and other such products if they take them in small amounts or eat other food at the same time. Others can use lactase liquid or tablets to help digest the lactose. Even older women at risk for osteoporosis and growing children who must avoid milk and foods made with milk can meet most of their special dietary needs by eating greens, fish, and other calcium-rich foods that are free of lactose. A carefully chosen diet, with calcium supplements if the doctor or dietitian recommends them, is the key to reducing symptoms and protecting future health.

- instant potatoes, soups, and breakfast drinks

- margarine

- lunch meats (other than kosher)

- salad dressings

- candies and other snacks

- mixes for pancakes, biscuits, and cookies

- powdered meal-replacement supplements

Some products labeled nondairy, such as powdered coffee creamer and whipped toppings, may also include ingredients that are derived from milk and therefore contain lactose.

Smart shoppers learn to read food labels with care, looking not only for milk and lactose among the contents, but also for such words as whey, curds, milk by-products, dry milk solids, and nonfat dry milk powder. If any of these are listed on a label, the product contains lactose.

In addition, lactose is used as the base for more than 20 percent of prescription drugs and about 6 percent of over-the-counter medicines. Many types of birth control pills, for example, contain lactose, as do some tablets for stomach acid and gas. However, these products typically affect only people with severe lactose intolerance.

Chapter 47

Oral Health And Nutrition

What is the relationship between your mouth and good health? The links between oral health and nutrition are many. Just as oral diseases can affect diet and nutrition, diet and nutrition, in turn, may affect the development and progression of diseases of the oral cavity.

The Road To Good Health

The mouth is a window to your health that allows the skilled dental practitioner to make overall assessments. Regular dental examinations make it possible to screen for early warnings of eating disorders and precancerous conditions. Additionally, by administering a special x-ray of the carotid artery, the dentist can screen in advance for stroke indicators.

Taking care of your mouth is an important step on the road to good health. Eating habits, regular brushing, flossing, fluoride treatments, and checkups are all part of maintaining good health.

Caries Prevention Emphasis Shifts

For many years, the primary focus of oral health care was the prevention of cavities (dental caries) in children, with an emphasis on dietary influences

About This Chapter: From "Background on Oral Health and Nutrition," © 2005 International Food Information Council. All rights reserved. Reprinted with permission.

on caries formation. In today's world, however, prevention focuses on fluoride, the use of sealants, frequency of eating, and good oral hygiene. With evolving science, specific foods no longer are being singled out as major risk factors for caries.

Nevertheless, eating patterns and food choices can be important factors in tooth decay. Everything eaten passes through the mouth, where carbohydrates can be used by the bacteria in plaque to produce acids capable of damaging tooth enamel. Plaque is an almost invisible deposit of bacteria and their byproducts that constantly forms on everyone's teeth. Plaque holds the acids on the teeth. In time, the tooth enamel may break down, forming a cavity.

Factors involved in plaque build-up or acid production include the following:

- **Frequency of eating:** Each time carbohydrate-containing foods are consumed, acids are released on teeth for about 20 to 40 minutes. The greater the frequency of eating, the more opportunity for acid production.

- **Food characteristics:** Some foods tend to cling or stick to the teeth. While one might not think of them as sticky, cooked starches such as chips and crackers rank higher on the list of sticky foods than candy bars and toffee. A food's characteristics affect the time that it remains in the mouth. Foods that are slow to dissolve, such as cookies and granola bars, are in longer contact with the teeth, providing more time for the acids to damage enamel, as opposed to foods that dissolve quickly such as caramels and jelly beans.

- **Whether or not the food is eaten as part of a meal:** Saliva production is increased during a meal to help neutralize acid and clear food from the mouth.

- **Starches can cause caries, too:** Starches in general—from bread to crackers to sugars from fruit, milk, honey, molasses, corn sweeteners, and refined sugar—can all produce the acids that damage teeth.

Dental Caries—A Disease In Decline

Far and away the most important factor in reducing caries has been the widespread introduction of fluoride into water supplies as well as fluoridation of toothpaste. Precisely how fluoride works to treat and, in effect, prevent formation of dental cavities is still being studied; but the evidence of effectiveness is overwhelming.

Widespread use of fluoride is credited with a dramatic decline in dental caries during recent decades, according to a survey by the National Institute of Dental Research (NIDR). The number of cavity-free children in the U.S. doubled during this period, with more than six out of ten having no cavities in their primary teeth. An increase in the number of people who regularly visit their dentist and overall improved diet are also cited as factors in the improvement reported by the NIDR.

✔ Quick Tip

What can people do to protect and enhance oral health?

- Incorporate balance, variety and moderation in food choices—important guidelines for oral health as well as for good nutrition.

- Clean teeth with fluoride toothpaste at least twice a day.

- Floss regularly, or use an interdental brush (particularly useful for braces, bridges, or hard-to-reach places).

- Visit the dentist regularly.

- Limit eating occasions to regular meals and no more than two to three snacking occasions daily.

Chapter 48

Sports Nutrition

What diet is best for athletes?

It's important that an athlete's diet provides the right amount of energy, the 50-plus nutrients the body needs and adequate water. No single food or supplement can do this. A variety of foods are needed every day. But, just as there is more than one way to achieve a goal, there is more than one way to follow a nutritious diet.

Do the nutritional needs of athletes differ from non-athletes?

Competitive athletes, sedentary individuals and people who exercise for health and fitness all need the same nutrients. However, because of the intensity of their sport or training program, some athletes have higher calorie and fluid requirements. Eating a variety of foods to meet increased calorie needs helps to ensure that the athlete's diet contains appropriate amounts of carbohydrate, protein, vitamins and minerals.

Are there certain dietary guidelines athletes should follow?

Health and nutrition professionals recommend that 55–60% of the calories in our diet come from carbohydrate, no more than 30% from fat and the

About This Chapter: From "Questions Most Frequently Asked About Sports Nutrition," The President's Council on Physical Fitness and Sports, updated October 15, 2004.

remaining 10–15% from protein. While the exact percentages may vary slightly for some athletes based on their sport or training program, these guidelines will promote health and serve as the basis for a diet that will maximize performance.

Which is better for replacing fluids-water or sports drinks?

Depending on how muscular you are, 55–70% of your body weight is water. Being "hydrated" means maintaining your body's fluid level. When you sweat, you lose water which must be replaced if you want to perform your best. You need to drink fluids before, during and after all workouts and events.

> ♣ **It's A Fact!!**
> **How many calories do I need a day?**
>
> This depends on your age, body size, sport and training program. For example, a 250-pound weight lifter needs more calories than a 98-pound gymnast. Exercise or training may increase calorie needs by as much as 1,000 to 1,500 calories a day. The best way to determine if you're getting too few or too many calories is to monitor your weight. Keeping within your ideal competitive weight range means that you are getting the right amount of calories.

Whether you drink water or a sports drink is a matter of choice. However, if your workout or event lasts for more than 90 minutes, you may benefit from the carbohydrates provided by sports drinks. A sports drink that contains 15–18 grams of carbohydrate in every 8 ounces of fluid should be used. Drinks with a higher carbohydrate content will delay the absorption of water and may cause dehydration, cramps, nausea or diarrhea. There are a variety of sports drinks on the market. Be sure to experiment with sports drinks during practice instead of trying them for the first time the day of an event.

What are electrolytes?

Electrolytes are nutrients that affect fluid balance in the body and are necessary for our nerves and muscles to function. Sodium and potassium are the two electrolytes most often added to sports drinks. Generally, electrolyte replacement is not needed during short bursts of exercise since sweat is approximately 99% water and less than 1% electrolytes. Water, in combination with a well-balanced diet, will restore normal fluid and electrolyte levels in the body. However, replacing electrolytes may be beneficial during continuous activity of longer than two hours, especially in a hot environment.

What are carbohydrates?

Carbohydrates are sugars and starches found in foods like breads, cereals, fruits, vegetables, pasta, milk, honey, syrups, and table sugar. Carbohydrates are the preferred source of energy for your body. Regardless of origin, your body breaks down carbohydrates into glucose that your blood carries to cells to be used for energy. Carbohydrates provide 4 calories per gram, while fat provides 9 calories per gram. Your body cannot differentiate between glucose that comes from starches or sugars. Glucose from either source provides energy for working muscles.

Is it true that athletes should eat a lot of carbohydrates?

When you are training or competing, your muscles need energy to perform. One source of energy for working muscles is glycogen which is made from carbohydrates and stored in your muscles. Every time you work out, you use some of your glycogen. If you don't consume enough carbohydrates, your glycogen stores become depleted, which can result in fatigue. Both sugars and starches are effective in replenishing glycogen stores.

When and what should I eat before I compete?

Performance depends largely on the foods consumed during the days and weeks leading up to an event. If you regularly eat a varied, carbohydrate-rich diet you are in good standing and probably have ample glycogen stores to fuel activity. The purpose of the pre-competition meal is to prevent hunger and to provide the water and additional energy the athlete will need during competition. Most athletes eat two to four hours before their event. However, some athletes perform their best if they eat a small amount 30 minutes before competing, while others eat nothing for six hours beforehand. For many athletes, carbohydrate-rich foods serve as the basis of the meal. However, there is no magic pre-event diet. Simply choose foods and beverages that you enjoy and that don't bother your stomach. Experiment during the weeks before an event to see which foods work best for you.

Will eating sugary foods before an event hurt my performance?

In the past, athletes were warned that eating sugary foods before exercise could hurt performance by causing a drop in blood glucose levels. Recent studies, however, have shown that consuming sugar up to 30 minutes before an event does not diminish performance. In fact, evidence suggests that a sugar-containing pre-competition beverage or snack may improve performance during endurance workouts and events.

What is carbohydrate loading?

Carbohydrate loading is a technique used to increase the amount of glycogen in muscles. For five to seven days before an event, the athlete eats 10–12 grams of carbohydrate per kilogram body weight and gradually reduces the intensity of the workouts. (To find out how much you weigh in kilograms, simply divide your weight in pounds by 2.2.) The day before the event, the athlete rests and eats the same high-carbohydrate diet. Although carbohydrate loading may be beneficial for athletes participating in endurance sports which require 90 minutes or more of non-stop effort, most athletes needn't worry about carbohydrate loading. Simply eating a diet that derives more than half of its calories from carbohydrates will do.

♣ **It's A Fact!!**
What do muscles use for energy during exercise?

Most activities use a combination of fat and carbohydrate as energy sources. How hard and how long you work out, your level of fitness and your diet will affect the type of fuel your body uses. For short-term, high-intensity activities like sprinting, athletes rely mostly on carbohydrate for energy. During low-intensity exercises like walking, the body uses more fat for energy.

As an athlete, do I need to take extra vitamins and minerals?

Athletes need to eat about 1,800 calories a day to get the vitamins and minerals they need for good health and optimal performance. Since most athletes eat more than this amount, vitamin and mineral supplements are needed only in special situations. Athletes who follow vegetarian diets or who avoid an entire group of foods (for example, never drink milk) may need a supplement to make up for the vitamins and minerals not being supplied by food. A multivitamin-mineral pill that supplies 100% of the recommended dietary allowance (RDA) will provide the nutrients needed. An athlete who frequently cuts back on calories, especially below the 1,800 calorie level, is not only at risk for inadequate vitamin and mineral intake, but also may not be getting enough carbohydrate. Since vitamins and minerals do not provide energy, they cannot replace the energy provided by carbohydrates.

Will extra protein help build muscle mass?

Many athletes, especially those on strength-training programs or who participate in power sports, are told that eating a ton of protein or taking protein supplements will help them gain muscle weight. However, the true secret to building muscle is training hard and consuming enough calories. While some extra protein is needed to build muscle, most American diets provide more than enough protein. Between 1.0 and 1.5 grams of protein per kilogram body weight per day is sufficient if your calorie intake is adequate and you're eating a variety of foods. For a 150-pound athlete, that represents 68–102 grams of protein a day.

Why is iron so important?

Hemoglobin, which contains iron, is the part of red blood cells that carries oxygen from the lungs to all parts of the body, including muscles. Since your muscles need oxygen to produce energy, if you have low iron levels in your blood, you may tire quickly. Symptoms of iron deficiency include fatigue, irritability, dizziness, headaches and lack of appetite. Many times, however; there are no symptoms at all. A blood test is the best way to find out if your iron level is low. It is recommended that athletes have their hemoglobin levels checked once a year.

The RDA for iron is 15 milligrams a day for women and 10 milligrams a day for men. Red meat is the richest source of iron, but fish and poultry also are good sources. Fortified breakfast cereals, beans and green leafy vegetables also contain iron. Our bodies absorb the iron found in animal products best.

Should I take an iron supplement?

Taking iron supplements will not improve performance unless an athlete is truly iron deficient. Too much iron can cause constipation, diarrhea, nausea and may interfere with the absorption of other nutrients such as copper and zinc. Therefore, iron supplements should not be taken without proper medical supervision.

Why is calcium so important?

Calcium is needed for strong bones and proper muscle function. Dairy foods are the best source of calcium. However, studies show that many female athletes who are trying to lose weight cut back on dairy products. Female athletes who don't get enough calcium may be at risk for stress fractures and, when they're older, osteoporosis. Young women between the ages of 11 and 24 need about 1,200 milligrams of calcium a day. After age 25, the recommended intake is 800 milligrams. Low-fat dairy products are a rich source of calcium and also are low in fat and calories.

Chapter 49

Foodborne Illnesses

The Causes Of Foodborne Illness

This information is reprinted from "Foodborne Illness: A Constant Challenge" with permission from the Partnership for Food Safety Education's Fight BAC!® website, http://www.fightbac.org. © 2005 Partnership for Food Safety Education.

Because harmful microorganisms are present everywhere in the environment, any food can become contaminated if not properly handled before consumption. Consider these facts:

• The Centers for Disease Control and Prevention (CDC) lists four sources of foodborne illness: disease-causing bacteria, viruses, parasites, and toxins. A few of these are very common and account for the majority of reported illness cases.

• Half of all foodborne outbreaks reported to CDC have no identifiable cause. However, most of the outbreaks are due to microorganisms in food. At least 30 pathogens are commonly associated with foodborne illness.

About This Chapter: This chapter contains excerpts from several fact sheets produced by the Partnership for Food Safety Education which are cited individually within the text; "Cooking Safely in the Microwave Oven," is from *Food Safety Facts* series, U.S. Department of Agriculture, November 2000; Food Safety Tips for Outdoor Eating is from a *Constituent Update* produced by the Center for Food Safety and Applied Nutrition, U.S. Food and Drug Administration (FDA), 2005.

- CDC has targeted four bacterial pathogens—*E. coli O157:H7*, *Salmonella enteritidis*, *Listeria monocytogenes*, and *Campylobacter jejuni*—as those of greatest concern. Also of concern to CDC are other bacterial pathogens, such as *Vibrio vulnificus*, *Yersinia enterocolitica*, *Clostridium perfringens*, and *Staphylococcus aureus*.

- Bacteria in food can cause infections when the microorganism is eaten and established in the body, usually multiplying inside the intestinal tract and irritating the lining of the intestines. Two well-known bacteria that can cause these types of infections are *Salmonella* and *Campylobacter*.

- Other microorganisms in food may produce harmful or deadly toxins while growing in the intestinal tract. Two pathogens that work this way are *Clostridium botulinum* and *Staphylococcus aureus*.

- Viral pathogens are often transmitted by infected food handlers or through contact with sewage. Only a few viral pathogens, such as Hepatitis A and Norwalk viruses, have been proven to cause foodborne illnesses.

- Parasites, such as *Trichinella spiralis*, which causes trichinosis, can occur in microscopic forms, such as eggs and larvae.

- CDC experts report that many of the intestinal illnesses commonly referred to as stomach flu are actually caused by foodborne pathogens. People do not associate these illnesses with food because the onset of symptoms often occurs two or more days after the contaminated food was eaten.

- Natural toxins may occur in some fish or other foods, such as scombroid toxin in tuna, mackerel, or bluefish that have not been properly refrigerated.

- Most cases of foodborne illness in healthy adults are self-limiting and of short duration. Diarrhea, cramps, and vomiting are the most common acute symptoms of many foodborne illnesses, which can range from mild to severe.

Fridge Facts

This information is reprinted from "Fridge Fact Sheet" with permission from the Partnership for Food Safety Education's Fight BAC!® website, http://www.fightbac.org. © 2005 Partnership for Food Safety Education.

Refrigerate Promptly

Bacteria grow most rapidly in the danger zone—the unsafe temperatures between 40° F and 140° F, so it's key to keep foods out of this temperature range. And since cold temperatures keep most harmful bacteria from growing and multiplying—be sure to refrigerate foods quickly!

The Cool Rules

- **Use This Tool To Keep It Cool:** Use a refrigerator thermometer to be sure the temperature is consistently 40° F or below.

- **The Chill Factor:** Refrigerate or freeze perishables, prepared foods, and leftovers within two hours of purchase or use. Always marinate foods in the refrigerator.

- **The Thaw Law:** Never defrost food at room temperature. Thaw food in the refrigerator. For a quick thaw, submerge in cold water in an airtight package or thaw in the microwave if you will be cooking it immediately.

- **Divide and Conquer:** Separate large amounts of leftovers into small, shallow containers for quicker cooling in the refrigerator.

- **Avoid the Pack Attack:** Do not over-stuff the refrigerator. Cold air must circulate to keep food safe.

- **Rotate Before It's Too Late:** Use or discard chilled foods as recommended in the USDA Cold Storage Chart found online at http://www.foodsafety.gov/~fsg/f01chart.html.

- **Don't Go Too Low:** As you approach 32° F ice crystals can begin to form and lower the quality of some foods such as raw fruits, vegetables, and eggs. A refrigerator thermometer will help you determine whether you are too close to this zone.

Serve And Preserve

When serving cold food at a buffet, picnic, or barbecue, keep the following "chilling tips" in mind.

- Cold foods should be kept at 40° F or colder.

- Keep all perishable foods chilled right up until serving time.

- Place containers of cold food on ice for serving to make sure they stay cold.

- It's particularly important to keep custards, cream pies, and cakes with whipped-cream or cream-cheese frostings refrigerated. Don't serve them if refrigeration is not possible.

✎ What's It Mean?

Campylobacter: Most common bacterial cause of diarrhea in the United States. Sources include raw and undercooked meat and poultry, raw milk, and untreated water.

Clostridium botulinum: This organism produces a toxin which causes botulism, a life-threatening illness that can prevent the breathing muscles from moving air in and out of the lungs. Sources include home-prepared foods and herbal oils; honey should not be fed to children less than 12 months old.

E. coli O157:H7: A bacterium that can produce a deadly toxin and causes approximately 73,000 cases of foodborne illness each year in the U.S. Sources include meat, especially undercooked or raw hamburger, produce, and raw milk.

Listeria monocytogenes: Causes listeriosis, a serious disease for pregnant women, newborns, and adults with a weakened immune system. Sources include soil and water. It has been found in dairy products including soft cheeses as well as in raw and undercooked meat, in poultry and seafood, and in produce.

Norovirus: This virus is the leading cause of diarrhea in the United States. Any food can be contaminated with norovirus if handled by someone who is infected with this virus.

The Big Thaw

Foods must remain at a safe temperature while thawing. Now is the perfect time to learn about the DOs and DON'Ts of defrosting.

Defrosting DOs

- Defrost food in the refrigerator. This is the safest method for all foods.

- Short on time? Thaw meat and poultry in airtight packaging in cold water. Change the water every 30 minutes, so the food continues to thaw.

- Defrost food in the microwave only if it will be cooked immediately.

Salmonella: Most common cause of foodborne deaths. Responsible for millions of cases of foodborne illness a year. Sources include raw and undercooked eggs, undercooked poultry and meat, dairy products, seafood, fruits, and vegetables.

Staphylococcus aureus: This bacterium produces a toxin that causes vomiting shortly after ingesting. Sources include cooked foods high in protein (for example, cooked ham, salads, bakery products, dairy products.)

Shigella: Causes an estimated 300,000 cases of diarrhea illnesses. Poor hygiene causes *Shigella* to be easily passed from person to person. Sources include salads, milk and dairy products, and unclean water.

Toxoplasma gondii: A parasite that causes toxoplasmosis, a very severe disease that can produce central nervous system disorders particularly mental retardation and visual impairment in children. Pregnant women and people with weakened immune systems are at higher risk. Sources include meat, primarily pork.

Vibrio vulnificus: Causes gastroenteritis or a syndrome known as primary septicemia. People with liver diseases are especially at high risk. Sources include raw or undercooked seafood.

Source: From "Foodborne Illness: Ten Least Wanted Foodborne Pathogens;" this information is reprinted with permission from the Partnership for Food Safety Education's Fight BAC!® website, http://www.fightbac.org. © 2005 Partnership for Food Safety Education.

✎ What's It Mean?

Bacteria: Living single-celled organisms. They can be carried by water, wind, insects, plants, animals, and people. Bacteria survive well on skin and clothes and in human hair. They also thrive in scabs, scars, the mouth, nose, throat, intestines, and room-temperature foods.

Biological hazard: Refers to the danger of food contamination by disease-causing microorganisms (bacteria, viruses, parasites, or fungi) and their toxins and by certain plants and fish that carry natural toxins.

Contamination: The unintended presence of potentially harmful substances, including microorganisms in food.

Cross-contamination: The transfer of harmful substances or disease-causing microorganisms to food by hands, food-contact surfaces, sponges, cloth towels, and utensils that touch raw food, are not cleaned, and then touch ready-to-eat foods. Cross-contamination can also occur when raw food touches or drips onto cooked or ready-to-eat foods.

Foodborne illness: A disease that is carried or transmitted to humans by food containing harmful substances. Examples are the disease salmonellosis, which is caused by *Salmonella* bacteria and the disease botulism, which is caused by the toxin produced by the bacteria *Clostridium botulinum*.

Food contact surface: Any equipment or utensil which normally comes in contact with food or which may drain, drip, or splash on food or on surfaces normally in contact with food. Examples: cutting boards, knives, sponges, countertops, and colanders.

Fungi: A group of microorganisms that includes molds and yeasts.

• You can thaw food as part of the cooking process, but make sure food reaches its safe internal temperature.

Defrosting DON'Ts

• Avoid keeping foods in the danger zone—the unsafe temperatures between 40° F and 140° F.

Incidence: The number of new cases of foodborne illness in a given population during a specified period of time (for example, the number of new cases per 100,000 population per year).

Microorganism: A small life form, only seen through a microscope, that may cause disease. For example, bacteria, fungi, parasites, or viruses.

Outbreak: An incident in which two or more people experience the same illness after eating the same food.

Parasite: A microorganism that needs a host to survive. Examples: *Cryptosporidium*, *Toxoplasma*.

Pathogen: A microorganism that is infectious and causes disease.

Spore: A thick-walled protective structure produced by certain bacteria and fungi to protect their cells. Spores often survive cooking, freezing, and some sanitizing measures.

Toxins: Poisons that are produced by microorganisms, carried by fish, or released by plants. For example, botulism caused by the toxin from *Clostridium botulinum*, scombroid poisoning from the naturally occurring scombroid toxin in some improperly refrigerated fish, such as mackerel and tuna.

Virus: A protein-wrapped genetic material which is the smallest and simplest life-form known. For example, Norwalk virus, hepatitis A.

Source: "Foodborne Illness: A Constant Challenge, Food Safety Glossary;" this information is reprinted with permission from the Partnership for Food Safety Education's Fight BAC!® website, http://www.fightbac.org. © 2005 Partnership for Food Safety Education.

- Don't defrost food in hot water.

- Don't thaw food on the counter. Food that's left out at room temperature longer than two hours is not within a safe temperature range and may not be safe to eat.

Cooking Safely In The Microwave Oven

Microwave ovens can play an important role at mealtime, but special care must be taken when cooking or reheating meat, poultry, fish, and eggs to make sure they are prepared safely. Microwave ovens can cook unevenly and leave "cold spots," where harmful bacteria can survive. For this reason, it is important to use the following safe microwaving tips to prevent foodborne illness.

Microwave Oven Cooking

• Arrange food items evenly in a covered dish and add some liquid if needed. Cover the dish with a lid or plastic wrap; loosen or vent the lid or wrap to let steam escape. The moist heat that is created will help destroy harmful bacteria and ensure uniform cooking. Cooking bags also provide safe, even cooking.

• Do not cook large cuts of meat on high power (100%). Large cuts of meat should be cooked on medium power (50%) for longer periods. This allows heat to reach the center without overcooking outer areas.

• Stir or rotate food midway through the microwaving time to eliminate cold spots where harmful bacteria can survive, and for more even cooking.

✔ Quick Tip
Hit The Road

When traveling with food be aware that time, temperature, and a cold source are key. Here are some tips to help keep your travels cool.

• Keep frozen foods in the refrigerator or freezer until you're ready to go.

• Always use ice or cold packs and fill your cooler with food. A full cooler will maintain its cold temperatures longer than one that is partially filled.

• When traveling, keep the cooler in the air-conditioned passenger compartment of your car, rather than in a hot trunk.

• If you've asked for a doggie bag to take home from a restaurant, it should be refrigerated within two hours of serving.

Source: This information is excerpted and reprinted from "Fridge Fact Sheet" with permission from the Partnership for Food Safety Education's Fight BAC!® website, http://www.fightbac.org. © 2005 Partnership for Food Safety Education.

- When partially cooking food in the microwave oven to finish cooking on the grill or in a conventional oven, it is important to transfer the microwaved food to the other heat source immediately. Never partially cook food and store it for later use.

- Use a food thermometer or the oven's temperature probe to verify the food has reached a safe temperature. Place the thermometer in the thickest area of the meat or poultry—not near fat or bone—and in the innermost part of the thigh of whole poultry. Cooking times may vary because ovens vary in power and efficiency. Check in several places to be sure red meat is 160° F, whole poultry is 180° F, and egg casseroles are 160° F. Fish should flake with a fork. Always allow standing time, which completes the cooking, before checking the internal temperature with a food thermometer.

- Cooking whole, stuffed poultry in a microwave oven is not recommended. The stuffing might not reach the temperature needed to destroy harmful bacteria.

Microwave Defrosting

- Remove food from packaging before defrosting. Do not use foam trays and plastic wraps because they are not heat stable at high temperatures. Melting or warping may cause harmful chemicals to migrate into food.

- Cook meat, poultry, egg casseroles, and fish immediately after defrosting in the microwave oven because some areas of the frozen food may begin to cook during the defrosting time. Do not hold partially cooked food to use later.

Reheating In The Microwave Oven

- Cover foods with a lid or a microwave-safe plastic wrap to hold in moisture and provide safe, even heating.

- Heat ready-to-eat foods such as hot dogs, luncheon meats, fully cooked ham, and leftovers until steaming hot.

- After reheating foods in the microwave oven, allow standing time. Then, use a clean food thermometer to check that food has reached 165° F.

♣ It's A Fact!!
Containers And Wraps

- Only use cookware that is specially manufactured for use in the microwave oven. Glass, ceramic containers, and all plastics should be labeled for microwave oven use.

- Plastic storage containers such as margarine tubs, take-out containers, whipped topping bowls, and other one-time use containers should not be used in microwave ovens. These containers can warp or melt, possibly causing harmful chemicals to migrate into the food.

- Microwave plastic wraps, wax paper, cooking bags, parchment paper, and white microwave-safe paper towels should be safe to use. Do not let plastic wrap touch foods during microwaving.

- Never use thin plastic storage bags, brown paper or plastic grocery bags, newspapers, or aluminum foil in the microwave oven.

Source: U.S. Department of Agriculture, November 2000.

Meat, Poultry, And Seafood

This information is reprinted from "Food Safety For Meat, Poultry, and Seafood Lovers!" with permission from the Partnership for Food Safety Education's Fight BAC!® website, http://www.fightbac.org. © 2005 Partnership for Food Safety Education.

We all know that meat, poultry, and seafood provide great sources of protein and other essential vitamins, but mishandling them may not be so healthful. Remember that all perishable foods, like meat, poultry, eggs, and seafood, need to be handled properly to prevent foodborne illness.

Cook It Right

- Cook ground meat to at least 160° F. Ground poultry should be cooked to 165° F.

- Cook roasts and steaks to an internal temperature of at least 145° F for medium rare or to 160° F for medium.

- Whole poultry should be cooked to 180° F—measure the temperature in the thigh. Poultry breasts should be cooked to 170° F.

- Cook fish until it's opaque and flakes easily with a fork.

Should I wash raw meat, poultry or seafood before cooking it?

Washing raw poultry, beef, pork, lamb, veal, or seafood before cooking is not necessary. Although washing these raw foods may get rid of some of the pathogens on the surface of these foods, it may allow the pathogens to spread around the kitchen. Cooking these foods to a safe internal temperature will destroy any bacteria that may be present in the food. Use a clean food thermometer to make sure food has reached the proper temperature.

If cooked meat and poultry look pink, does it mean that the food is not done?

The color of cooked meat and poultry is not a sure sign of its degree of doneness. For instance, hamburgers and fresh pork can remain pink even after cooking to temperatures of 160° F or higher. Smoked poultry remains pink, no matter how cooked it is. Only by using a food thermometer can you accurately determine that meat and poultry have reached safe internal temperatures.

The Centers for Disease Control and Prevention does not recommend eating undercooked or raw meat, poultry, and seafood as these can be associated with a higher risk of foodborne illness.

Is it safe to eat sushi, the Japanese raw fish specialty?

People in the at-risk groups (young children, pregnant women, senior citizens, and people with weakened immune systems) should not eat raw or undercooked fish or shellfish. People with liver disorders or weakened immune systems are especially at risk for getting sick. Foods made with raw fish are more likely to contain parasites or *Vibrio* species than foods made from cooked fish. Always cook fish until it's opaque and flakes easily with a fork.

Outdoor Eating Food Safety Tips

To protect yourself, your family, and friends from foodborne illness, practice safe food handling techniques when eating outdoors. Keep these tips in mind when preparing, storing, and cooking food for picnics and barbecues.

When You Transport Food

- Keep cold food cold. Place cold food in a cooler with ice or frozen gel packs. Cold food should be held at or below 40° F.

- Consider packing beverages in one cooler and perishable foods in another.

- Meat, poultry, and seafood may be packed while it is still frozen so that it stays colder longer. Be sure to keep raw meat, poultry, and seafood securely wrapped so their juices don't contaminate cooked foods or foods eaten raw such as fruits and vegetables. And don't forget to rinse raw fruits and vegetables in water before packing them.

- Rinse fresh fruits and vegetables under running tap water, including those with skins and rinds that are not eaten. Packaged fruits and vegetables labeled "ready-to-eat," "washed," or "triple washed" need not be washed.

- Rub firm-skin fruits and vegetables under running tap water or scrub with a clean vegetable brush while rinsing with running tap water.

- Dry fruits and vegetables with a clean cloth towel or paper towel.

- Keep the cooler in the air-conditioned passenger compartment of your car, rather than in a hot trunk. Limit the times the cooler is opened.

Before You Begin

- Food safety begins with hand-washing even in outdoor settings. And it can be as simple as using a water jug, some soap, and paper towels.

✔ Quick Tip

- Don't forget to wash your hands with soap and warm water before and after preparing raw meat, poultry, and seafood.

- Use a clean food thermometer to make sure raw meat and poultry have been cooked to a safe internal temperature. Wash the food thermometer in hot, soapy water between uses.

Combating Cross-Contamination

- **S-e-p-a-r-a-t-i-n-g is essential:** To prevent raw juices from contaminating ready-to-eat foods, separate raw meat, poultry, and seafood from other foods in your grocery store shopping cart and in your refrigerator.

- **Take 2:** Consider using one cutting board for raw meat, poultry, and seafood products and another one for fresh fruits and vegetables. In addition, don't forget to wash your hands with soap and warm water and your cutting boards, dishes, and utensils with hot, soapy water after they come in contact with raw meat, poultry, and seafood.

- **Clean your plate:** Place cooked food on a clean platter. If you put cooked food on an unwashed platter that previously held raw meat, poultry, or seafood, bacteria from the raw food could contaminate the safely cooked food.

- **Seal it up:** To prevent juices from raw meat, poultry, or seafood from dripping onto other foods in your refrigerator, place these raw foods in sealed containers, plastic bags, or on a plate or tray. Then store them on the bottom shelf, so they don't drip onto foods below them.

- **Marinating mandate:** Don't use sauce that was used to marinate raw meat, poultry, or seafood on cooked foods, unless you boil it before applying. Never taste marinade or sauce that was used to marinate raw meat, poultry, or seafood unless it was heated to the boiling point first.

Source: This information is excerpted and reprinted from "Food Safety For Meat, Poultry, and Seafood Lovers!" with permission from the Partnership for Food Safety Education's Fight BAC!® website, http://www.fightbac.org. © 2005 Partnership for Food Safety Education.

- Consider using moist disposable Towelettes for cleaning your hands.

- Keep all utensils and platters clean when preparing food.

Safe Grilling Tips

- Marinate foods in the refrigerator, not on the counter or outdoors. If some of the marinade is to be used as a sauce on the cooked food, reserve a portion separately before adding the raw meat, poultry, or seafood. Don't reuse marinade.

- Don't use the same platter and utensils that previously held raw meat or seafood to serve cooked meats and seafood.

- If you partially cook food in the microwave, oven, or stove to reduce grilling time, do so immediately before the food goes on the hot grill.

♣ It's A Fact!!
Safe-Cooking Temperature Chart

Beef/Pork

- Cook beef roasts and steaks to 145° F for medium rare or to 160° F for medium.

- Cook ground beef to at least 160° F.

- Cook raw sausages to 160° F.

- Reheat ready-to-eat sausages to 165° F.

- Cook pork roasts, chops, or ground patties to 160° F for medium, or 170° F for well done.

Poultry

- Cook whole poultry to 180° F.

- Cook ground poultry to 165° F.

- Cook chicken breasts to 170° F.

- Cook stuffing to 165° F.

- When it's time to cook the food, cook it thoroughly. Use a food thermometer to be sure.

  - Beef, veal, and lamb steaks and roasts: 145° F for medium rare, 160° F for medium, and 170° F for well done.

  - Ground pork and ground beef: 160° F.

  - Ground poultry: 165° F.

  - Poultry breasts: 170° F.

  - Whole poultry (take measurement in the thigh): 180° F.

  - Fin fish: 145° F or until the flesh is opaque and separates easily with a fork.

  - Shrimp, lobster, and crabs: the meat should be pearly and opaque.

Eggs

- Cook eggs until the yolks and whites are firm.

- Don't use recipes in which eggs remain raw or only partially cooked.

Fish

- Cook fish until it's opaque and flakes easily with a fork.

- Avoid eating raw oysters or raw shellfish. People with liver disorders or weakened immune systems are especially at risk for getting sick.

Leftovers

- When reheating leftovers, heat them thoroughly to at least 165° F.

Source: This information is excerpted and reprinted from "Food Safety For Meat, Poultry, and Seafood Lovers!" with permission from the Partnership for Food Safety Education's Fight BAC!® website, http://www.fightbac.org. © 2005 Partnership for Food Safety Education.

- Clams, oysters, and mussels: until the shells are open.

- Grilled food can be kept hot until served by moving it to the side of the grill rack, just away from the coals where it can overcook.

When You Serve Food

- Keep cold foods cold and hot foods hot.

- Do not use a plate that previously held raw meat, poultry, or seafood for anything else unless the plate has first been washed in hot, soapy water.

- Hot food should be kept hot, at or above 140° F. Wrap well and place in an insulated container.

- Foods like chicken salad and desserts in individual serving dishes can also be placed directly on ice, or in a shallow container set in a deep pan filled with ice. Drain off water as ice melts and replace ice frequently.

- Don't let perishable food sit out longer than two hours.

- Food should not sit out for more than one hour in temperatures above 90° F.

☞ Remember!! Clean: Wash Hands And Surfaces Often

Bacteria can spread throughout the kitchen and get onto cutting boards, utensils, sponges, and counter tops. Here's what you can do:

- Wash your hands with hot soapy water before handling food and after using the bathroom, changing diapers, and handling pets.

- Wash your cutting boards, dishes, utensils, and counter tops with hot soapy water after preparing each food item and before you go on to the next food.

- Use plastic or other non-porous cutting boards. These boards should be run through the dishwasher—or washed in hot soapy water—after use.

- Consider using paper towels to clean up kitchen surfaces. If you use cloth towels, wash them often in the hot cycle of your washing machine.

Source: Excerpted from "Fight BAC! Four Simple Steps to Food Safety," this information is reprinted with permission from the Partnership for Food Safety Education's Fight BAC!® website, http://www.fightbac.org. © 2005 Partnership for Food Safety Education.

Part Five

If You Need More Information

Chapter 50

Cooking Tips and Resources

Ever wish you could head into the kitchen and whip up a delicious dinner? The good news is that if you've read this far, you'll have no problem at all—because if you can read, you can cook! The trick is knowing some kitchen basics, what kinds of recipes are best, and where to find inspiration for making mouth-watering meals. Read on for some ideas about how to get started.

Kitchen 101: The Basics

Even world-class chefs have to start somewhere. Here are some basic tips for getting off on the right foot in the kitchen.

- Choose recipes that aren't too complicated when you first start cooking. You don't want to be overwhelmed by a recipe that has unusual ingredients or difficult steps, or that is time consuming. Try one- or two-pot dishes, and be sure to check out the KidsHealth recipe section (http://www.kidshealth.org/teen/recipies) for some simple meal ideas.

About This Chapter: This chapter begins with information provided by TeensHealth, one of the largest resources online for medically reviewed health information written for parents, kids, and teens. For more articles like this one, visit www.TeensHealth.org, or www.KidsHealth.org. © 2004 The Nemours Center for Children's Health Media, a division of The Nemours Foundation. The information under "Cooking Resources" was compiled from many sources deemed accurate; all contact information was verified in December 2005. Items listed under "Cookbooks" were excerpted from "Food and Nutrition Fun for Children," Food and Nutrition Information Center, National Agricultural Library, U.S. Department of Agriculture, January 2002, with updates made by the editor in 2005.

- Read the recipe through from beginning to end before you start. Do you have all the right ingredients? Utensils? Appliances?

- Make sure you understand all the directions.

- Check the clock and make sure you have enough time to make the recipe. You don't want to spend tons of time in the kitchen—and with the right recipe, you won't need to. If you have to get dinner on the table for a certain time, figure out when you'll need to start in order to have the meal ready. Most recipes include the amount of time it takes to prepare them in the instructions. It might be a good idea to add 10 or 15 minutes to that time when you first try to conquer the kitchen— just to be on the safe side.

- Assemble all your ingredients in one place before you start. Some chefs like to measure out each ingredient ahead of time before cooking. Pull out the utensils, measuring cups, and spoons you'll be using and keep them handy, so you won't need to run all over the kitchen.

- An apron is a good idea if you want to keep your clothes from getting dirty. (You can skip the chef's hat, but it's smart to tie back long hair.)

- Always wash your hands before any kind of food preparation. You may need to wash your hands several times as you cook, especially after touching raw meat, poultry (chicken and turkey), fish, and egg products.

- Never put cooked or ready-to-serve foods on plates, cutting boards, counters, or other places you have placed raw meat, poultry, fish, or egg products without washing these surfaces first.

- Don't cook without a parent's permission.

Recipes: Where To Find 'Em

If you've never actually looked for recipes, you've probably never taken notice of them. But once you start keeping an eye out for recipes, you'll find them everywhere! Here's a list of some places you can find fantastic recipes:

- your family (does your uncle have a world-famous pasta salad or have you always loved your grandmother's spicy chicken? You'll probably find that they're flattered when you ask.)

- cookbooks (in bookstores or on library shelves, where you can photo-copy them)

- food, fitness, and women's magazines

- newspapers (there is a dining section in the Sunday edition of many newspapers)

- supermarkets (check by the meat, produce, and fish sections)

- food packages (the box or bag may have a recipe on or inside the package)

- send-away offers (some foods have a send-away offer; if you send a proof of purchase, they send you a small book of recipes)

- TV cooking shows

- the internet

- cooking class at school

- your friends

Keep your recipes in one place—a recipe box, folder, or notebook is fine. As you start to collect recipes, you can even organize them according to their category (for example, salads, chicken dishes, or pasta).

Getting Creative in the Kitchen

Once you get the hang of reading recipes and mastering some meals, you can get creative in the kitchen! Let loose and:

- Try experimenting with different ingredients—substitute beans for meat, or crunchy green beans for carrots, for example.

- Learn to use herbs and spices.

- Bring out your artistic side in the kitchen by experimenting with different colors and textures in meals.

- Focus on one type of dish and learn lots of variations.

- Try recipes from cultures or ethnicities other than our own.

- Invent your own recipes and try them out on family members and friends.

Most of all, don't be afraid to fail a few times. Cooking is like anything else—it takes practice. So even if no one likes your banana tacos, just remember: delicious meals come out of creative (and adventurous) minds.

Cooking Resources

5 A Day: Recipes
Centers for Disease Control and Prevention
http://www.cdc.gov/nccdphp/dnpa/5aday/recipes

Allrecipes.com
http://allrecipies.com

Cooking Light
http://cookinglight.com

DASH Recipes
National Heart, Lung, and Blood Institute
http://hin.nhlbi.nih.gov/NHBPEP_Kit/recipes.htm

Eat 5 To 9 A Day
National Cancer Institute
http://5aday.nci.nih.gov/recipes/index.html

Food Network
http://www.foodtv.com

Food, Family, and Fun
Food and Nutrition Service, U.S. Department of Agriculture
http://www.fns.usda.gov/tn/Students/Food_Family/index.html

Healthy Kids Corner
Wisconsin Department of Health and Family Services
http://dhfs.wisconsin.gov/kids/nutrition.htm

Healthy Potato
U.S. Potato Board
http://www.healthypotato.com

Meals for You
http://www.mealsforyou.com

Meals Matter
http://www.mealsmatter.org

Pork4Kids
National Pork Board
http://www.pork4kids.com/FoodList.aspx?id=3

Sample Reduced-Calorie Menus
National Heart, Lung, and Blood Institute
http://www.nhlbi.nih.gov/health/public/heart/obesity/lose_wt/
sampmenu.htm

U.S. Department of Agriculture
Recipes and Tips for Healthy, Thrifty Meals
http://www.cnpp.usda.gov/Pubs/Cookbook/thriftym.pdf

Cookbooks

Better Homes and Gardens New Junior Cookbook
Jennifer Dorland Darling, Better Homes and Gardens Books, 1997
ISBN: 0696207087

Everything Kids' Cookbook
Sandra K. Nissenberg, Adams Media Corporation, 2002
ISBN: 1580626580

Fannie Farmer Junior Cookbook
Joan Scobey, Little Brown and Company, 2000
ISBN: 0316776173

Good Housekeeping Illustrated Children's Cookbook
Marianne Zanzarella, Hearst Books, 2004
ISBN: 1588164241

Good Soup Attracts Chairs: A First African Cookbook for American Kids
Fran Osseo-Asare, Pelican Publishing Co., 2002
ISBN: 156554918X

Healthy Body Cookbook
Joan D'Amico and Karen Drummond, J. Wiley and Sons, 1998
ISBN: 0471188883

Holidays of the World Cookbook for Students
Lois Sinaiko Webb, Greenwood Publishing Group, Inc., 1995
ISBN: 0897748840

Honest Pretzels: And 64 Other Amazing Recipes for Cooks Ages 8 and Up
Mollie Katzen, Red Leaf Press, 1999
ISBN: 1883672860

Kid's Cookbook: Educational and Edible Delights
Carol Kurzweg and Kimble Mead, Celebration Press, 1994
ISBN: 0673360652

Mix-it-up Cookbook
Staff of American Girl, Pleasant Company Publications, 2003
ISBN: 1584857420

Quick Meals for Healthy Kids and Busy Parents
Sandra Nissenberg, R.D., Margaret Bogle, R.D., and Audrey Wright, R.D.,
J. Wiley and Sons, 1995
ISBN: 0471346985

Science Chef: 100 Fun Food Experiments and Recipes for Kids
Joan D'Amico and Karen Eich Drummond, J. Wiley and Sons, 1994
ISBN: 047131045X

Chapter 51

Resources For Dietary Information

Academy for Eating Disorders

60 Revere Drive, Suite 500
Northbrook, IL 60062-1577
Phone: 847-498-4274
Fax: 847-480-9282
Website: http://www.aedweb.org

American Dietetic Association

120 South Riverside Plaza
Suite 2000
Chicago, IL 60606-6995
Toll-Free: 800-877-1600
Website: http://www.eatright.org

American Heart Association

National Center
7272 Greenville Avenue
Dallas, TX 75231
Toll-Free: 800-242-8721
Website: http://www.americanheart.org

American Obesity Association

1250 24th Street, NW, Suite 300
Washington, DC 20037
Phone: 202-776-7711
Fax: 202-776-7712
Website: http://www.obesity.org
E-mail: executive@obesity.org

About This Chapter: The resources listed in this chapter were compiled from multiple sources deemed reliable. All contact information was verified in December 2005.

Anorexia Nervosa and Related Eating Disorders, Inc.

Phone: 541-344-1144
Website: http://www.anred.com

Center for Food Safety and Applied Nutrition

U.S. Food and Drug Administration
5100 Paint Branch Parkway
College Park, MD 20740
Toll-Free: 888-SAFEFOOD (888-723-3663)
Website: www.cfsan.fda.gov

Center for Science in the Public Interest

1875 Connecticut Ave., NW
Suite 300
Washington, DC 20009-5728
Phone: 202-332-9110
Fax: 202-265-4954
Website: http://www.cspinet.org
E-mail: cspi@cspinet.org

Center for Young Women's Health

Children's Hospital Boston
300 Longwood Avenue
Boston, MA 02115
Phone: 617-730-0192
Fax: 617-730-0192
Website: http://www.youngwomenshealth.org
E-mail: cywh@childrens.harvard.edu

Centers for Disease Control and Prevention

1600 Clifton Rd., MS D-31
Atlanta, GA 30333
Phone: 404-639-3311
Toll-Free: 800-311-3435
Website: http://www.cdc.gov

Children's Nutrition Research Center

Baylor College of Medicine
1100 Bates Street
Houston, TX 77030
Phone: 713-798-6767
Website: http://kidsnutrition.org
E-mail: cnrc@bcm.tmc.edu

Cooperative Extension Services Webpage

U. S. Department of Agriculture
Child Care Nutrition Program
Website: http://www.nal.usda.gov/childcare/Resources/cooperative_extension.html

Dairy Council of California

1101 National Dr., Suite B
Sacramento, CA 95834-1901
Toll-Free Outside CA: 866-572-1359
Toll-Free In CA: 877-324-7901
www.dairycouncilofca.org/globals/glob_sear_main.htm (click on "Learning Tools")

Dietary Guidelines for Americans

U.S. Department of Agriculture
Website: http://www.health.gov/
dietaryguidelines

European Food Information Council.

http://www.foodstudents.net

Food Allergy News for Kids/ Food Allergy News for Teens

Website: http://www.fankids.org

Food Allergy and Anaphylaxis Network

11781 Lee Jackson Hwy., Suite 160
Fairfax, VA 22033-3309
Toll-Free: 800-929-4040
Fax: 703-691-2713
Website: http://www.foodallergy.org
E-mail: faan@foodallergy.org

Food and Nutrition Service

U.S. Department of Agriculture
3101 Park Center Drive
Alexandria, VA 22302
Website: http://www.fns.usda.gov

Food Marketing Institute

655 15th Street, NW
Washington, DC 20005
Phone: 202-452-8444
Fax: 202-429-4519
Website: http://www.fmi.org
E-mail: fmi@fmil.org

Food Research and Action Center

1875 Connecticut Ave., NW
Suite 540
Washington, DC 20009
Phone: 202-986-2200
Fax: 202-986-2525
Website: http://www.frac.org

4Girls Health

The National Women's Health
Information Center
Attention: GirlsHealth.gov
8270 Willow Oaks Corporate Dr.,
Suite 301
Fairfax, VA 22031
Website: http://www.4girls.gov

Go Ask Alice!

Fitness and Nutrition Section
Columbia University's Health
Education Program
Website: http://
www.goaskalice.columbia.edu/
Cat3.html

International Food Information Council

1100 Connecticut Avenue, NW,
Suite 430
Washington, DC 20036
Phone: 202-296-6540
Fax: 202-296-6547
Website: http://www.ific.org
E-mail: foodinfo@ific.org

International Foundation for Functional Gastrointestinal Disorders, Inc.
P.O. Box 170864
Milwaukee, WI 53217-8076
Toll-Free: 888–964–2001
Phone: 414–964–1799
Fax: 414–964–7176
Website: http://www.iffgd.org
E-mail: iffgd@iffgd.org

Kellogg's Nutrition University
One Kellogg Square
Battle Creek, MI 49016
Toll-Free: 800-962-1413
Website: http://
www.kelloggsnu.com

Kidnetic
International Food Information
Council Foundation
Website: http://www.kidnetic.com

Kids Food Cyber Club
Website: http://www.kidfood.org

Mayo Clinic Food and Nutrition Center
Website: http://
www.mayoclinic.com/health/
food-and-nutrition/NU99999

Milk Matters
P.O. Box 3006
Rockville, MD 20847
Phone: 800-370-2943
TTY: 888-320-6942
Fax: 301-984-1473
http://www.nichd.nih.gov/milk/
milk.cfm
E-mail: NICHDinformation
ResourceCenter@mail.nih.gov

National Association of Anorexia Nervosa and Associated Disorders
Box 7
Highland Park, IL 60035
Phone: 847-831-3438
Website: http://www.anad.org

National Cholesterol Education Program
National Heart, Lung, and Blood
Institute Information Center
P.O. Box 30105
Bethesda, MD 20824-0105
Phone: 301-592-8673
Fax: 301-592-8563
Website: http://www.nhlbi.nih.gov/
about/ncep

National Eating Disorders Association

603 Stewart Street, Suite 803
Seattle, WA 98101
Toll-Free: 800-931-2237
Phone: 206-382-3587
Fax: 206-829-8501
Website: http://
www.nationaleatingdisorders.org
E-mail:
info@nationaleatingdisorders.org

National Institute of Child Health and Human Development

P.O. Box 3006
Rockville, MD 20847
Toll-Free: 800-370-2943
TTY: 888-320-6942
Fax: 301-984-1473
Website: http://www.nichd.nih.gov
E-mail: NICHDInformation
ResourceCenter@mail.nih.gov

Nutrition and Physical Activity

Centers for Disease Control and
Prevention
1600 Clifton Rd., MS D-31
Atlanta, GA 30333
Toll-Free: 800-311-3435
Phone: 404-639-3311
Website for Nutrition Topics: http://
www.cdc.gov/nccdphp/dnpa/
nutrition.htm
Website for Healthy Weight
Topics: http://www.cdc.gov/
nccdphp/dnpa/nutrition/
nutrition_for_everyone/
healthy_weight/index.htm

Nutrition Cafe

Pacific Science Center and
Washington State Dairy Council
Website: http://exhibits.pacsci.org/
nutrition

Nutrition Explorations

National Dairy Council
10255 W. Higgins Road, Suite 900
Rosemont, IL 60018
Phone: 847-803-2000
Fax: 847-803-2077
Website: http://
www.nutritionexplorations.org

Nutrition.gov
National Agricultural Library
Food and Nutrition Information
Center
Nutrition.gov Staff
10301 Baltimore Avenue
Beltsville, MD 20705-2351
Website: http://www.nutrition.gov

Nutrition Information Line
American Dietetic Association
Toll-Free: 800-366-1655

Obesity Education Initiative
National Heart, Lung, and Blood
Institute
NHLBI Information Center
P.O. Box 30105
Bethesda, MD 20824-0105
Phone: 301-592-8573
Website: http://rover.nhlbi.nih.gov/
health/public/heart/obesity/lose_wt

**Partnership for Food Safety
Education**
http://www.fightbac.org

**Tufts University Health and
Nutrition Letter**
P.O. Box 420235
Palm Coast, FL 32142-0235
Toll-Free: 800-274-7581
Website: http://
www.healthletter.tufts.edu

**U.S. Food and Drug
Administration**
5600 Fishers Lane
Rockville, MD 20857-0001
Toll-Free: 888-463-6332
Website: http://www.fda.gov

Vegetarian Resource Group
P.O. Box 1463
Baltimore, MD 21203
Phone: 410-366-VEGE
Website: http://www.vrg.org
E-mail: vrg@vrg.org

**Weight-Control Information
Network**
1 Win Way
Bethesda, MD 20892-3665
Toll-Free: 877-946-4627
Fax: 202-828-1028
Website: http://win.niddk.nih.gov
E-mail: win@info.niddk.nih.gov

Chapter 52

Resources For Fitness Information

Aerobics and Fitness Association of America

15250 Ventura Blvd., Suite 200
Sherman Oaks, CA 91403
Toll-Free: 877-YOURBODY (877-968-7263)
Phone: 818-9050040
Fax: 818-990-5468
Website: http://www.afaa.com
E-mail: contactAFAA@afaa.com

Amateur Athletic Union

National Headquarters
1910 Hotel Plaza Blvd.
P.O. Box 22409
Lake Buena Vista, FL 32830
Toll-Free: 800-AAU-4USA
Phone: 407-934-7200
Fax: 407-934-7242
Website: http://www.aausports.org

American Alliance for Health, Physical Education, Recreation and Dance

1900 Association Dr.
Reston, VA 20191-1598
Toll-Free: 800-213-7193
Phone: 703-476-3400
Website: http://www.aahperd.org
E-mail: info@aahperd.org

American College of Sports Medicine

401 W. Michigan Street
Indianapolis, IN 46206-1440
Phone: 317-637-9200
Fax: 317-634-7817
Website: http://www.acsm.org/index.asp
E-mail: publicinfo@acsm.org

About This Chapter: The resources listed in this chapter were compiled from multiple sources deemed reliable. All contact information was verified in December 2005.

American Council on Exercise

4851 Paramount Drive
San Diego, CA 92123
Toll-Free: 800-825-3636
Phone: 858-279-8227
Fax: 858-279-8064
Website: http://www.acefitness.org
E-mail: support@acefitness.org

American Running Association

4405 East West Highway
Suite 405
Bethesda, MD 20814
Toll-Free: 800-776-2732
Phone: 301-913-9517
Website: http://
www.americanrunning.org
E-mail: run@americanrunning.org

Aquatic Exercise Association

201 Tamiami Trail, S., Suite 3
Nokomis, FL 34275
Toll-Free: 888-AEA-WAVE
Phone: (941) 486-8600
Fax: 941-486-8820
Website: http://aeawave.com
E-mail: info@aeawave.com

BAM! (Body and Mind)

Centers for Disease Control and
Prevention
1600 Clifton Road, MS C-04
Atlanta, GA 30333
Toll-Free: 800-311-3435
Website: http://www.bam.gov
E-mail: bam@cdc.gov

Body Positive

http://www.bodypositive.com

Eat Smart Play Hard

Food and Nutrition Service
U.S. Department of Agriculture
Website: http://www.fns.usda.gov/
eatsmartplayhard

Fire FitKids

City of Phoenix
Phoenix City Hall
200 W. Washington St.
Phoenix, AZ 85003
Website: http://phoenix.gov/FIRE/
fitkids.html

Idea, Inc.

10455 Pacific Center Court
San Diego, CA 92121-4339
Toll-Free: 800-999-4332
Phone: 858-535-8979
Fax: 858-535-8234
Website: http://www.ideafit.com

National Association for Fitness Certification
Bodybasics Fitness Training
P.O. Box 67
Sierra Vista, AZ 85636
Toll-Free: 800-324-8315
Phone: 520-452-8712
Website: http://
www.body-basics.com

National Association for Girls and Women in Sports
1900 Association Drive
Reston, VA 20191-1598
Toll-Free: 800-213-7193
Phone: 703-476-3452
Website: http://www.aahperd.org/
nagws

National Collegiate Athletic Association
700 W. Washington Street
P.O. Box 6222
Indianapolis, IN 46206-6222
Phone: 317-917-6222
Fax: 317-917-6888
Website: http://www.ncaa.org

National High School Athletic Coaches Association
Website: http://www.hscoaches.org
E-mail: office@hscoaches.org

President's Challenge
501 N. Morton, Suite 104
Bloomington, IN 47404
Toll-Free: 800-258-8146
Fax: 812-855-8999
Website: http://
www.presidentschallenge.org
E-mail: preschal@indiana.edu

President's Council on Physical Fitness and Sports
200 Independence Ave. SW
Room 738-H
Washington, DC 20201-0004
Phone: 202-690-9000
Fax: 202-690-5211
Website: http://www.fitness.gov

Shape Up America!
Website: http://www.shapeup.org
E-mail: customer-care@shapeup.org

Special Olympics
1133 19th Street, NW
Washington, DC 20036
Phone: 202-628-3630
Fax: 202-824-0200
Website: http://
www.specialolympics.org
E-mail: info@specdialolympics.org

Women's Sports Foundation
Eisenhower Park
East Meadow, NY 11554
Toll-Free: 800-227-3988
Phone: 516-542-4700
Fax: 516-542-4716
Website: http://
www.womenssportsfoundation.org
E-mail: wfs@
womenssportsfoundation.org

Young Men's Christian Association
101 N. Wacker Dr.
Chicago, IL 60606
Phone: 312-977-0031
Website: http://www.ymca.net

Young Women's Christian Association
1015 18th St., NW, Suite 1100
Washington, DC 20036
Phone: 202-467-0801
Fax: 202-467-0802
Website: http://www.ywca.org
E-mail: info@ywca.org

Index

Index

Page numbers that appear in *Italics* refer to illustrations. Page numbers that have a small 'n' after the page number refer to information shown as Notes at the beginning of each chapter. Page numbers that appear in **Bold** refer to information contained in boxes on that page (except Notes information at the beginning of each chapter).

O

P